HUMAN OBESITY

ANNALS OF THE NEW YORK ACADEMY OF SCIENCES
Volume 499

HUMAN OBESITY

Edited by Richard J. Wurtman and Judith J. Wurtman

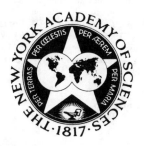

The New York Academy of Sciences
.New York, New York
1987

Library of Congress Cataloging-in-Publication Data

Human obesity.

(Annals of the New York Academy of Sciences, ISSN
0077-8923 ; v. 499)
Based on the Conference on Human Obesity, held in New
York City on June 19-21, 1986, by the New York Academy
of Sciences.
Includes bibliographies and index.
1. Obesity—Congresses. I. Wurtman, Richard J.,
1936-   . II. Wurtman, Judith J. III. Conference on
Human Obesity (1986 : New York, N.Y.) IV. New York
Academy of Sciences. V. Series. [DNLM: 1. Obesity—
congresses. W1 AN626YL v.499 / WD 210 H918 1986]
Q11.N5 vol. 499   500 s   87-14201
[RC628]   [616.3'98]
ISBN 0-89766-393-4
ISBN 0-89766-394-2 (pbk.)

BCP/PCP
Printed in the United States of America
ISBN 0-89766-393-4 (cloth)
ISBN 0-89766-394-2 (paper)
ISSN 0077-8923

ANNALS OF THE NEW YORK ACADEMY OF SCIENCES

Volume 499
June 15, 1987

HUMAN OBESITY[a]

Editors and Conference Organizers
RICHARD J. WURTMAN AND JUDITH J. WURTMAN

CONTENTS

---

[a] This volume is the result of a conference entitled Conference on Human Obesity, held in New York City on June 19-21, 1986, by the New York Academy of Sciences.

Financial assistance was received from:

- BIORESEARCH S.P.A.
- BRISTOL-MYERS COMPANY
- CENTER FOR BRAIN SCIENCES AND METABOLISM
  CHARITABLE TRUST
- CIBA-GEIGY, BASEL
- THE COCA-COLA COMPANY
- ELI LILLY AND COMPANY
- FIDIA
- ISF PHARMACEUTICALS
- JOHNSON & JOHNSON
- LES LABORATOIRES SERVIER
- MEDICAL RESEARCH DIVISION OF THE AMERICAN CYANAMID
  COMPANY (LEDERLE LABORATORIES)
- THE NUTRASWEET COMPANY
- SQUIBB CORPORATION
- THOMPSON MEDICAL COMPANY, INC.
- UNILEVER

Introduction

RICHARD J. WURTMAN AND JUDITH J. WURTMAN

Massachusetts Institute of Technology
Cambridge, Massachusetts 02139

This conference, the first on human obesity to be sponsored by the New York Academy of Sciences, differs in focus and, we hope, outcome, from most prior meetings devoted to this endemic disorder. These differences may enable us to accelerate the disappointingly slow growth of knowledge about the causes of obesity and its clinical management. This meeting also differs from many of its precedessors in outlook: It is optimistic in design and has been planned based on the beliefs that obesity will become a treatable disease and that advances in research will make it so.

This volume, resulting from the conference, has as its focus the nature and the prime manifestations of ordinary obesity in America. It considers the various theories that have been proposed to explain the etiology and pathophysiology of obesity and evaluates the extent to which these formulations actually describe the behavioral and metabolic patterns that characterize people who already are obese, or are in the process of becoming so. This monograph similarly evaluates the animal models that often are used to test hypotheses about the pathogenesis of obesity, or the efficacy of new drugs or diets proposed for its treatment, particularly from the standpoint of how faithfully these experimental preparations actually do model the human condition.

Although the number of clinical investigators and basic scientists working on obesity is not small, it seems no exaggeration to state that this disorder remains poorly understood and, for the most part, unsuccessfully managed. Surprisingly little information is available, even about its epidemiology and natural history, with many key questions like the following remaining unresolved: Do the clinical histories of obese people (not suffering from distinct disease entities like the Prader-Willi syndrome) indicate that they constitute a single population, with common signs and symptoms, a common course, and, ultimately, a common etiology and therapy? Or is it more likely that several distinct processes can generate ordinary obesity? Can evidence be obtained that a genetic predisposition for obesity operates in a significant fraction of patients, or, conversely, is the main contribution that a family usually makes to the development of obesity in its offspring its style of eating and exercising? Do obese people accumulate their excess weight seasonally, in relation to changes in their psychosocial milieu, or more or less continuously until a high plateau is reached? Are the obesities seen in old people, in prepuberal children, or adolescents, separate clinical entities from those of adults? Are periods of weight gain commonly associated with clinical signs of depression or with other behavioral disorders? During periods of weight gain, do obese people overeat all types of foods, only those that are rich in carbohydrates (or perhaps proteins or fats), or just those that are sweet? Do some really not overeat at all, while concurrently gaining weight?

The information that is available about the epidemiology and clinical course of obesity is discussed in this volume, and that which is unavailable is noted, perhaps thereby helping to motivate investigators to fill in the gaps.

Research on human obesity has often used animal models that share with obese humans only the fact of excess body weight (or body fat), and not obesity's behavioral or metabolic concomitants. Biochemical and cellular disturbances discovered in these animals have sometimes been proposed as also having an analogous etiologic role in human obesity, without adequate distinction made between disturbances that are primary, antedating and perhaps causing the obesity, and those that are secondary to the obese state, for example, insulin resistance. Attempts to develop new antiobesity drugs using these animal models have largely been unsuccessful, perhaps reflecting the inadequacies of the models themselves, or the ways that they have been used. For example, the anorexic effects of drugs are usually tested using animals given access to a single food containing fixed proportions of carbohydrates, protein, and fat; this experimental design obviates the very brain mechanisms that normally control nutrient choice, and that appear to be abnormal in certain types of obesity. Animals may be required to work (using an operant-conditioning apparatus) to "earn" their food, thus interposing a test of motivation, and even of physical capacity, between the decision to eat and the process of eating. They may be given access to food for only a few hours of each day, or during a time of day (the daylight period) when they normally choose not to eat. The animals themselves may have endocrine or metabolic disturbances, not present in human obesity, which impair nutrient utilization. By contrast, natural animal models that show cycles of fat deposition and weight loss (e.g., the King Penguin) tend to be underused in obesity research. Here, we discuss criteria for acceptable animal models of human obesity.

It now seems clear that human obesity is a heterogeneous disorder, and data presented in this Annal show that a large subgroup of obese individuals also suffers from characteristic disturbances of mood (or from other psychiatric disturbances), especially during periods when they are gaining their excess weight. One major focus, using the approaches of psychiatry, is the development of a classification of obesity syndromes based on their association with specific behavioral disturbances (like bipolar or seasonal depressions), and the formulation of hypotheses concerning the brain mechanisms that might underlie the concurrent appetitive and affective symptoms seen in such patients. (In this context, we also include considerable discussion of the brain mechanisms that normally control appetites for calories and for particular macronutrients, like carbohydrates and proteins.) Perhaps a better understanding of the association between appetitive and mood disorders seen in the seasonal affective disorder (SAD) syndrome or in carbohydrate-craving obesity will provide us with insights into such other appetitive/psychiatric disorders as bulimia, anorexia nervosa, and the Kleine-Levin syndrome. This volume also considers metabolic derangements that might contribute to the development or the persistence of obesity (e.g., abnormalities in energy utilization, in the mass or distribution of fat cells, and in plasma amino acid metabolism, secondary to insulin resistance). Finally, this monograph evaluates the therapies that currently are used in the United States to treat obesity and related appetitive disorders (drugs, diets, surgery, and behavioral modification), and considers the logic underlying proposed new types of therapies.

This Annal incorporates the advice of 30 leading investigators in obesity research. Other members of the organizing committee were Dr. Silvio Garattini, Director of the Mario Negri Institute in Milan, Italy, Dr. Harris Lieberman, of the Department of Psychology at MIT, and Dr. Trevor Silverstone, of the Medical Colleges of St. Bartholomew's and the London Hospitals, London, England. It is interesting, and perhaps symptomatic of the field of obesity, that our letters soliciting suggestions about this program evoked almost as many proposals as to the identity of the key to obesity as the total number of replies. Some people proposed that the meeting focus on the distribution and number of fat cells. Others saw obesity as, variously, a behavioral disorder (*e.g.*, too rapid a rate of eating or too little chewing per mouthful); a consequence of impaired energy utilization; a hedonic disease, perhaps involving opiates or other brain peptides; the result of a faulty set-point for body weight; a passive-aggressive behavioral strategy for manipulating one's associates; an enzyme deficit; or as a vestige of earlier periods in humanity's evolutionary history when food supplies were abundant for only a part of the year. (It should perhaps be noted that some of these formulations are intrinsically pessimistic about the possibility that obesity can ever be treated effectively. For example, if lean adults are constantly made to feel hungry because "empty" fat cells, a holdover from their fat babyhood, are somehow "telling" the brain to feed them, overeating becomes inevitable. Fortunately, there is little evidence that fat cells "tell" the brain anything, that is, that chemicals secreted from these cells enter the brain and modify neurotransmission.) This variety in formulations about obesity's etiology and persistence are mirrored in a corresponding abundance of largely unsuccessful ideas about its treatment. Current therapies now include, among others, destructive surgery (jaw wiring and stomach stapling), hypnosis, meticulous record-keeping of food ingestion, fasting or near-fasting, use of drugs to increase fecal loss or to accelerate the breakdown of fat, diets rich in carbohydrate or containing no carbohydrate at all, tieing a gold cord around the waist, and a very small number of old drugs to suppress the appetite. Perhaps as more information accumulates about the natural history of obesity, about what and when obese people eat (and overeat) while they are in the process of gaining weight, and about how eating affects how they feel, it will be easier to develop effective therapies for obesity.

Characteristics of Obesity: An Overview

ARTEMIS P. SIMOPOULOS[a]

Nutrition Coordinating Committee
National Institutes of Health
Bethesda, Maryland 20892

INTRODUCTION

A number of definitions of obesity exist and have been reviewed and discussed.[1] The most recent one was included in a statement on the Health Implications of Obesity developed by an NIH panel: "The evidence is now overwhelming that obesity, defined as excessive storage of energy in the form of fat, has adverse effects on health and longevity."[2] The question is, What is an excessive storage of energy? and In relation to what outcome? that is, In relation to morbidity or in relation to mortality? The association of obesity with reduced life expectancy was first noted by Hippocrates, who said, "Sudden death is more common in those who are naturally fat than in the lean."[3]

In 1982, the National Institutes of Health (NIH) Nutrition Coordinating Committee (NCC) and the Centers for Disease Control held a workshop entitled Body Weight, Health and Longevity.[1] Its purpose was to clarify the terminology used in defining overweight and obesity; to formulate concepts relating body weight to health and longevity; and to precisely define the health implications of obesity. It was concluded that "In the United States . . . below-average weights tend to be associated with the greatest longevity, if such weights are not associated with concurrent illness or a history of significant medical impairment. Overweight persons tend to die sooner than average-weight persons, particularly those who are overweight at younger ages. The effect of obesity on mortality is delayed, so that it is not seen in short-term studies . . . the interpretation of studies on body weight, morbidity, and mortality must also carefully consider 1) the definition of obesity used, 2) preexisting illnesses in persons, 3) the length of follow-up, and 4) any confounding risk factors."

PREVALENCE OF OBESITY IN THE UNITED STATES

In any discussion of the prevalence of obesity—that is, the number of overweight or obese individuals in existence at a given time within a population—it is important to discuss the type of data used to calculate the prevalence. The prevalence of obesity varies, and is less when normative data collected in cross-sectional surveys are used, rather than data from long-term prospective studies that relate body weight to risks for developing diseases.[4]

Data generated by the National Center for Health Statistics (NCHS) are normative data based on a national probability sample. TABLE 1 indicates the trends in the weights of the U.S. population 18 to 74 years of age in 1960–62, 1971–74, and 1976–80. These data are cross-sectional and were generated by three surveys:

---

[a] Present address: Director, Nutritional Sciences, ILSI Research Foundation, 1126 Sixteenth St., N.W., Washington, D.C. 20036.

4

the National Health Examination Survey (NHES), 1960–62; and the National Health and Nutrition Examination Surveys (NHANES) I, 1971 to 1974, and II, 1976 to 1980.[5–7]

As can be seen in TABLE 1, a comparison of mean heights and weights of adults ages 18 to 74 years in the three surveys shows that both men and women were taller and heavier in 1971 to 1974 and 1976 to 1980 than they were in 1960 to 1962. The average weight for height of the population is continuing to rise, suggesting that the population is continuing to become more overweight.

Not only is the U.S. population getting heavier, but the average energy intake has increased. The most recent survey on food intake was carried out by the USDA on 1503 women 19 to 50 years of age and 548 of their children 1 to 5 years of age in the 48 coterminous states as part of the continuing Survey of Food

TABLE 1. Mean Weights and Heights by Age and Sex in Three Populations[a]

	Men			Women		
Age Group	NHES	NHANES I	NHANES II	NHES	NHANES I	NHANES II
Weight, kg						
18–24 yrs	71.7	74.8	73.9	57.6	59.9	60.8
25–34 yrs	76.7	79.8	78.5	60.8	63.5	64.4
35–44 yrs	77.1	80.7	80.7	64.4	67.1	67.1
45–54 yrs	77.1	79.4	80.7	65.8	67.6	68.0
55–64 yrs	74.4	77.6	78.9	68.0	67.6	68.0
65–74 yrs	71.7	74.4	74.8	65.3	66.2	66.7
18–74 yrs	75.3	78.0	78.0	63.5	64.9	65.3
Height, m						
18–24 yrs	1.74	1.77	1.77	1.62	1.63	1.63
25–34 yrs	1.76	1.77	1.77	1.62	1.63	1.63
35–44 yrs	1.74	1.76	1.76	1.61	1.63	1.63
45–54 yrs	1.73	1.75	1.75	1.60	1.62	1.61
55–64 yrs	1.71	1.73	1.74	1.58	1.60	1.60
65–74 yrs	1.70	1.71	1.71	1.56	1.58	1.58
18–74 yrs	1.73	1.75	1.76	1.60	1.62	1.62

[a] The three populations are from the National Health Examination Survey (NHES), 1960 to 1962, and the National Health and Nutrition Examination Surveys (NHANES) I, 1971 to 1974, and II, 1976 to 1980. Two pounds were deducted from NHES data to allow for weight of clothing; total weight of all clothing for NHANES I and II ranged from 0.1 to 0.3 kg and was not deducted from weights in table. Height was measured without shoes. Data are preliminary. Age-adjusted mean values and estimates of variations (standard error) are not currently available.[1]

Intakes by Individuals.[8] The data were collected from April 1, 1985, to June 1985 using a one-day recall in a personal interview. These data were compared with data collected in a comparable manner for individuals of the same ages in the Nationwide Food Consumption Survey 1977–78, spring quarter (April through June). TABLES 2 and 3 indicate that there was a decrease in the mean intake of meat, poultry, and fish by both children and women in 1985 in comparison with 1977 regardless of income, and an increase in calories over the same time period. Thus, overall excess intake has increased over the past 8 years. There are no data available on energy expenditure.

The three NCHS surveys have defined overweight as a condition in which the body mass index (BMI) is equal to or higher than the 85th percentile of BMI for men (28 kg/m^2) and women (34 kg/m$^{1.5}$), ages 20 to 29 years, who were studied

TABLE 2. Mean Intakes of Meat, Poultry, and Fish Per Individual in 1977 and 1985: All Income Levels[a]

		Mean Intake (g/day)	
Group	Age (yr)	1977	1985
Children	1–3	99	98
	4–5	128	114
	All	112	104
Women	19–34	184	179
	35–50	188	185
	All	186	181

[a] Data collected and compiled by the USDA/Human Nutrition Information Service Nationwide Food Consumption Survey.[8] Data collected in the spring of 1977 and 1985.

between 1976 and 1980.[9] Severe overweight is defined as a BMI (32 kg/m^2 for men and 42 kg/m$^{1.5}$ for women) at or higher than the 95th percentile of the same 20- to 29-year-old reference group. By the NHANES BMI criteria, 32.6 million adult Americans are overweight, whereas 11.5 million are severely overweight. The rationale underlying the use of the 20- to 29-year-old reference population is that young adults are relatively lean, and the increase in body weight that usually occurs as men and women age is due almost entirely to fat accumulation. It is well known, however, that the U.S. population at ages 20–29 is not necessarily lean; therefore, any calculation based on this rationale underestimates the prevalence of obesity. Furthermore, the criteria (85th or 95th percentile) are defined statistically; they are not derived from morbidity or mortality experience of the survey population. The use of 1.5 instead of 2 as a factor in the calculation of BMI for women underestimates further the prevalence of obesity in women.

Data relating body weight to morbidity or to risks from cardiovascular disease (CVD) as well as mortality have been obtained from the Framingham Heart Study. This is the longest prospective study to date. Data over a 26- to 30-year follow-up indicate that small increases in body weight above 110 percent of the Metropolitan Relative Weight (MRW) or a BMI of 24.4 kg/m^2 are associated with increased risk from cardiovascular disease. Thus, if instead of using normative data generated by cross-sectional surveys, we calculate the prevalence of obesity

TABLE 3. Mean Food Energy Intake Per Individual in 1977 and 1985: All Income Levels[a]

		Mean Intake (kcal/day)	
Group	Age (yr)	1977	1985
Children	1–3	1210	1372
	4–5	1486	1564
	All	1335	1446
Women	19–34	1617	1707
	35–50	1514	1602
	All	1573	1661

[a] Data collected and compiled by the USDA/HNIS Nationwide Food Consumption Survey.[8] Data collected in the spring of 1977 and 1985.

on the basis of the work of Garrison et al.[10] and Hubert et al.[11] using criteria that relate obesity to morbidity and mortality from cardiovascular disease, 80 percent of men and 70 percent of women over 40 years of age in the Framingham Heart Study are above the desirable weight range (MRW > 110 percent; kg/m^2 > 24.4) and are at increased risk for cardiovascular disease.[1]

Mean BMI values for men and women aged 30–39, 40–49, and 50–62 years have been calculated for the following study populations: NHES, NHANES I and II, Build and Blood Pressure Study 1959, Build Study 1979, American Cancer Society Study, and the Framingham Heart Study; the values are shown in TABLES 4–6. As can be seen in these tables, the mean desirable BMI is 22.0 for men and 21.5 for women, and the range is 20–25 for men and 19–26 for women. A BMI of 28, as advocated by those who use normative data for treatment of obesity, is

TABLE 4. Mean Body Mass Index (BMI) for Men and Women Aged 30–39 Years in Various Study Populations[a]

Study	Men kg/m^2(1 SD)	Women kg/m^2(1 SD)
NHES[b]	25.2 (3.84)	24.1 (5.12)
NHANES I[c]	26.0 (4.40)	24.7 (5.71)
NHANES II[d]	25.6 (3.96)	24.9 (5.79)
BBP-59[e]	24.3	23.1
BS-79[f]	25.0	22.7
ACS[g]	24.6	22.6
FRAM[h]	25.8 (3.7)	24.2 (4.3)
Desirable BMI mean[i]	22.0	21.5
Desirable BMI range[i]	20–25	19–26
Olympic sprinters	23.	
Olympic marathon runners	20.	

[a] Tabulated values are the means of the populations studied.
[b] NHES = National Health Examination Survey
[c] NHANES I = National Health and Nutrition Examination Survey I
[d] NHANES II = National Health and Nutrition Examination Survey II
[e] BBP-59 = Build and Blood Pressure Study, 1959
[f] BS-79 = Build Study 1979
[g] ACS = American Cancer Society Study
[h] FRAM = Framingham Heart Study
[i] From Metropolitan Life Insurance Company 1959 Desirable Weight Table (mean of midpoint of medium frame; range of all heights and frames for all ages.)

indicative of an already obese state that is difficult to treat and leads to a lifestyle of repeated episodes of weight gain and weight loss. Of interest is the fact that none of the groups included in the major studies depicted in TABLES 4–6 are at the desirable BMI, except for the women in the age group 30 to 39 years in the Build Study 1979[12] and the American Cancer Society study,[13] whose mean BMI (22.7 and 22.6 kg/m^2, respectively) approaches the desirable BMI (21.5 kg/m^2). In all other groups, including women in the older age groups (40 to 49 and 50 to 62 years), the mean BMI exceeds the desirable BMI. It is, of course, known that overweight at younger ages has deleterious effects on life expectancy. The participants in the American Cancer Society study and the Build Study 1979 are not representative of the U.S. population, because blacks and persons of lower socio-economic groups were underrepresented in the American Cancer Society study

TABLE 5. Mean Body Mass Index (BMI) for Men and Women Aged 40–49
Years in Various Study Populations[a]

Study	Men kg/m²(1 SD)		Women kg/m²(1 SD)
NHES	25.5 (3.78)		25.2 (5.49)
NHANES I	26.1 (3.93)		25.7 (5.61)
NHANES II	26.4 (3.93)		25.7 (6.07)
BBP-59	24.9		24.2
BS-79	25.4		23.6
ACS	24.9		23.5
FRAM	26.1 (3.5)		25.7 (4.6)
Desirable BMI mean[b]	22.0		21.5
Desirable BMI range[b]	20–25		19–26
Olympic sprinters		23.	
Olympic marathon runners		20.	

[a] Tabulated values are the means of the populations studied.
[b] From Metropolitan Life Insurance Company 1959 Desirable Weight Table (mean of midpoint of medium frame; range of all heights and frames for all ages.)

and insured persons are of higher socioeconomic levels. Yet only in these two studies did women 30–39 years of age have body weights close to the desirable BMI.

Studies have shown that the weights of the Framingham Heart Study cohort are similar to those in the general population of the U.S. Because of the importance of taking morbidity statistics into consideration in defining desirable body weight, the Dietary Guidelines for Americans[14] use desirable body weight, based on the 1959 Metropolitan Life Insurance table without distinction of size frame (TABLE 7), rather than the tables developed by NCHS, which are based on normative data.

At present we do not have standards for children and adolescents that are based either on morbidity statistics or on data that define obesity as an antecedent

TABLE 6. Mean Body Mass Index (BMI) for Men and Women Aged 50–62
Years in Various Study Populations[a]

Study	Men kg/m²(1 SD)		Women kg/m²(1 SD)
NHES	25.5 (4.03)		26.7 (5.24)
NHANES I	25.9 (4.36)		26.4 (5.69)
NHANES II	26.2 (3.91)		26.5 (5.56)
BBP-59	25.1		25.2
BS-79	25.5		24.3
ACS	24.9		24.4
FRAM	26.3 (3.5)		27.5 (5.0)
Desirable BMI mean[b]	22.0		21.5
Desirable BMI range[b]	20–25		19–26
Olympic sprinters		23.	
Olympic marathon runners		20.	

[a] Tabulated values are the means of the populations studied.
[b] From Metropolitan Life Insurance Company 1959 Desirable Weight Table (mean of midpoint of medium frame; range of all heights and frames for all ages.)

to adult disease. Therefore, for these populations, U.S. investigators are using statistical definitions based on normative data.

A large survey based on a national sample of characteristics of the growth of children in the United States, carried out by NCHS, has produced data that led to the development of tables and charts. The children studied represented a cross section of ethnic and socioeconomic groups; as a result, genetic, ethnic, and socioeconomic differences are all part of the final data. For this reason, they are used as reference standards, rather than body weight standards, for the evaluation of growth and development of children in the United States. The charts depict the course of normal growth. Although there is evidence that ethnic differences depend mostly upon differences in the prevalence of malnutrition and infectious diseases in various parts of the world, there can be no universal standard.

TABLE 7. Desirable Body Weight Ranges[a]

Height Without Shoes	Weight Without Clothes	
	Men (pounds)	Women (pounds)
4 10		92–121
4 11		95–124
5 0		98–127
5 1	105–134	101–130
5 2	108–137	104–134
5 3	111–141	107–138
5 4	114–145	110–142
5 5	117–149	114–146
5 6	121–154	118–150
5 7	125–159	122–154
5 8	129–163	126–159
5 9	133–167	130–164
5 10	137–172	134–169
5 11	141–177	
6 0	145–182	
6 1	149–187	
6 2	153–192	
6 3	157–197	

[a] For women 18–25 years of age, subtract one pound for each year under 25. Adapted from the 1959 Metropolitan Desirable Weight Table. TABLE reproduced from 1985 Dietary Guidelines.[14]

Dietz et al.[15] have shown that obesity is epidemic in the pediatric population, and emphasize the need for more effective therapy and prevention of childhood obesity. Obesity in the adult may be preceded by obesity during childhood, but only a few studies of this association[16–18] have been reported. Furthermore, reliable longitudinal data from childhood to adulthood are difficult to obtain. Genetics, rather than environment, appears to be of greater importance in determining adult body weight.[19]

OVERWEIGHT, MORBIDITY, AND MORTALITY

Data from national cross-sectional surveys and epidemiological studies show that the following: Both men and women were taller and heavier in 1971 to 1974 and 1976 to 1980 than they were in 1960 to 1962. Women below the poverty line have a much higher prevalence of overweight between ages 25 and 55 years than women above the poverty line. Race and poverty status are independent predictors of overweight in women. Overweight increases with age. In women, overweight peaks in the late fifties and early sixties, whereas in men, overweight peaks in the early forties. In overweight persons the relative risk for diabetes, hypertension, and hypercholesterolemia is greater at ages 20 to 45 years than at ages 45 to 75 years.

Analyses of a 26-year follow-up of the Framingham Heart Study population[10,11,20,21] were recently performed, using the 1959 Metropolitan Life Insurance Company Table as a reference standard. The analyses validated the concept of desirable body weight as defined by the 1959 Metropolitan Life Insurance Company Table and suggested that elevated mortality in low-weight American men results from the mortality risks associated with cigarette smoking. It showed that cigarette smoking is a potential confounder of the relationship between relative weight and long-term mortality (statistical control for this factor requires careful consideration) and suggested that obesity is an independent risk factor for cardiovascular disease. It also indicated that weight gain after the young adult years conveys an increased risk of cardiovascular disease in both sexes." A change in MRW after the young adult years made an independent contribution to the prediction of CVD. The characteristic most strongly related to lipoprotein and blood pressure changes in both sexes was a change in Quetelet's index (QI). A unit change in QI (<3 kg/m^2), for example, resulted in a change in low density lipoprotein of about 3 mg/dl in young men.

Ashley and Kamel[22] showed that an increase in MRW from 100 to 110 percent would predict a rise in systolic blood pressure of 7 mm Hg. Weight loss of 8.3 kg led to a drop of 14/13 mm Hg in blood pressure.[23] Garrison et al.[24] stated: "Adiposity stands out as a major controllable contributor to hypertension. Changes in body fat over 8 years were mirrored by changes in both systolic and diastolic pressure. Markedly obese women in their fourth decade were 7 times more likely to develop hypertension than lean women the same age." Westlund and Nicholaysen,[25] in a prospective study, showed that in moderate obesity, risk of diabetes was increased about 10-fold. In those whose weights exceeded the standard by 45 percent or more, risk was increased about 30-fold.

Most of the work on the relationship of obesity to reduced life expectancy has been carried out in relation to cardiovascular disease. Studies on the relationship of obesity to cancer have not been carried out to the same extent. Certainly no long-term prospective studies comparable in scope to the Framingham Heart Study, which has a 30-year follow-up period, have been performed to examine the relationship between obesity and cancer, although the American Cancer Society conducted a long-term prospective study during the period 1959–1972.[13] Data from the American Cancer Society Study show that risk of cancer increases with weight. Cancer mortality was elevated among those 40 percent or more overweight. Cancer of the colon and rectum were the principal causes of excess cancer mortality among men, whereas cancer of the gallbladder and biliary passages, breast, cervix, endometrium, uterus, and ovary were the major causes of excess mortality among women.

Obese individuals have increased levels of prolactin, androgens, estrogens, and cortisol. A number of studies have pointed to estrogen as having a role in the development of cancers of the reproductive system such as cancers of the endometrium, cervix, breast, and ovaries.[26] These cancers account for half of all cancers in women. Adipose tissue is the major source of estrogen formation in postmenopausal women, and it is derived by aromatization of androstenedione into estrone.[27] The increase in estrogen formation as a function of obesity is probably due to increased numbers of adipose cells, rather than to an increase in the specific activity of aromatase in those cells. Stromal cells are more active than adipocytes in converting androstenedione into estrone,[28] and weight reduction does not decrease the efficacy of the conversion.[29]

The finding by Siiteri et al.[29] that weight reduction does not decrease the efficacy of converting androstenedione into estrone emphasizes the need to prevent the development of obesity in order to avoid any possible deleterious endocrine effects of estrogens during the postmenopausal period. Although it is known that weight loss decreases blood pressure, improves the glucose tolerance of the diabetic, and decreases insulin requirements, it is not known how weight (gain or loss) exerts its effects on human metabolism. Therefore, in the analyses of prospective studies, the effects of weight gain and weight loss on cancer incidence need to be evaluated.

Studies relating obesity to cancer—particularly cancer of the breast and endometrium—have not been based on longitudinal data from representative samples; they have not considered measures of weight and loss, the duration of obesity, time of onset, nor type of obesity (android or gynoid).[26] The distinction between the latter two types might be important, because the android type is associated with diabetes and other metabolic changes, whereas the gynoid type is not.[30]

SUMMARY

Obesity is considered to be a major nutritional disorder in the U.S. and in many parts of the industrialized world. The physiology of the obese and their propensity for chronic disease has been of growing interest over the past few years, and an extensive literature has begun to accumulate. Obesity is a heterogeneous disorder. When viewed in the broadest sense, it has been considered a disorder of energy balance. The development of obesity in humans is of complex etiology, involving genetic and environmental components that affect regulatory and metabolic events.

The prevalence of overweight and obesity in a population depends on the particular reference or standard of desirable weight selected for use. A trend toward increasing height and weight has been evident among adults for several centuries, and among children as early as the 7th year of life in developed countries.

Overweight persons are at increased risk for coronary artery disease, high blood pressure, diabetes mellitus, and cancer. The degree of overweight that carries additional risk without affecting mortality needs to be defined. Overweight most likely contributes in varying degrees to morbidity in different societies, because the risk for most common chronic diseases is multifactorial. In defining overweight and obesity, morbidity, in addition to mortality, ought to be taken into consideration.

The multidisciplinary approach to the study of obesity—borrowing concepts and techniques from endocrinology, neurobiology, genetics, and nutrition—should yield new insights into how environmental factors such as diet and physical expenditure interact to influence energy metabolism and body composition.

REFERENCES

1. SIMOPOULOS, A. P. & T. B. VAN ITALLIE. 1984. Body weight, health, and longevity. Ann. Intern. Med. **100:** 285–295.
2. 1985. Health Implications of Obesity. National Institutes of Health Consensus Conference Statement. Vol. 5. No. 9. U.S. Department of Health and Human Services, Bethesda, MD.
3. CHADWICK, J. & W. N. MANN. 1950. Medical Works of Hippocrates. 154. Blackwell. Oxford.
4. SIMOPOULOS, A. P. 1985. Dietary control of hypertension and obesity and body weight standards. J. Am. Diet. Assoc. **85:** 419–422.
5. 1966. Weight by Height and Age of Adults, United States, 1960–1962. Vital and Health Statistics, Series 11, No. 14. National Center for Health Statistics, Hyattsville, MD.
6. ABRAHAM, S., C. L. JOHNSON & M. F. NAJJAR. 1979. Weight and Height of Adults 18–74 Years of Age, United Staes, 1971–1974. DHEW Publication No. (PHS) 79-1659, Vital and Health Statistics, Series 11, No. 211. National Center for Health Statistics, Hyattsville, MD.
7. 1981. Plan and operation of the National Health and Nutrition Examination Survey, 1976–1980. DHHS Publication No. (PHS) 81-1317, Vital and Health Statistics, Series 1, No. 15. National Center for Health Statistics, Hyattsville, MD.
8. 1985. Nationwide Food Consumption Survey: Continuing Survey of Food Intakes by Individuals. Women 19–50 Years and Their Children 1–5 Years, 1 Day, 1985. U.S. Department of Agriculture, Nutrition Monitoring Service, NFCS, CSFII Report No. 85-1.
9. VAN ITALLIE, T. B. & S. ABRAHAM. 1985. Some hazards of obesity and its treatment. In Recent Advances of Obesity Research. IV. Proceedings of the IV International Congress on Obesity. J. Hirsch and T. B. Van Itallie, Eds. John Libby & Company. London.
10. GARRISON, R. J., M. FEINLEIB, W. P. CASTELLI & P. M. McNAMARA. 1983. Cigarette smoking as a confounder of the relationship between relative weight and long-term mortality: the Framingham Heart Study. J. Am. Med. Assoc. **249:** 2199–2203.
11. HUBERT, H. B., M. FEINLEIB, P. M. McNAMARA & W. P. CASTELLI. 1983. Obesity as an independent risk factor for cardiovascular disease: a 26-year follow-up of participants in the Framingham Heart Study. Circulation **67:** 968–977.
12. Build Study. 1979. Society of Actuaries and Association of Life Insurance Medical Directors. Chicago.
13. LEW, E. A. & L. GARFINKEL. 1979. Variations in mortality by weight among 750,000 men and women. J. Chronic Dis. **32:** 563–576.
14. Nutrition and Your Health. 1985. Dietary Guidelines for Americans, 2nd Edition. U.S. Department of Health and Human Services and U.S. Department of Agriculture, Washington, DC. Home and Garden Bulletin No. 232.
15. DIETZ, W. H., S. L. GORTMAKER, A. M. SOBOL & C. A. WEHLER. 1985. Trends in the prevalence of childhood and adolescent obesity in the United States. Pediatr. Res. **19:** 527 (Abstr).
16. ABRAHAM, S. & M. NORDSIECK. 1960. Relationship of excess weight in children and adults. Public Health Rep. **75:** 263–273.
17. CHARNEY, E., H. C. GOODMAN & M. McBRIDE. 1976. Childhood antecedents of adult obesity. Do chubby infants become obese adults? N. Engl. J. Med. **295:** 6–9.
18. MULLINS, A. G. 1958. The prognosis in juvenile obesity. Arch. Dis. Child. **33:** 307–314.
19. STUNKARD, A. J., T. I. A. SORENSEN, C. HANIS, T. W. TEASDALE, R. CHAKRABORTY, W. J. SCHULL & F. SCHULSINGER. 1986. An adoption study of human obesity. N. Engl. J. Med. **314:** 193–198.
20. SIMOPOULOS, A. P. 1985. The health implications of overweight and obesity. Nutr. Rev. **43:** 33–40.
21. HUBERT, H. B., W. P. CASTELLI & R. J. GARRISON. 1983. Longitudinal study of coronary heart disease risk factors in young adults: the Framingham offspring study. Am. J. Epidemiol. **118:** 443.

22. ASHLEY JR., F. W. & W. B. KAMEL. 1974. Relationship of weight change to changes in atherogenic traits: the Framingham Study. J. Chronic Dis. **27:** 103–114.
23. MACMAHON, S. W., D. E. L. WILCKEN & G. J. MACDONALD. 1986. The effect of weight reduction on left ventricular mass. A randomized controlled trial in young, overweight hypertensive patients. N. Engl. J. Med. **314:** 334–339.
24. GARRISON, R. J., W. B. KANNEL, J. STOKES III & W. P. CASTELLI. 1985. Incidence and precursors of hypertension in young adults. The Framingham Offspring Study. Cardiovascular Disease Epidemiology Newsletter, March.
25. WESTLUND, K. & R. NICHOLAYSEN. 1972. Ten-year mortality and morbidity related to serum cholesterol: a follow-up of 3,751 men aged 40–49. Scand. J. Clin. Lab. Invest. **127** (Suppl): 1–24.
26. SIMOPOULOS, A. P. 1985. Fat intake, obesity, and cancer of the breast and endometrium. Med Oncol. Tumor Pharmacother. **2:** 125–135.
27. CLELAND, W. H., C. R. MENDELSON & E. R. SIMPSON. 1985. Effects of aging and obesity on aromatase activity of human adipose tissue. J. Clin. Endocrinol. Metab. **60:** 174.
28. SIMPSON, E. R., G. E. ACKERMAN, M. E. SMITH & C. R. MENDELSON. 1981. Estrogen formation in stromal cells of adipose tissue of women: induction by glucocorticosteroid. Proc. Natl. Acad. Sci. USA **78:** 5690–5694.
29. SIITERI, P. K., J. E. WILLIAMS & N. K. TAKAKI. 1976. Steroid abnormalities in endometrial and breast carcinoma: a unifying hypothesis. J. Steroid Biochem. **7:** 897–903.
30. KISSEBAH, A. H., N. VYDELINGUM, R. MURRAY et al. 1982. Relation of body fat distribution to metabolic complications of obesity. J. Clin. Endocrinol. Metab. **54:** 254–260.

Overweight Is Risking Fate

Definition, Classification, Prevalence, and Risks

GEORGE A. BRAY

Section of Diabetes and Clinical Nutrition
University of Southern California
University of Southern California School of Medicine
Los Angeles, California 90033

INTRODUCTION

Obesity is a major problem for the affluent nations. Estimates of its prevalence range from 10 to 50% or most of the adult population. These differing estimates depend in large part on the definitions and standards used to identify and segregate the population at risk. Overweight individuals are those with an increase of body weight above some arbitrary standard defined in relation to height. To be obese, on the other hand, means to have an abnormally high proportion of body fat. In order to determine whether an individual is obese or simply overweight due to increased lean body mass (*i.e.*, athletes), one needs techniques and standards for quantitating body fat.

DEFINING OBESITY

Both the direct and indirect methods have been used to evaluate the composition of the human body.

Direct Analysis of Body Composition

Measurement of body composition by analysis of individual cadavers has been performed several times in this century.[1] Water was the major body component, accounting for about 60–65 percent. Fat and protein each account for about 15% of the body weight of these individuals. Women have more fat than men,[2] and when adipose tissue is dissected free, the other components have similar proportion between men and women.[2] Because direct analysis cannot be performed under normal circumstances, most attention has been turned to indirect methods for measuring body fat.

Indirect Analysis of Body Composition

Visual Observation

Superficial analysis of fatness may be done by self-examination or through visual examination by another person. Increased bulging of skinfolds or excessive roundness in most instances suggests increased fatness. Although such observa-

14

tions provide a good individual guide, they are not quantitative. One solution to this problem is the assignment of body types using photographs taken without clothing. With this technique, called somatotyping, the degree of endomorphy (roundness), mesomorphy (muscularity), and ectomorphy (leanness) can be given numerical values.[1]

Anthropometric Measurements

Height and Weight. Height and weight can each be measured with considerable reliability and are the most widely available data from life insurance examinations and health surveys. Based on life insurance statistics relating height and weight to the likelihood of survival, the Metropolitan Life Insurance Company has proposed tables of desirable weights in 1959 and again in 1983. FIGURE 1 plots the

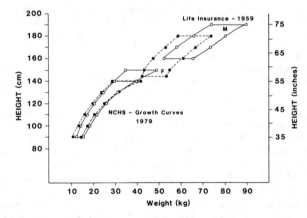

FIGURE 1. Relationship of height and weight from two data bases. Data from the National Center for Health Statistics (NCHS)[3] were used to plot the height and weight relationships between the 10th and 90th percentiles for both growing boys and girls. The adult data were taken from the height and weight relationships for adults from the 1959 Metropolitan Life Insurance Co. table, plotting the lowest small frame and highest large frame data. Note the discontinuity between the height for weight among young adults from the NCHS data and the insurance company tables. This discontinuity suggests that the weights in the 1959 tables were too high for short and younger women. These discrepancies would be even greater if the newer life insurance tables had been used.

recommended weight ranges in relation to height for men and women age 25 to 65 as published in 1959. Also plotted on this figure are the 10 to 90th percentile of weight for height in children obtained from the National Center for Health Statistics.[3] The discontinuity in these two sets of data is obvious and would be even more exaggerated if the proposed 1983 Metropolitan data had been used. At entry into adulthood, actual weights for height are lower than the recommended adult ranges for short men and women. Extrapolation of data for height in relation to weight suggests that, in addition, the life insurance recommendations for taller men and women may be too low. Finally, the nearly identical weight for height patterns of males and females during growth suggests that the subsequent separation of weight tables into one for men and one for women, as recommended in life insurance tables, may be both artificial and inaccurate.

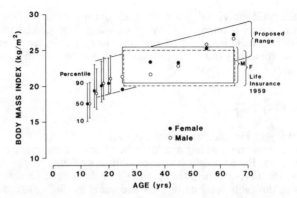

FIGURE 2. Relationship of BMI to age from three studies. The rectangles are the 1959 life insurance tables that are recommended for ages 20–65. The data under 20 were plotted from the calculated BMI for 10th and 90th percentile height and weight data for 16- to 20-year olds. The open circles for men and the closed circles for women were calculated by Andres[5] from the minimum death rate figures published by the Society of Actuaries in the 1979 Build Study.[6] Note that there is an increasing average BMI from these latter data, which suggest, along with the data of those under 20, that the BMI should be adjusted for age.

An alternative approach to developing recommendations for appropriate ranges of body weight in relation to height can be developed using the body mass or Quetelet index. The body mass index (BMI) as used here is body weight (in kg) divided by the square of the height (in meters)(BMI = kg/m^2). The correlation of BMI with body fat measured from body density is between 0.7 and 0.8.[4] Of these, the BMI (W/H^2) has the best correlation with body fat and is thus preferred.[1,4] FIGURE 2 shows the BMI (kg/m^2) in relation to age. The range of body mass indices for adults was taken from the upper and lower limits of weight for height from the life insurance data of 1959 shown in FIGURE 1. I have not used the ranges of weight in the 1983 life insurance tables because the calculated BMI for so-called large frame individuals is above the levels where a recent consensus conference of the National Institutes of Health expressed the concern for health risks. Since the life insurance data are recommendations for all adults, age 25 to 70, these limits do not change with age and are presented for men and women as open rectangular boxes. The range of body mass indices for growing children are also depicted in FIGURE 2 and show a discontinuity with the adult data. From these two presentations of the life insurance data, it is clear that these tables are inappropriate for general use by the American public.

In an analysis of the life insurance data, Andres[5] has further concluded that age-adjustment is desirable. Using the life insurance data published in 1980,[6] he calculated the BMI at which the minimum mortality occurred for both men and women at each decade in life. The data for both men and women rise with age, and there is no sex difference. On the basis of this analysis, a new set of age-related ranges for BMI is presented in TABLE 1. The body mass or Quetelet index is not only a useful way of relating body weight to height, it can also be used to assess the magnitude of potential health risks associated with overweight and as a guide to therapy.

Circumference. Both measurements of circumference and skinfolds have been used to obtain additional information about body fat and its distribution.

Circumferences can be measured more reliably than skinfolds[7] and provide valuable insight into regional fat distribution. In women, fat tends to be distributed more on the thighs and buttocks to give a gynoid, lower body, or centripetal pattern. In men, on the other hand, body fat is more often located on the abdomen or chest, giving an android, central, or upper body distribution. These regional differences for both sexes can be quantitated by the ratio of the circumference at the waist to the circumference of the hips. This waist-hips ratio (WHR) has proven to be an important predictor of risk associated with obesity. In both sexes, a higher waist to hips ratio (WHR) is associated with increased risk of hypertension, diabetes, stroke, and death.[7,8] For men, a WHR above 1.0 and for women a WHR above 0.9 indicates substantially increased risk.

Skinfolds. The thickness of skinfolds can be used to assess obesity. The accuracy for measurement of skinfolds is considerably less than for height and weight or circumference.[9] These problems are made worse in obese individuals. One difficulty with measuring skinfold thickness is that body fat increases with age even though skinfold thickness may not change. This implies that the accumulation of fat with age occurs in large part at sites other than subcutaneous ones. There are also sex and ethnic differences in skinfold measurements. The subscapular skinfold, as a single measure appears to provide a better index of fatness than the triceps skinfold; it is preferable, however, to obtain data on both a truncal (subscapular) and extremity (triceps) skinfold. Based on the anthropometric measures, overweight may be defined as BMI from top of normal to less than 5 kg/m^2 above normal for age or body weight between the upper limit of normal and 20% above that limit. Obesity may be defined as BMI greater than 5 kg/m^2 above the upper limit of normal, triceps plus subscapular skinfold of $\geq$45 mm (males) and $\geq$69 mm (females), body weight more than 20% above the upper limit for height, or body fat $\geq$25% in males or $\geq$30% in females.

Other Techniques

Another approach for estimating body composition is to use one of several dilutional techniques. The most direct is the use of a fat soluble substance such as cyclopropane whose distribution can be related to total fat. The equilibration time is long, however, and special equipment is needed. The second approach is to calculate body fat from measurements of body water by the distribution of tritiated water[1,10] or antipyrine,[1] which equilibrates with body water. Body cell mass can also be quantitated by measuring the amount of the naturally occurring isotope of potassium (40K) in the body.[1,10]

TABLE 1. Recommendations for Age-Adjusted Levels of the Body Mass Index

Age Group (yr)	Body Mass Index (kg/m^2)
19–24	19–24
25–34	20–25
35–44	21–26
45–54	22–27
55–64	23–28
65+	24–29

Measurement of body density provides a quantitative technique for measuring body fat. Density is determined from the specific gravity, that is, the weight of the body in and out of water.[1,10] In this procedure, individuals are weighed underwater and out of water, and the residual volume of the lungs is determined. With this information, it is possible to fractionate the body into its fat and fat-free components because fat is lighter than water and other tissues are heavier than water. The method is relatively easy if appropriate facilities are available, but it remains primarily a research method.

Ultrasound waves applied to the skin will be reflected by the fat-muscle interface and can be more reproducible than skinfold measurements. Electromagnetic conductivity can be used to quantitate lean tissue and fat due to differences in their ability to conduct electromagnetic waves.[11] Computerized tomographic scans and nuclear magnetic resonance scans can provide pictures from which the thickness of fat can be calculated. Finally, neutron activation can activate various chemical components of the body that can be identified by their emission spectra.[12]

In summary, body fat can be estimated in many ways, but the most accurate are not widely available or are the most expensive. From a practical point of view, methods involving measurement of height and weight, preferably expressed as the BMI (W/H^2) and measurement of a ratio of the circumference of the waist to the hips would appear to provide the most useful approaches for determining who are the obese and estimating the degree of risk associated with obesity.

PREVALENCE OF OBESITY

The prevalence of overweight and/or obesity depends upon the criteria that are used to define obesity. The massively obese are readily recognized, but represent only a small segment of the population. Using the 95th percentile for the BMI, 5.8% of men and 8.3% of women in the United States are obese. Using the criterion of 20% or more overweight as the criterion, we can compare the figures obtained in 1960–62 and again in 1971–74 in relation to age and sex (TABLE 2). More females than males are obese at all ages, but there was no consistent trend to increasing overweight during this decade. The frequency of overweight also increases in older age groups of both sexes. After 55–64, there is a decline in the percent of the population that is overweight.[14]

The patterns of body weight in males and females are changing. Data supplied by the Selective Service show that men inducted into the Army in the 1950s were heavier than those men of the same height in 1943. The 1943 inductees were in turn heavier in relation to height than those inducted in 1918.[1] On the average, American men have become progressively heavier during the century. During the past decade both men and women of the same height are 2 to 8 pounds heavier.[13]

Racial differences in body weight also exist.[1] The prevalence of overweight in all races increases in both sexes with age, and averages 24.2% for males and 27.1% for females. More black women, however, are overweight at all ages than white women, but among the males, this racial effect is only present between ages 35 and 54.[15] Socioeconomic conditions also play an important role in the development of obesity. Excess body weight is 7–12 times more frequent in women from lower social classes than in women from the upper social classes.[1] Among males, social class has a significant but much smaller relationship to overweight. Cultural

TABLE 2. Prevalence of Overweight in 1960–1962 and 1971–1974[a]

	Men		Women	
Age	1960–1962	1971–1974	1960–1962	1971–1974
20–74	14.5%	14.0%	25.1%	23.8%
20–24	9.6	7.4	9.1	9.6
25–34	13.3	13.6	14.8	17.1
35–44	14.9	17.0	23.2	24.3
45–54	16.7	15.8	28.9	27.8
55–64	15.8	15.1	38.6	34.7
65–74	14.6	13.4	38.8	31.5

[a] The percent of the population deviating by 20 percent or more from desirable weight is estimated from the regression equation of weight over height for men and women ages 20–29 years obtained from the Health and Nutrition Examination Survey I: 1960–62, and the Health and Nutrition Examination, National Center for Health Statistics.

background also seems to affect the development of obesity. Individuals from Eastern Europe living in the United States have a higher frequency of obesity than those who originated in Western Europe. Recent immigrants to the United States have a higher frequency of obesity than do fourth generation Americans from the same heritage.

Using the body mass or Quetelet index, it is possible to compare the prevalence of obesity in three English-speaking countries[16] (TABLE 3). The prevalence of individuals with a BMI of 25–30 kg/m^2 is almost identical in the three populations. The prevalence of those with a BMI above 30 kg/m^2, however, is higher in the United States. Although prevalence data exist for many other populations, the use of a variety of criteria make comparison difficult.

Overweight Is Risking Fate

Mortality and Obesity

Life insurance statistics published in 1979,[6] as well as those assembled earlier,[1] showed that excess weight was associated with increased mortality for both men and women. This effect is shown in FIGURE 3, which plots relative mortality for various deviations of body weight. The minimal mortality for both men and women occurs among individuals 10% below average weight. Deviations in body

TABLE 3. Percent of Overweight and Obese People in Three English-Speaking Countries[16]

Country	Age	Overweight[a]		Obese[b]	
		M	F	M	F
Australia	25–64	34%	24%	7%	7%
Britain	16–65	34%	24%	6%	8%
United States	20–74	31%	24%	12%	12%

[a] Overweight = body mass index of 25–30 kg/m^2
[b] Obese = body mass index above 30 kg/m^2

weight above or below this are associated with an increase in mortality. The effect on life expectancy of small deviations in body weight, however, is small. Based on the 1979 data, a body weight that is 10% above average weight is accompanied by an 11% increase in excess mortality for men and a 7% increase for women. If body weight is 20% above average weight, the excess mortality rises to 20% for men and 10% for women. This relationship of BMI to health risks can also be used to provide guidelines for treatment of obesity.[17]

Prospective Studies of Obesity and Mortality

The Pooling Project. As the title of this section suggests the data from several prospective studies have been brought together and the data pooled for analytical

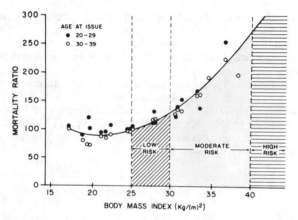

FIGURE 3. Relationship of BMI to excess mortality. There is a curvilinear increase in excess mortality with rising BMI. With this relationship, arbitrary dividing lines for low, moderate, and high risk from obesity have been drawn. These provide a framework in which to consider the various treatment options for obesity.[17]

purposes. The reason for the decision by the various principal investigators to do this was to increase the number of individuals on whom data would be available.[18] At the time this project began, there were eight studies underway on the factors involved in the development of coronary artery disease. For analytical purposes, three industrial studies (Albany Civil Servants, Chicago Gas Co., Chicago Western Electric Co.) and two community-based studies (Framingham, MA and Tecumseh, MI) were pooled. Because the number of non-white men were small, the data were only analyzed for white males. Similarly, because the number of individuals under 40 years of age was small, the entry data on men age 40–64 were selected for analysis. The data after ten years of follow-up were used for this analysis. Body weight was obtained in most studies with men in their underclothes and expressed as a relative weight using the 1959 Metropolitan Life Insurance Co. table. Height was recorded to the nearest inch and weight was divided into five-pound intervals. In this study 8422 men were included in the analysis of these five studies, with a mean length of follow-up of 8.6 years. The mean percentage of desirable weight at entry for these men was 116.7 percent. A high relative weight was associated with an increased risk of a first major coronary event for men only in their forties. For the older groups there was no effect of age on the risk of developing coronary heart disease. The data were examined in terms of relative risk by comparing the quintiles of weight at five-year age intervals. When this was done, there was a relative risk of 2.1 in the men (ages 40–44), which had fallen to 116 for the men ages 45–49. That means that an individual, aged 40–44, in the highest quintile for relative weight was 2.1 times as likely of developing a first coronary event within an average of 3.6 years as an individual in the lowest quintile. In the men over 55, this gradient with quintiles of weight was largely gone. The major risk factors for coronary artery disease identified in this pooling project and in the individual prospective studies were high blood pressure, high serum cholesterol, and smoking. An increase in relative weight was only significant in the younger men (ages 40–49).

There are three major limitations of the pooling project. First the total number of men available for analysis, even after pooling the data, is small. Second, the duration of average follow-up was only 8.6 years, and third, the number of individuals under 40 years of age was too small for analysis. The importance of long-term follow-up has been noted in the Manitoba study.[19] The observation of greater impact on younger individuals is noted by Drenick (see below) and again in the Framingham study.

The Framingham Study. More than 5000 residents of Framingham, Massachusetts have been examined periodically for epidemiologic clues to the development of heart disease and other ailments. After 26 years of following this group, there have been 870 deaths among the men and 688 deaths among the women.[20] Relative weight at entry into the study was found to be an independent predictor of cardiovascular disease, particularly in women. The 26-year incidence of coronary artery disease, the death rate from coronary artery disease, and the likelihood of developing heart failure in men were predicted from the initial degree of overweight. The predictive effect of the initial measurement of overweight was independent of age, cholesterol level, systolic blood pressure, cigarette smoking, or glucose intolerance. The conclusion from this study is that obesity is an important long-term predictor of cardiovascular disease, particularly among younger individuals. In women, only age and blood pressure were more powerful predictors. For the 2223 men, the minimum mortality over 30 years of age for both smokers and nonsmokers occurred at a relative weight of 100% to 109% of the Metropolitan 1959 table. From the data collected in Framingham, the investigators estimated that "if everyone were at optimal weight, there would be 25% less coronary heart disease and 35% less congestive heart failure and brain infarction."[21]

The American Cancer Society Study. The American Cancer Society has also published data on mortality in relation to body weight for more than 750 000 individuals studied prospectively between 1959 and 1972.[22] Relative death rates among subgroups that deviated above or below the average body weight were compared to the death rate for the group who had an average weight of 90–109 percent. As the weight increased, the overall mortality rate increased. The data for men and women have a J or U shape similar to the curve plotted in FIGURE 3. This study separated smokers from nonsmokers. A smoker of normal body weight has an increased mortality ratio comparable to a nonsmoker with a BMI of 30–35

kg/m^2. A major factor in this extra mortality is cardiovascular disease. There is no increase in mortality until the BMI reaches 25 kg/m^2.[22] Above this point the increase in relative mortality is almost linear for both sexes. These findings are similar to the increase observed in both the Build Study of 1979[6] and in the Framingham Study.[20] There was also a pronounced effect of excess weight on death from diabetes mellitus and gall bladder disease. Cancer also showed a significant association with weight status. As the BMI increased, there was an increase in death from cancer. This effect, however, is much smaller than the other causes of death, reaching a maximum of 1.5 times average when the BMI is 35 kg/m^2. Overweight males experience significantly higher rates of prostatic and colorectal cancer. For overweight women, cancers of the gall bladder, breast, cervix, endometrium, uterus, and ovary all showed increased rates with excess weight.[22]

The Scandinavian Studies. a. The Göteborg Study. A prospective study from Göteborg, Sweden provided additional information about the health consequences of moderate obesity.[7,8] In men, the BMI and the ratio of waist to hip circumference were positively correlated in those who developed strokes.[7] That is, men in the highest tertile for waist/hip ratio and the highest tertile for BMI had a 20.8% risk for developing strokes compared to a 5.6% risk for men in the lowest tertile of the BMI and waist-to-hips ratio. For cardiovascular disease, a different relationship was detected. The highest risk was in the group with the highest hips-to-waist ratio and the lowest BMI (kg/m^2). Thus, carrying extra fat around the waist is particularly risky for individuals who are not much overweight.[7]

A similar set of relationships apply to women as well.[8] Among 14 462 women, aged 38–60, living in Göteborg, Sweden, the 12-year age-specific incidence rates for myocardial infarction, stroke, and overall death were related to the waist-to-hips ratio. Among the highest quintile, the relative risk of myocardial infarction was increased 8.2 times that for those in the lowest quintile. For stroke and overall death rate, the relative risk increased 3.8 and 2.0 for those in the highest quintile for waist-to-hips circumference. When the women in the top 5% of the waist-to-hips ratio were compared to the women in the lowest quintile, the risk of having a myocardial infarction was increased 14.8 times; the risk of having a stroke was increased 11.0 times, and the risk of dying was increased 4.8 times. Both increasing BMI and higher waist to hips ratio enhanced the risk of developing coronary artery disease.

b. The Norwegian Study. The availability of height and weight measurements for a majority of the Norwegian population obtained during mass X ray screening conducted between 1963 and 1975 provided the basis for this prospective study.[23] A total of 1 717 000 men and women aged 15–90 were followed with a total of 176 574 deaths occurring during the years 1963 to 1979. The body weight was measured without shoes in over 95% of the cases and with the upper body undressed in preparation for the X rays. Height and weight were analyzed using the BMI (kg/mg^2).

There was a U-shaped relationship between mortality and BMI. The minimal mortality rates for males and females occurred at a BMI of 23. There was a steep increase in death rate when the BMI was less than 23. Between BMI 23 and 27, relative mortality showed little change. As the BMI increased above 27 kg/m^2 there was a curvilinear increase in excess mortality. There was also a strong negative association between mortality and height. That is, mortality experience was lower in tall individuals than in short ones. The principal causes of excess mortality in the shorter individuals was tuberculosis, obstructive lung diseases, and cancer of the stomach and lung. Among the overweight individuals, the principal causes of death were cerebrovascular diseases, cardiovascular diseases, diabetes mellitus, and cancer of the colon. From his analysis, Waaler concludes that "if everybody obtained the low mortality at the optimal W/H^2 (body mass index) level, the total mortality would be reduced by an additional 15%".[23]

Age and Risk from Obesity

Previous studies have suggested that the effects of excess weight may well be of more importance in younger individuals than in those who develop obesity later in life. In the men who are overweight early in life, the extra mortality may be partially dissipated by the time they reach the age of 50 to 60. Abraham *et al.*[24] related the changes in weight status between childhood and adult life to the incidence of hypertensive and cardiovascular renal disease in 715 males. Childhood weight status was determined from school records when these men were aged 9 to 13. Follow-up weights were taken at an average age of 48. The highest prevalence for both conditions occurred in the men with the lowest childhood weight who became overweight as adults. Drenick *et al.*[25] have also provided insight into the effects of gross obesity on life expectancy. They reviewed 200 morbidly obese men whose average weight was 143.5 kg when admitted for a weight control program. They were followed for an average period of 7.5 years. Of these men, 185 were followed until death or termination of the study. The age range was 23 to 70 years with a mean of 42.7 years. The mortality rate was higher at all ages when compared with the mortality expected for the general population of U.S. males. In men aged 25–34, the excess mortality was 1200 percent! In those aged 35–44, the excess mortality had declined to 550%, and in men 45–54, it was still 300%. In men 55–64 the excess mortality was only double that of the normal-weight U.S. population. This study shows that the excess mortality associated with obesity is greatly increased in the younger age groups and that excess mortality is substantially higher in grossly obese persons.

Both the insurance companies[16] and the Framingham Study[20,21] have also provided retrospective data that suggests that weight reduction may prolong life. In both men and women who successfully lose and maintain a lower weight, mortality was reduced to within normal limits based on sex and age. From the data obtained in Framingham, it was observed that a 10% reduction in the body weight of men would produce an anticipated 20% decrease in the incidence of coronary artery disease.

Morbidity and Obesity

Hypertension. The relation of hypertension to obesity has been widely recognized.[1,26] Blood pressure measured with a standard blood pressure cuff may be higher or lower than values obtained by direct intraarterial measurement.[1] The major source of error occurs when the bladder of the blood pressure cuff does not adequately encircle the arm. To quantitate this relationship, Maxwell *et al.*[27] have compared 84 000 measurements of blood pressure in 1240 obese subjects using cuffs of three different sizes. Arm circumference was correlated with standard body weight in both males (r = .79) and females (r = .84). The values for both diastolic and systolic blood pressure were highest with the regular cuff and lowest with the large cuff or the thigh cuff. As arm circumference increases, the comparative blood pressure also rises with decreasing cuff size. From their data the authors estimate that in subjects with arm circumferences between 33 and 41 cm (large arms) nearly 37% of those found to be hypertensive with normal cuffs may actually be normotensive.

A reduction in blood pressure usually follows weight loss.[29] During periods of caloric deprivation in World War II hypertension was almost nonexistent. A number of clinical studies correlating changes in blood pressure with weight reduction have shown that 50 to 70% of those who lose weight show a fall in blood pressure. One explanation for this fall in blood pressure might be the reduced intake of salt that is associated with reduced caloric intake. Reisin et al.[28] and Tuck et al.[29] showed, however, that the reduction in blood pressure occurred even when salt intake was held constant. This latter group went on to suggest that the lower caloric intake may reduce blood pressure by lowering the activity of the sympathetic nervous system.

Obesity and Pulmonary Function. Measurement of pulmonary function in the obese individual shows a number of abnormalities.[30,31] At one extreme are the patients with the Pickwickian syndrome named after Joe, the fat boy in Dickens' *Pickwick Papers*. The Pickwickian syndrome or the obesity-hypoventilation syndrome is characterized by somnolence, obesity, and hypoventilation. At the other extreme are the impairments in work capacity and pulmonary function that are due to obesity itself. Significant alterations in pulmonary function in obesity are observed primarily in the massively obese or in those with obesity and some other respiratory or cardiovascular problem. In a careful study of 29 obese women and 14 obese men, we noted that there was a progressive decrease in expiratory reserve volume as the weight/height (cm/kg) ratio increased. On the other hand, vital capacity, inspiratory capacity, residual volume, and diffusion capacity remained fairly constant until the weight/height ratio exceeded 1.0 (*i.e.* massive obesity).[30]

Respiratory muscles may also function abnormally in obese patients, and there may be a disturbance in ventilation and perfusion. The most significant pulmonary problem in the obese patient, however, is the Pickwickian or obesity-hypoventilation syndrome. Although obesity is common, this syndrome is not. There is a growing body of literature that suggests that the symptoms of the obesity-hypoventilation syndrome may result largely from sleep apnea.[30] Sharp et al.[30] believe that the hypoxemia and hypercapnia that occur during part of the day may eventually adversely affect the control of ventilation during the rest of the day. Patients with the obesity-hypoventilation syndrome have markedly impaired ventilatory responses to breathing carbon dioxide (CO_2). The hypoxia associated with the obstructive or mixed sleep apnea produces hypoxia that worsens as the obesity progresses. The hypoxia in turn blunts the hypoxemic drive. Sleep is disturbed and compensatory sleep occurs during the day (diurnal hypersomnolence). With time, the hypoxemia is followed by hypercapnia that eventually leads to cor pulmonale and right-sided heart failure.[30] Patients with the Pickwickian or obesity-hypoventilation syndrome may require intensive care in a hospital to treat respiratory or cardiac failure.

Obesity and Gallbladder Diseases. The association of obesity with gallbladder disease has been documented in several studies. The life insurance statistics show that obesity increases the risk of dying from gallbladder disease.[16] Digestive diseases were 40% above the normal level in those 15–35% overweight and nearly

150% above normal among those who were 25% or more overweight. Increased mortality from digestive diseases is also evident in the American Cancer Society study.[22] In an autopsy study, Sturdevant et al.[32] found that the body weight of men without gallstones was significantly less than in men with gallstones. In a cross-sectional study of 62 739 respondents to a questionnaire developed by the self-help group called TOPS (Take Off Pounds Sensibly), Bernstein et al.[33] found that the risk of gallbladder disease increases with age, body weight, and parity. Within any age group, the frequency of gallbladder disease increases with the level of body weight. For women aged 25 to 34 years who are 100% or more overweight, 18% had gallbladder disease compared to nearly 35% of the women aged 45 to 55 who were 100% or more overweight. In this study, 88% of the variation in frequency of gallbladder disease was accounted for by weight, age, and parity, with weight being the most important variable. Obese women between 20 and 30 years of age had a sixfold increase in the risk of developing gallbladder disease compared to normal weight women. By age 60 nearly one-third of obese women can expect to develop gallbladder disease. In the Framingham Study, individuals who were at least 20% above the median weight for their height had about twice the risk of developing gallbladder disease as those who were less than 90% of the median weight for height.[34]

Increased cholesterol production and secretion provides one explanation for the increased risk of gallbladder disease in obesity. First, there is a significant correlation between the degree of fatness and cholesterol. Second the cholesterol production rate is correlated with body weight. For each extra kg of body weight, cholesterol production increased 20–22 mg per day.[35] Third, the bile of obese patients is more saturated with cholesterol than in nonobese controls.[36] Finally, the hepatic secretion of cholesterol was higher before weight loss than afterward, although neither phospholipids nor bile salt secretion changed. Thus the increased biliary excretion of cholesterol in obesity is the likely cause of the increased risk of gallstones.

Obesity and Diabetes. Obesity appears to aggravate the development of diabetes, and weight loss appears to reduce the risk of this disease. Drenick[37] followed a group of obese men none of whom were initially diabetic. During the six years of follow-up, the percentage of those with frank diabetes increased steadily to become more than 40% of the total. An additional 40% showed impaired glucose tolerance, meaning that during the six years of follow-up, more than 80% of the group showed a deterioration in glucose tolerance. In a similar vein, Toeller et al.[38] have reported a follow-up of 60 subjects, including 11 men and 49 women, who received glucose tolerance tests at the beginning and again at two five-year intervals for 10 years. Five of the subjects were initially diabetic and remained that way during the 10-year study. The remaining 55 patients fell into groups with either normal or impaired glucose tolerance. After five years, 19 of the original 26 with normal glucose tolerance tests fell into this group, and by 10 years only 9 still had normal glucose tolerance. By 10 years, 9 of those with initially normal glucose tolerance had become diabetic, and 7 showed impaired glucose tolerance. Of the 29 patients who initially had impaired glucose tolerance, 14 showed normal glucose tolerance five years later, and 4 retained this status after 10 years. Those who maintained a normal glucose tolerance showed a steady decrease in the degree of overweight during the 10-year time interval, falling from an initial value of 68% overweight to 62% overweight at five years and 53% overweight at 10 years. These data as a whole show the importance of both the duration and the severity of obesity as factors in the development of diabetes.

The importance of weight loss in improving glucose tolerance and insulin secretion cannot be emphasized too strongly. Drenick[39] studied three groups of subjects before and after weight loss and again after regaining part of the weight loss. When glucose tolerance was initially normal, the insulin response to glucose improved with weight loss and then deteriorated when weight was regained. In subjects who initially had only mild impairment of glucose tolerance, the improvement in insulin secretion with weight loss was more evident, and the deterioration of insulin secretion when weight was regained was associated with a marked worsening of glucose tolerance. In the final group, with minimal insulin response initially, and much higher initial body weights, the impact of weight loss on insulin secretion was most evident. The fact that obese subjects with normal glucose tolerance can develop clinical diabetes and even diabetic ketoacidosis requiring hospital care cannot be overlooked, simply because they are obese.[40]

SUMMARY

In this paper I have defined obesity and indicated its prevalence, as well as its risks. Body fat and its relation to other body components can be quantitated in many ways. From a practical point of view, the use of body mass or Quetelet index, defined as the ratio of weight (kg) divided by the square of the height (m^2) is the most useful. Overweight is defined as a BMI of 25 to 30 kg/m^2 and obesity as a BMI above 30 kg/m^2. The WHR can provide additional information about the risk of obesity. Using BMI, the prevalence of overweight in the English-speaking countries of Australia, Great Britain, and the United States is almost identical at 24% of women and 31 to 34% of men. In the obese category, there are more Americans (12%) than in the other two countries (6–8%). There is a U-shaped relationship between weight and risk of death. When body weight is increased 20% above average, the extra mortality rises to 20% for men and 10% for women. This extra mortality is associated with an increased death rate from heart disease, hypertension, diabetes mellitus, digestive diseases, and cancer. In addition to an increased risk of death, overweight individuals demand more from their heart, lungs, and musculoskeletal and digestive systems.

REFERENCES

1. BRAY, G. A. 1976. The Obese Patient. Major Problems in Internal Medicine. Vol. 9: 1–450. W. B. Saunders Company. Philadelphia, PA.
2. CLARYS, J. P., A. D. MARTIN & D. T. DRINKWATER. 1984. Gross tissue weight in the human body by cadaver dissection. Hum. Biol. 56: 459–473.
3. HAMILL, P. V., T. A. DRIZD, C. L. JOHNSON, R. B. REED, A. F. ROCHE & W. M. MOORE. 1979. Physical growth: National Center for Health Statistics percentiles. Am. J. Clin. Nutr. 32: 607–629.
4. BENN, R. T. 1970. Indices of height and weight as measures of obesity. Br. J. Prev. Soc. Med. 24: 64.
5. ANDRES, R., D. ELAHI, J. D. TOBIN, D. C. MULLER & L. BRANT. 1985. Impact of age on weight goals. Ann. Intern. Med. 103(6 pt2): 1030–1033.
6. Society of Actuaries. Build Study of 1979. Society of Actuaries and Association of Life Insurance Medical Directors of America.
7. LARRSON, B. K., L. SVARDSUUD, L. WELIN, L. WILHELMSE, P. BJORNTORP & G. TIBBLIN. 1984. Abdominal adipose tissue distribution, obesity, and risk of cardiovas-

cular disease and death: 13 year follow-up of participants in the population study of women in Gothenburg, Sweden. Br. Med. J. **289:** 1257–1261.

8. LAPIDUS, L., C. BENGTSSON, B. LARSSON, K. PENNERT, E. RYBO & L. SJOSTROM. 1984. Distribution of adipose tissue and risk of cardiovascular disease and death: a 12 year follow-up of participants in the population study of women in Gothenberg, Sweden. Br. Med. J. **289:** 1257–1261.

9. BRAY, G. A., F. L. GREENWAY, M. MOLITCH, W. T. DAHMS, R. L. ATKINSON & K. HAMILTON. 1978. Use of anthropometric measures to assess weight loss. Am. J. Clin. Nutr. **31:** 769–773.

10. GARROW, J. S. 1978. Energy balance and obesity in man. 2nd edit. North Holland Biomedical Press. Amseterdam.

11. SEGAL, K. R., B. GUTIN, E. PRESTA, J. WANG & T. B. VAN ITALLIE. Estimation of human body composition by electrical impedance methods: a comparative study. 1985. J. Appl. Physiol. **58:** 1565–1571.

12. COHN, S. H., D. VARTSKY, S. YASUMURA, A. SAWITSKY, I. ZANIZI, A. VASWANI & K. ELLIS. 1980. Compartmental body composition based on total body nitrogen, postassium, and calcium. Am. J. Physiol. **239:** E524.

13. ABRAM S., M. D. CARROLL, M. F. NAJJAR & M. F. ROBINSON. 1983. Obese and overweight adults in the United States, Vital and Health Statistics USDHHS, Publ No. (PHS) 83-1680 PHS NCHS. Series 11. No. 230.

14. BRAY, G. A., Ed. 1979. Obesity in America. DHEW Publication No. (NIH), Washington. D.C.

15. VAN ITALLIE, T. B. 1985. Health implications of overweight and obesity in the United States. Ann. Intern. Med. **103:** 983–988.

16. BRAY, G. A. 1985. Obesity: Definition, diagnosis, and disadvantages. Aust. J. Med. **142**(Suppl. 7): S2–S8.

17. BRAY, G. A. 1985. Complications of obesity. Ann. Intern. Med. **103:** 1052–1062.

18. The Pooling Project Research Group. 1978. Relationship of blood pressure, serum cholesterol, smoking habits, relative weight and ECG abnormalities to incidence of major coronary events: final report of the pooling project. J. Chronic Dis. **31:** 201–206.

19. RABKIN, S. W., F. MATHEWSON & P. HAN. 1977. Relation of body weight to development of ischemic heart disease in a cohort of young North American men after a 26 year observation period: the Manitoba Study. Am. J. Cardiol. **39:** 452–458.

20. HUBERT, H. B., N. FEINLEIB, P. MCNAMARA & W. CASTELLI. 1983. Obesity as an independent risk factor for cardiovascular disease: a 26-year follow-up of participants in the Framingham Heart Study. Circulation **67**(5): 968–977.

21. KANNEL, W. B. & T. GORDON. 1979. Physiological and medical concomitants of obesity: The Framingham study. In Obesity in America. G. A. Bray, Ed: 125–153.

22. LEW, E. A. & L. GARFINKEL. 1979. Variations in mortality by weight among 750,000 men and women. J. Chronic Dis. **32:** 563–576.

23. WAALER, H. T. 1983. Weight and mortality: The Norwegian experience. Acta Med. Scand. **679:** 1–55.

24. ABRAHAM, S., G. COLLINS & M. NORDSIECK. 1971. Relationship of childhood weight status to morbidity in adults. HSMHA Health Reports **86:** 273–384.

25. DRENICK, E. J., G. S. BALE, F. S. A. SELTZER & D. G. JOHNSON. 1980. Excessive mortality and causes of death in morbidy obese men. J. Am. Med. Assoc. **243:** 443–445.

26. Report of the Hypertension Task Force. 1979. Vol. 9. Washington D.C. U.S. Department of Health, Education and Welfare. NIH publication No. 79-1631: 59–77.

27. MAXWELL, M. H., A.U. WAKS, P. C. SCHROTH, M. KARAM & L. P. DORNFELD. 1982. Error in blood pressure due to incorrect cuff size in obese patients. Lancet **2:** 33–36.

28. REISIN, E., R. ABEL, M. MODAN, D. S. SILVERBERG, H. E. ELIAHOU & B. MODAN. 1978. Effect of weight loss without salt restriction on reduction of blood pressure in overweight hypertensive patients. N. Engl. J. Med. **298:** 1–6.

29. TUCK, M. L., J. SOWERS, L. DORNFELD, G. KLEDZIK & M. MAXWELL. 1981. The effect of weight reduction on blood pressure, plasma renin activity, and plasma aldosterone levels in obese patients. N. Engl. J. Med. **304:** 933.

30. SHARP, J. T., M. BARROCAS & S. CHOKROVERTY. 1983. The cardiorespiratory effects of obesity on respiratory function. Am. Rev. Respir. Dis. **128:** 501–506.
31. RAY, C. S., D. Y. SUE, G. A. BRAY, J. E. HANSEN & K. WASSERMAN. 1983. Effect of obesity on respiratory function. Am. Rev. Respir. Dis. **128:** 501–506.
32. STURDEVANT, R. A., M. L. PEARCE & S. DAYTON. 1973. Increased prevalence of cholelithiasis in men ingesting a serum cholesterol-lowering diet. N. Engl. J. Med. **288:** 24–27.
33. BERNSTEIN, R. A., E. E. GIEFER, J. J. VIEIRA, L. H. WERNER & A. A. RIMM. 1977. Gallbladder disease. II. Utilization of the life table method in obtaining clinically useful information: a study of 62,739 weight-conscious women. J. Chronic Dis. **30:** 529–541.
34. FRIEDMAN, G. D., W. B. KANNEL & R. R. DAWBER. 1966. The epidemiology of gallbladder disease: observations in Framingham study. J. Chronic Dis. **19:** 273–292.
35. NESTLE, P. J., P. H. SCHREIBMAN & E. H. AHRENS. 1973. Cholesterol metabolism in human obesity. J. Clin. Invest. **52:** 2389–2397.
36. BENNION, L. T. & S. M. GRUNDY. 1978. Risk factors for the development of cholelithiasis in man (part 2). N. Engl. J. Med. **229:** 1221–1227.
37. DRENICK, E. J. 1979. Definition and health consequences of morbid obesity. Surg. Clin. North Am. **59**(6): 963–975.
38. TOELLER, M., F. A. GRIES & K. DANNEHL. 1982. Natural history of glucose intolerance in obesity: A ten year observation. Int. J. Obesity **6**(Suppl 1): 145–149.
39. DRENICK, E. J., A. S. BRICKMAN & E. M. GOLD. 1972. Dissociation of the obesity-hyperinsulinism relationship following dietary restriction and hyperalimentation. Am. J. Clin. Nutr. **25:** 746–755.
40. DRENICK, E. J. & D. JOHNSON. 1975. Evolution of diabetic ketoacidosis in gross obesity. Am. J. Clin. Nutr. **28:** 264–272.

An Anthropological Perspective on Obesity

PETER J. BROWN AND MELVIN KONNER

Department of Anthropology
Emory University
Atlanta, Georgia 30322

An anthropological approach to human obesity involves both an evolutionary and a cross-cultural dimension. That is, it attempts to understand how the human predisposition to obesity so evident in modern affluent societies may have been determined during our species' long evolutionary history as hunters and gatherers, as well as the variation in obesity prevalence in different societies, social classes, or ethnic groups.

The evolutionary success of *Homo sapiens* is best understood by reference to the operation of natural selection on our dual system of inheritance; that is, on genes and culture, but also, and perhaps especially, on their interaction. Human biology and culture are the product of adaptation to environmental constraints; traits that enhance an individual's ability to survive and reproduce should become common in human societies. In this view, the health and illness of a population can be conceived as measures of biocultural adaptation to a particular ecological setting. Changing patterns of morbidity and mortality, such as the epidemiological transition from infectious to chronic diseases, are the result of historical changes in lifestyle (*i.e.* culture) that affect health.

It is valuable to view obesity from this evolutionary perspective because of its great historical scope. The first appearance of the genus *Homo* occurred over two million years ago, and the first anatomically modern humans (*Homo sapiens sapiens*) became predominant about 40 000 years ago.[1] From either prehistoric point of departure, during most of human history, the exclusive cultural pattern was one of hunting and gathering. This original human lifestyle is rare, but a few such groups have been the subject of detailed anthropological study.[2]

Culture, in an anthropological sense, entails learned patterns of behavior and belief characteristic of a particular society. This second dimension of the anthropological perspective includes variables demonstrably related to the prevalence of obesity in a particular group—material aspects of lifestyle, like diet and productive economy—as well as more idealistic variables, the relationship of which to obesity is more speculative—such as aesthetic standards of ideal body type or the symbolic meaning of fatness.

Cross-cultural comparison thus serves two purposes, one relating to each of the two dimensions. First, technologically simple or primitive societies provide ethnographic analogies to amplify our understanding of prehistoric periods, or to test hypotheses about biocultural evolution. Such societies provide useful analogies to prehistoric societies, particularly in terms of economic production and diet. Second, cross-cultural comparison allows us to see our own society's health problems and cultural beliefs about health in a new way. In a heterogeneous society like the United States, where particular social groups have markedly high prevalences of obesity, attention to cultural variation in beliefs and behaviors has practical value for medicine. Going beyond the U.S. to the numerous cultural varieties in the anthropological record gives us a fascinating range of further variation for systematic analysis. Such analysis is likely to reveal relationships that may not appear in other approaches, and attention to this wider range of cultures becomes even more relevant as obesity becomes a factor in international health.

In this paper we argue that throughout most of human history, obesity was never a common health problem, nor was it a realistic possibility for most people. This was because, despite the qualitative adequacy of their diet, most primitive societies have been regularly subjected to food shortages. Scarcity has been a powerful agent of natural selection in human biocultural evolution. Both genes and cultural traits that may have been adaptive in the context of past food scarcities today play a role in the etiology of maladaptive adult obesity in affluent societies. Following this evolutionary argument about the origins of obesity, we turn our attention to the cross-cultural range of beliefs about ideal body characteristics and the social meanings of obesity. A prerequisite for both discussions is a review of some basic facts concerning the social epidemiology of obesity.

HUMAN OBESITY: THREE SOCIAL EPIDEMIOLOGICAL FACTS

Humans are among the fattest of all mammals;[3] the proportion of fat to total body mass ranges from approximately 10 percent in the very lean to over 35 percent in the obese.[4] In other mammals, the primary function of fat deposits is insulation from cold, but in humans, it is now widely accepted that much (but not all) fat serves as an energy reserve. The social distribution of adiposity within and between human populations is not random, and that distribution provides a key to understanding obesity. Three widely recognized social epidemiological facts about obesity are particularly salient for this discussion: (1) higher levels of fatness and risk of obesity in females represents a fundamental aspect of sexual dimorphism in *Homo sapiens*; (2) obesity is rare in unacculturated primitive populations, but the prevalence often increases rapidly during modernization; and (3) the prevalence of obesity is related to social class, usually positively; but among females in affluent societies, that relationship is inverted.

Obesity and Gender

Differences in fat deposition are an important aspect of sexual dimorphism in *Homo sapiens*.[5] Sexual dimorphism is found in many primate species, and it is more pronounced in terrestrial, polygynous species. Humans are only mildly dimorphic in morphological variables like stature; a survey of human populations around the world reveals a range of dimorphism in stature from 4.7 to 9.0 percent.[6] The most significant aspects of sexual dimorphism reside predominantly in soft tissue. On average for young adults in an affluent society, adipose tissue constitutes approximately 15 percent of body weight in males and about 27 percent in females.[4]

Fatness, particularly peripheral or limb body fat, is the most dimorphic of the morphological variables, as shown in FIGURE 1. Adult men are larger than women in stature (+8%) and total body mass (+20%), whereas women have more subcutaneous fat as measured in skinfold thicknesses. Bailey's analysis of sex differences in body composition using data from white Americans in Tecumseh, Michigan show greater female skinfolds in 16 of 17 measurement sites (the exception is the suprailiac). In general, adult limb fatness was much more dimorphic than trunk fatness: trunk: −7.5% (mean of 5 measures); arms: −35.4% (mean of 4 measures); and legs/thighs: −46.7% (mean of 5 measures).[4]

It is noteworthy that peripheral body fat does not have the same close association with chronic diseases (*i.e.* Type II diabetes mellitus or hypertension) as centripetal or trunk fatness. Thus the sexual dimorphism in fat deposition may be

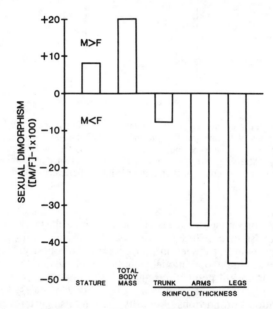

FIGURE 1. Sexual dimorphism in stature, body mass, and fat measures among white Americans aged 20 to 70 in Tecumseh, Michigan. Sexual dimorphism calculated by comparing male versus female means by ([M/F]-1×100); positive figures refer to greater male measures. Data are from Bailey.[4] Skinfold thicknesses are means of 4 sites (trunk) or 5 sites (arms and legs/thighs); the mean sexual dimorphism in all 17 fat measures is −19%.

unrelated to the dimension of obesity that most affects health. The developmental course of this dimorphism is also of interest. It is present in childhood, but increases markedly during adolescence, due to greatly increased divergence in the rate of fat gain.[7] Thus this divergence occurs at the time of reproductive maturation.

Although there is some population-specific variation in fat distribution, human sexual dimorphism in overall fat and peripheral fat appears to be universal. Although very small in stature and extremely lean by worldwide standards, the !Kung San, a hunting and gathering society of the Kalahari desert, show a similar pattern of sexual dimorphism, with a pronounced difference in measures of subcu-

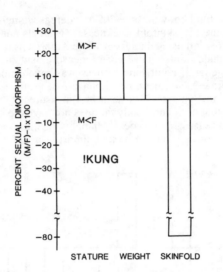

STATURE   WEIGHT   SKINFOLD

FIGURE 2. Sexual dimorphism in stature, weight, and mid-triceps skinfolds among !Kung San hunter-gatherers of Botswana. Sample includes 527 men and women, aged 10–80, all living in a traditional lifestyle. Sexual dimorphism calculated by comparing male versus female means by ([M/F]-1×100); positive figures refer to greater male measures. Note the larger male/female difference in fat than among white Americans shown in FIGURE 1.

taneous fat for women (see FIG. 2). The sexual dimorphism of the !Kung San is about +6.7% for stature, +20% in weight, and −80% in midtriceps skinfolds.[8]

Sex differences are also seen in the prevalence of obesity. Despite methodological differences in the operational definition of obesity and in sampling frameworks, data from the 14 populations shown in FIGURE 3 show that in all of the surveys, females have a higher prevalence of obesity than males. Variations in the male/female ratio of proportions of obesity seen in this figure reveal a new regularity that remains to be explained—namely, that more affluent western populations have more equivalent male/female ratios of obesity prevalence than poor populations in the underdeveloped world.

Obesity and Modernization

The second social epidemiological fact regards culture change and the origins of obesity. It is significant that anthropometric studies of traditional hunting and gathering populations report no obesity. By contrast, numerous studies of traditional societies undergoing the process of modernization (or Westernization) report rapid increases in the prevalence of obesity.[9–12] A classic natural experiment study by Prior and colleagues compared the diet and health of Polynesian islanders at different stages of acculturation: the prevalence of obesity in the most traditional island (Pukapuka) was 15.4%; for a rapidly modernizing population (Rarotonga), it was 29.3%; and for urban Maoris it was 35.4 percent.[13] Trowell and Burkitt, whose recent volume contains 15 case studies of societies experiencing increased obesity and associated Western diseases during modernization, conclude that obesity is the first of these diseases of civilization to appear.[14]

Change in diet appears to be a primary cause for the link between modernization and obesity. More precisely, westernization of traditional diets involves decreased intake of fiber and increased intake of fats and sugar. The seeming inevitability of this change toward a less healthy diet is impressive but not well understood. We suspect that more is involved in this dietary change than the simple imitation of prestigous western foodways: the quick shift from primitive to high fat, high sugar diets with the advent of affluence may have evolutionary roots.

Obesity and Social Class

The third and possibly most important fact concerning the social epidemiology of obesity is its association with social class and ethnicity. Research primarily by Stunkard and colleagues have shown that social class and obesity are inversely related, at least in heterogenous and affluent societies like the United States.[15,16] The inverse correlation of social class and obesity is very strong, particularly for females. A few studies, however, have found a weak association of class and

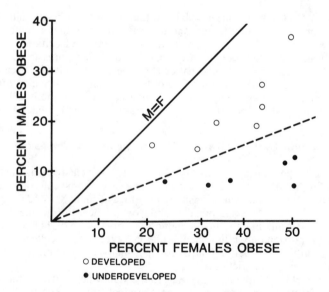

O DEVELOPED

● UNDERDEVELOPED

FIGURE 3. Gender differences in prevalence of obesity in 14 populations by general economic development. Only complete society prevalences were used, and underdeveloped populations were limited to groups with a significant degree of obesity. Operational definitions of obesity differ between studies. Populations include: Pukapuka, Rarotonga and New Zealand urban Maori,[13] Capetown Bantu, Guyana, Lagos (Nigeria), Puerto Rico, Germany, London,[12] U.S. Blacks, and U.S. Whites.[16] The unbroken line demarcates equal male/female obesity rates. The broken line indicates an apparent division between the proportion of gender difference in obesity between developed and underdeveloped countries.

obesity for groups including men, children, and certain ethnic groups.[17] But there is no doubt that social factors play a role in the epidemiology of obesity, and that the high prevalence of obesity for lower class women reflects that, "obesity may always be unhealthy, but it is not always abnormal."[15]

The association between socioeconomic class and obesity among adult women, therefore, merits special attention. This association is not constant through the life cycle. Garn and Clark describe a pattern of growth called "the socioeconomic reversal of fatness in females": in childhood, middle and upper class girls (and boys) are consistently fatter than poorer girls; at around the time of puberty, the relative level of fatness in the two groups switches; and in adulthood, lower class women are consistently fatter than middle and upper class women.[18]

In the traditional societies typically studied by anthropologists, the social epidemiology of adult obesity is not well documented. The data indirectly suggest, however, that the relationship of obesity and social class is often a positive one. Surveys from developing countries show a positive association between social class and obesity prevalence and, as expected, an inverse correlation between class and protein-calorie malnutrition.[19]

EVOLUTION AND OBESITY: DIET, FOOD SCARCITIES, AND ADAPTATION

Both genes and lifestyle are involved in the etiology of obesity, although the relative importance of either factor, and the ways in which they interact, are not thoroughly understood.[20] We suggest that both genetic and cultural predispositions to obesity may be products of the same evolutionary pressures, involving two related processes: first, traits that cause fatness were selected because they improved chances of survival in the face of food scarcities, particularly for pregnant and nursing women; second, fatness may have been directly selected because it is a cultural symbol of social prestige and an index of general health.

Cultural Evolution from Food Foraging to Food Production

For 95 to 99 percent of our history, humans lived exclusively as hunters and gatherers. Studies of contemporary food foragers reveal some cultural and biological commonalities despite variation in their ecological context. Food foragers live in small, socially flexible, seminomadic bands; experience slow population growth due to prolonged nursing and high childhood mortality; enjoy high quality diets and spend proportionately little time directly involved in food collection; and are generally healthier and better nourished than many contemporary third world populations relying on agriculture.

The reality of food foraging life is to be found somewhere between the Hobbesian "nasty, brutish, and short" and the "original affluent society," a phrase popularized by some anthropologists during the 1960s.[21] It is important to dispel romantic notions of food foragers, like the !Kung San of Botswana, as innocents leading a carefree existence; they suffer from a 50 percent child mortality rate, a low life expectancy at birth, and even a homicide rate that rivals that of many metropolitan areas. Yet, given the length of time that it has survived, food-foraging must be considered a successful strategy of adaptation.

Approximately 12 000 years ago, some human groups shifted from a food foraging economy to one of food production. This shift required the domestication of plants and animals, an evolutionary process in which humans acted as agents of selection for domestic phenotypes. This economic transformation, known as the neolithic revolution, may be considered the most important event in human history because it allowed population growth and the evolution of complex societies and civilization. The current consensus among archeologists is that the new economy based on agriculture was something that people were effectively forced to adopt because of ecological pressures from population growth and food scarcities.[22] Nearly everywhere it has been studied, the switch from food foraging to agriculture is associated with osteological evidence of nutritional stress, poor health, and diminished stature.[23]

It is important to note that the beginning of agriculture is linked to the emergence of social stratification. Civilization was made possible by the political, economic, and military power of urban elites over agricultural surpluses collected in the form of tribute. For members of the ruling class, social stratification has numerous advantages, the most important of which is guaranteed access to food during periods of relative food scarcity. In state level societies, nutritional stress is never evenly distributed across the social spectrum. Functionally, the poor insulate the rich from the threat of starvation.

Obesity is thus not simply a disease of civilization. It is common only in certain kinds of civilized societies—ones with an absolute level of affluence so that even the poor have access to enough food to become obese. Trowell has suggested that obesity became common in Europe, first in elites and then the rest of society, only about 200 years ago.[24]

The Adequacy of Preindustrial Diets

The adequacy of the diet of food foragers, and by close analogy that of our prehistoric ancestors, has been the subject of considerable interest. New analytical techniques now being applied to skeletal populations by archeologists are expanding our knowledge of prehistoric diet.[25] A recent analysis of the nutritional components of the Paleolithic diet,[26] shown in TABLE 1, suggests that the diet of prehistoric food foragers was high in protein, fiber, and vegetable carbohydrates and low in sugar and saturated fats. There are striking similarities of this reconstructed stone age diet and the daily nutritional requirements recommended by

TABLE 1. Late Paleolithic, Contemporary American, and Currently Recommended Dietary Composition[26]

	Late Paleolithic Diet	Contemporary American Diet	Current Recommendations
Total dietary energy (percent)			
Protein	34	12	12
Carbohydrate	45	46	58
Fat	21	42	30
P:S ratio[a]	1.41	0.44	1.00
Cholesterol (mg)	591	600	300
Fiber (gm)	45.7	19.7	30–60
Sodium (mg)	690	2300–6900	1100–3300
Calcium (mg)	1580	740	800–1200
Ascorbic Acid (mg)	392.3	87.7	45

[a] Polyunsaturated: saturated fat ratio.

the U.S. Senate Select Committee, in all areas except cholesterol intake. With this exception, the Paleolithic diet could be considered a model preventive diet, more stringent and thus probably more healthy even than the currently recommended one. But this fact reflects limitations in the availability and choice of foods rather than some primitive wisdom about a nutritionally optimal diet. Studies of culture change have repeatedly shown that when traditional populations with healthy diets have the opportunity, they readily switch to the less healthy (except in terms of abundance) Western diets.

Another method of estimation of the adequacy of the preindustrial diet is through cross-cultural comparison. Marjorie Whiting used ethnographic data from the Human Relations Area Files (HRAF) and nutritional studies to survey some major components of diet in a representative sample of 118 nonindustrial societies with economies based on food-foraging, pastoralism, simple horticulture, and agriculture.[27] (The HRAF is a compilation of ethnographic information on over 300 of the most thoroughly studied societies in the anthropological and historical record, cross-indexed for hundreds of variables. Subsamples of societies are chosen for representativeness of world areas and economic types.) In general, the quality of nonindustrial diets is high, the mean percent of calories derived from fat and carbohydrates falling within the recommended U.S. standards, and the percentage of protein nearly twice the recommended amount.[26] For the 84% of societies where food supply is adequate or plentiful, therefore, the diet seems superior to that of the United States. The major inadequacy of preindustrial diets and productive economies, however, is their susceptibility to food shortages.

The Ubiquity of Food Shortages

Food shortages have been so common in human prehistory and history that they could be considered a virtually inevitable fact of life in the past. Whiting's cross-cultural survey found some form of food shortages for all of the societies in the sample. FIGURE 4 illustrates the distribution of the frequency of shortages. In 28.7 percent of the societies, food shortages are rare, occurring every 10 to 15 years, whereas in 24.3 percent they happen every 2 to 3 years. Shortages occur annually or even more frequently in 47 percent of the societies. Half of these are annual shortfalls, which Whiting described as happening "a few weeks preceding harvest, anticipated and expected, recognized as temporary," and in the other 23.5 percent of the societies, shortages are more frequent than once a year. This distribution has great evolutionary significance.

The relative severity of these shortages is shown in FIGURE 5. For the 113 societies with adequate data, 29.3 percent had severe shortages that were characterized by the exhaustion of emergency foods, many people desperate for food, and starvation deaths—in short, a famine. Moderate shortages, in which food stores were used up, where emergency foods were used, and where people lost considerable weight, were found in 34.4 percent of the societies. Finally, 36.3 percent had mild food shortages, with fewer meals than usual, some weight loss, but no great hardships.[27] Two examples, one archeological and one ethnographic, will serve to illustrate these patterns and their relationship to the relative reliance on food foraging or food production.

The southwestern United States, where we today find Native American groups like the Pima, with endemic obesity and a high prevalence of type II

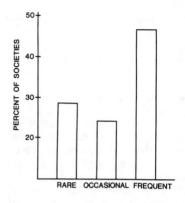

FIGURE 4. Frequency of food shortages in a sample of 115 preindustrial societies. Rare shortages occur every 5–10 years; occasional shortages occur every 2–3 years; and frequent shortages happen one or more times a year.[27]

diabetes,[28] was in the prehistoric past the frequent site of food shortages. Tree-ring analysis has been used to calculate the frequency of ecological stresses and resulting food shortages affecting these people, the builders of the impressive kivas and cliff dwellings. The data from southern New Mexico suggest that, between 600 and 1249 A.D., every other year had inadequate rainfall for dry farming, and that there was severe stress (more than two successive years of total crop failures) at least once every 25 years.[29] The complex agricultural societies of the prehistoric southwest expanded quickly during a period of uncharacteristically good weather. Despite a variety of social adaptations to food shortages, when lower rainfall pattern resumed, the complex chiefdomships could not be maintained: the population declined, and the culture devolved back to food foraging.

Medical studies of the !Kung San hunger-gatherers have found that adults were in generally good health, but exhibited periodic mild caloric undernutrition.[30] Seasonal variation in the availability of food resulted in an annual cycle of weight loss and weight gain in both food-foraging and food-producing societies. Agriculturalists, however, experience greater seasonal swings of weight loss and

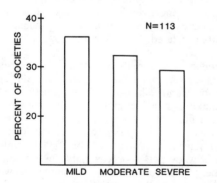

FIGURE 5. Severity of food shortages in a sample of 113 preindustrial societies.

gain. Seasonal weight loss among the !Kung, although it varied by ecological region and year, averaged between 1 and 2 percent of adult body weight.[8,31] Seasonal weight losses among African agriculturalists are more severe, averaging 4 to 6.5 percent of total body weight in typical years.[32]

Biological and Cultural Adaptations to Scarcity

Food shortages suggest a hypothesis of the evolution of obesity. Because shortages were ubiquitous for humans under natural conditions, selection favored individuals who could effectively store calories in times of surplus. For three-fourths of the societies, such stores would be depleted, or at least called on, every two to three years, and sometimes more frequently.

Medical data on famine victims show that, in addition to outright starvation, malnutrition from food shortages has a synergistic effect on infectious disease mortality, as well as decreasing birth weights and rates of child growth.[33] Females with greater energy reserves in fat have a selective advantage over their lean counterparts in withstanding the stress of food shortage, not only for themselves, but for their fetuses or nursing children. Humans have evolved to "save up" food energy for the inevitability of food shortages through the synthesis and storage of fat. Moreover, females, whose reproductive fitness depends upon their ability to withstand the nutritional demands of pregnancy and lactation, appear to have been selected for more slow-releasing peripheral body fat than males.

In this evolutionary context the usual range of human metabolic variation must have produced many individuals with a predisposition to become obese; yet they would, in all likelihood, never have the opportunity to do so. Furthermore, in this context there could be little or no natural selection against such a tendency. Selection could not provide for the eventuality of continuous surplus because it had simply never existed.

There is little evidence that obesity, at least moderate obesity, reduces Darwinian reproductive fitness. A follow-up study of participants to the Third Harvard Growth Study found a positive correlation between fatness and fertility when holding both social class and ethnicity constant.[34] The influence of social class is important and complex: in developed countries, fatness, lower social class, and fertility are all positively associated, whereas in underdeveloped countries, fatness and fertility are associated only in upper socioeconomic classes.[35] A minimal level of female fatness may increase lifetime reproductive success because of its association with regular cycling as well as earlier menarche. In preindustrial societies, social status is related, both symbolically and statistically, to fertility and fatness.

It is likely that under some conditions fatness is an adaptation to successful completion of pregnancy. Recommended weight gain during pregnancy is between 20 and 30 pounds, and failure to gain weight (which may be caused by inadequate caloric intake) is considered a clinically ominous sign.[36,37] Especially for women with lower gains and lower pregravid weight, weight gain is positively correlated with birth weight and negatively correlated with perinatal mortality. The energy cost of pregnancy is estimated to be 80 000 kcal (300 kcal/d), assuming no change in energy output[38]—a reasonable assumption for nonindustrial societies. Intrauterine growth retardation associated with working during pregnancy is greatest against the background of low pregravid weight and low pregnancy weight gain.[39] Failure to supplement usual intake adequately will result in a depletion of pregravid tissue reserves.

The ongoing energy cost of lactation, if milk is the sole primary infant food, is higher than that of pregnancy, and lactation in traditional societies may last up to four years and be superimposed on early pregnancy. Estimated needed supplements, converted to energy in milk with high efficiency (around 90%), range from 500 kcal/d in the early postpartum period to 1000 kcal/d by the end of the first year.[36,40] Well-fed women with high pregnancy weight gains can supplement less and safely attain a deliberately negative energy balance during lactation by drawing on prepartum fatty tissue reserves.[41] At the other extreme, experimental interventions in Gambia[42] and Guatemala[43] provided caloric supplementation to pregnant and lactating women. In the Gambian case, women readily took supplements larger than the above-mentioned estimates, and supplemented women who completed pregnancy in the lean season experienced a six-fold reduction of the proportion of low-birth-weight infants, ending up with an incidence typical of developed countries (4.7%). In both populations, supplements during lactation also increased the duration of postpartum infertility.

Using the figure 80 000 kcal for pregnancy, and a conversion rate of 9.1 kcal/g, pregnancy with no supplementation could be maintained by pregravid tissue reserves amounting to 8.8 kg of fat. Viewed from the perspective of the costs of shortage rather than the costs of pregnancy *per se*, an annual or less frequent shortage of the length and type experienced by the Gambian women, whether occurring during pregnancy or lactation, would be cushioned against by excess fat amounting to 15 to 20% of body weight. In as much as women in traditional societies spend the great majority of their reproductive lives either pregnant or nursing, an ideal of plumpness would be adaptive throughout that period. A custom such as the fattening hut for brides-to-be (see below) might provide a critical head-start on this lifelong reproductive energy drain.

Humans have also evolved other cultural mechanisms to minimize the effects of food shortages, including economic diversification, storage of foods, knowledge of possible famine foods, conversion of surplus food into durable valuables to be exchanged for food in emergencies, and cultivation of strong social relations with individuals in other regions.[44] These mechanisms act as buffers between environmental fluctuation and biological adaptation.

THE SOCIAL MEANING OF OBESITY: CROSS-CULTURAL COMPARISONS

Fatness is symbolically linked to psychological dimensions such as self-worth and sexuality in many societies of the world, including our own, but the nature of that symbolic association is not constant. In mainstream U.S. culture, obesity is socially stigmatized[45] even to the point of abhorrence. Weight loss is a major industry in the U.S., with annual expenditures of over five billion dollars. Most cultures of the world, by contrast, view fatness as a welcome sign of health and prosperity.

In an obesity-prevention campaign in a Zulu community outside of Durban,[46] one of the health education posters depicted an obese woman and an overloaded truck with a flat tire, with a caption "Both carry too much weight." Another poster showed a slender woman easily sweeping under a table next to an obese woman who is using the table for support; it has the caption "Who do you prefer to look like?" The intended message of these posters was misinterpreted by the community because of a cultural connection between obesity and social status. The woman in the first poster was perceived to be rich and happy, since she was not only fat, but had a truck overflowing with her possessions. The second poster was perceived as a scene of an affluent mistress directing her underfed servant.

Given the rarity of obesity in unacculturated preindustrial societies, it is not surprising that many groups have no ethnomedical definition of or concern with obesity. Given the frequency of food shortages, it is equally predictable that thinness, rather than fatness, will be deemed a serious medical symptom. The Tupinamba of Brazil have no descriptive term for fat people, but are reported to fear the symptom of thinness (angaiuare).[47] In the preindustrial context, thin people are to be pitied; this is the case for food foragers like the !Kung San, where culturally defined thinness (zham) is viewed as a symptom of starvation.

It may be large body size rather than obesity per se that in agricultural societies becomes an admired symbol of health, prestige, prosperity, or maternity. The agricultural Tiv of Nigeria, for example, distinguish between a very positive category, too big (kehe), and an unpleasant condition, to grow fat (ahon).[48] The first is a compliment—sign of prosperity that also refers to the seasonal weight gain of the early dry season when food is plentiful. The second term refers to a rare and undesirable condition.

Even in the industrialized U.S., there is ethnic variation in definitions of obesity. Some Mexican-Americans have coined a new term, gordura mala (bad fatness) because the original term gordura continues to have positive cultural connotations.[49] There has also been historical variation in clinical standardized definitions of obesity in American medicine. Between 1943 and 1980, definitions of ideal weights declined for women but not for men; more recently, upward revision of those standards has been proposed, due to an apparent disjunction in some data sets between cosmetically ideal weights and the weights at which mortality is minimized. This, however, remains controversial.[50,51] In any case, the definition of obesity is ultimately linked to cultural conceptions of normality, beauty, and health.

Cross-Cultural Variation in Ideal Body Type

In addition to the basic association between plumpness and health, culturally defined standards of beauty may have been a factor in the sexual selection for phenotypes predisposed to obesity. In a classic example, Malcom described the custom of fattening huts for the seclusion of elite Efik pubescent girls in traditional Nigeria.[52] A girl spent up to two years in seclusion before marriage, and at the end of this rite of passage she possessed symbols of womanhood and marriageability: a three-tiered hairstyle, clitoridectomy, and fatness. This fatness was a primary criterion of beauty as it was defined by the elites, who had the economic resources to participate in this custom. Similar fattening huts were found in other parts of West Africa.

Among the Havasupai of the American Southwest, if a girl at puberty is thin, a fat woman stands (places her foot) on the girl's back so that she will become attractively plump. In this society, fat legs, and to a lesser extent arms, are considered essential to beauty.[53] The Tarahumara of Northern Mexico, whose men are famous as long-distance runners, reportedly consider large, fat thighs as the first requisite of beauty; a good-looking woman is called a "beautiful thigh."[54] Among the Amhara of the Horn of Africa, thin hips are called "dog hips" in a typical insult.[55] A South African Bemba courting song has the following verse: "Hullo Mama, the beautiful one, let us go to town/You will be very fat, you girl, if you stay with me."[56]

But how common is such a cultural connection between beauty and fat? There has been no systematic cross-cultural survey of definitions of feminine beauty or ideal body type among the societies of the world. The lack of a survey reflects, in part, the failure of ethnographers and historians to report adequately on this cultural element. Of the 325 cultures coded by the Human Relation Area Files, only 58 have adequate data to estimate some characteristic of ideal female body type.

The data summarized in TABLE 2 must be considered cautiously for a number of reasons: Because of the paucity of ethnographic data, a representative sample is impossible. Although limited to sources rated good or better, there is potential ethnographer bias toward the exotic. Observations cover a wide historical time span, often characterized by substantial cultural changes. There is the problem of relative standards; given the endemic obesity in modern society, what we consider normal may be fat to members of a society where obesity is uncommon. There is no consideration of intracultural diversity. Because the unit of analysis is a culture, the HRAF data base is skewed toward demographically small and

TABLE 2. Cross-Cultural Standards of Female Beauty

	Number of Societies	Percent of Category
Overall Body		
Extreme Obesity	0	0
Plumpness/moderate fat	31	81
thin/abhorence of fat	7	19
Breasts		
Large or long	9	50
small/abhorence of large	9	50
Hips and Legs		
Large or Fat	9	90
Slender	1	10
Stature		
Tall	3	30
Moderate	6	60
Small	1	10

technologically simple societies; the HRAF data base does not include the U.S. or modern European societies.

Granting the weaknesses of the data base, some guarded generalizations still seem possible. Cultural standards of beauty seem to be based on the normal characteristics of the dominant group of a society; they do not refer to physical extremes. No society on record has an ideal of extreme obesity. On the other hand, the desirability of plumpness or being filled out is found in 81 percent of societies for which there is data. This standard, which probably includes the clinical categories of overweight and mild obesity, apparently refers to the desirability of subcutaneous fat deposits. For societies where data on ideal standards on hips and legs is available, it appears that plumpness in peripheral body fat is commonly preferred. Societies that favor plumpness as a standard of beauty are found in all of the major world culture areas, with the exception of Asia. There appears to be no trend in preference for breast-size or stature. Ethnographic discussion of beauty in other societies often emphasizes cultural enhancements to the body, such as scarification, clothes, body paint, jewelry, and other adornments, rather than attributes of the body itself.[57] Standards of sexual beauty are based upon images of nubile, postpubertal, young-adult years in virtually all societies.

Fatness may also be a symbol of maternity and nurturance. In traditional societies where a woman attains her proper status only through motherhood, this symbolic association increases the cultural acceptability of obesity. A fat woman, symbolically, is well taken care of, and she in turn takes good care of her children. Fellahin Arabs in Egypt describe the proper woman as an "envelope for conception," and therefore a fat woman is a desirable ideal because she has more room to bear the child, lactate abundantly, and give warmth to her children.[58]

Although there is cross-cultural variation in standards of beauty, this variation falls within a certain range. American ideals of thinness occur in a setting where it is easy to become fat, and preference for plumpness occurs in settings where it is easy to remain lean. In context, both standards require the investment of individual effort and economic resources; furthermore, each in its context involves a display of wealth. In poor societies the rich impress the poor by becoming fat, which the poor cannot do. In rich societies even the poor can become fat, and avidly do; therefore, the rich must impress by staying thin, as if to say, "We have so little doubt about where out next meal is coming from, that we don't need a single gram of fat store." Cultural relativism in feminine beauty standards, therefore, may be limited by evolutionarily determined human universals on the one hand and by lawful cross-cultural variation on the other.

The ethnographic record concerning body preferences in males is very weak. The HRAF data base includes only 12 societies with adequate information to gauge ideal male body type. In all of these societies, the expressed preference was for a muscular physique and for tall or moderately tall stature. Other characteristics mentioned include broad shoulders and being well filled out. One extreme in this admiration of large body size would be Japanese Sumo wrestlers whose program to build large bodies is really purposeful obesity; similar patterns of fattening young male wrestlers is found in Polynesia.[59] With few exceptions (e.g. the !Kung San)[8] human societies admire large body size, but not necessarily fatness, as an attribute of attractiveness in men. All of these physical characteristics can be considered as indicators of general health and nutritional status. Large body size and even obesity, however, are desirable because they symbolize economic success, political power, and social status in some societies.

Big Men, political leaders in tribal New Guinea, are described by their constituents in terms of their size and physical well-being (as well as other attributes). A Big Man may be described as a tall forest beech tree or as a man "whose skin swells with 'grease' [or fat] underneath".[60] Large body size may, in fact, be an index of differential access to food resources. This is seen in chiefdomships, as in ancient Polynesia, where hereditary political leaders sit at the hub of a redistribution system in which chiefly families are assured a portion of each family's harvest. The spiritual power (mana) and noble breeding of a Polynesian chief is expected to be seen in his physical appearance. One ethnographer in Polynesia was asked, "Can't you see he is a chief? See how big he is?"[61] The Bemba of South Africa believe that fatness in a man demonstrates not only his economic success but also his spiritual power in fending off the sorcery attacks.[62] A similar symbolic association can be assigned to deities. The corpulence of the seated Buddha, for example, symbolizes his divinity and otherworldliness.

Cultural variation in the meaning of fatness is also found among ethnic groups in the United States. Massara's ethnographic study of the cultural meanings of weight in a Puerto Rican community in Philadelphia[63] documents the positive associations and lack of social stigma of obesity. In addition, quantitative evidence[64] suggests that there are significant differences in ideal body preferences between this ethnic community and mainstream American culture. Positive evaluations of fatness may also occur in lower class Black Americans[65] and Mexican Americans.[17] There is also heterogeneity within these ethnic groups; upwardly mobile ethnics more closely resemble mainstream American culture in attitudes about obesity and ideal body shape.

In contrast to these ethnic minorities, and most of the cultures of the world, the ideal of female body shape in dominant middle/upper class America is thin. Studies suggest that females hold this cultural value more strongly than males,[66] who tend to be more satisfied with their own current body shape. Over the past three decades cosmetic ideals of female body shape have gotten thinner,[67] even thinner than medical ideals. Cultural beliefs about attractive body shape, therefore, place pressure on females to lose weight, and appear to be involved in the etiology of anorexia and bulimia. Neither the socioeconomic reversal of fatness in females nor the social history of symbolism of thinness has been adequately examined. Thinness, like tanning, is a contemporary symbol of economic status and leisure time for women. Both may be unhealthy, and both represent reversals of previous ideals.

Finally, although we have focused on the role of food shortages in human history, they are unfortunately not limited to the past. The drought and famine in the Horn of Africa and the Sahel have justifiably received world attention. Even in the United States, arguably the richest nation in human history, an estimated 20 million people are hungry.[68] This continuing worldwide epidemic of hunger presents a powerful and tragic counterbalance to our contemplation of the new epidemic of obesity and a reminder of the sometimes harsh realities of our history.

SUMMARY

An anthropological perspective on obesity considers both its evolutionary background and cross-cultural variation. It must explain three basic facts about obesity: gender dimorphism (women > men), an increase with modernization, and a positive association with socioeconomic status. Preindustrial diets varied in quality but shared a tendency to periodic shortages. Such shortages, particularly disadvantageous to women in their reproductive years, favored individuals who, for biological and cultural reasons, stored fat. Not surprisingly, the majority of the world's cultures had or have ideals of feminine beauty that include plumpness. This is consistent with the hypothesis that fat stores functioned as a cushion against food shortages during pregnancy and lactation. As obesity has increased, the traditional gap between males and females in its prevalence has narrowed. Under Western conditions of abundance, our biological tendency to regulate body weight at levels above our ideal cannot be easily controlled even with a complete reversal of the widespread cultural ideal of plumpness.

REFERENCES

1. PILBEAM, D. 1984. The descent of hominoids and hominids. Sci. Am. 250: 84–96.
2. LEE, R. B. & I. DEVORE, Eds. 1968. Man the Hunter. Aldine. Chicago, IL.
3. PITTS, G. C. & T. R. BULLARD. 1968. Some interspecific aspects of body composition in mammals. In Body Composition in Animals and Man. National Academy of Science, Washington D.C. Pub. No. 1598:45–70.

4. BAILEY, S. M. 1982. Absolute and relative sex differences in body composition. *In* Sexual dimorphism in *Homo sapiens*. R. L. Hall, Ed. Praeger Scientific. New York.
5. POND, C. M. 1978. Morphological aspects and the ecological and mechanical consequences of fat deposition in wild vertebrates. Ann. Rev. Ecol. Syste. **9:** 519–570.
6. STINI, W. A. 1978. Malnutrition, body size and proportion. Ecol. Food Nutr. **1:** 125–132.
7. TANNER, J. M. 1962. Growth at Adolescence. Blackwell Scientific. Oxford.
8. LEE, R. B. 1979. The !Kung San: Men, Women, and Work in a Foraging Society. Harvard University Press. Cambridge, MA.
9. PAGE, L. B., A. DAMON & R. C. MOELLERING. 1974. Antecedents of cardiovascular disease in six Solomon Islands societies. Circulation **49:** 1132–1146.
10. ZIMMET, P. 1979. Epidemiology of diabetes and its macrovascular manifestations in Pacific populations: the medical effects of social progress. Diabetes Care **2:** 144–153.
11. WEST, K. 1978. Diabetes in American Indians. *In* Advances in metabolic disorders. Academic Press. New York.
12. CHRISTAKIS, G. 1973. The prevalence of adult obesity. *In* Obesity in Perspective. G. Bray, Ed. **2:** 209–213. Fogarty International Center Series on Preventive Medicine.
13. PRIOR, I. A. 1971. The price of civilization. Nutr. Today **6**(4): 2–11.
14. TROWELL, H. C. & D. P. BURKITT. 1981. Western Diseases: Their Emergence and Prevention. Harvard University Press. Cambridge, MA.
15. GOLDBLATT, P. B., M. E. MOORE & A. J. STUNKARD. 1965. Social factors in obesity. J. Am. Med. Assoc. **192:** 1039–1044.
16. BURNIGHT, R. G. & P. G. MARDEN. 1967. Social correlates of weight in an aging population. Milbank Mem. Fund Q. **45:** 75–92.
17. ROSS, C. E. & J. MIROWSKY. 1983. Social epidemiology of overweight: a substantive and methodological investigation. J. Health Soc. Behav. **24:** 288–298.
18. GARN, S. M. & D. C. CLARK. 1976. Trends in fatness and the origins of obesity. Pediatrics **57:** 443–456.
19. ARTEAGA, P., J. E. DOS SANTOS & J. E. DUTRA DE OLIVEIRA. 1982. Obesity among school-children of different socioeconomic levels in a developing country. Int. J. Obesity **6:** 291–297.
20. STUNKARD, A. J., T. I. A. SORENSON, C. HANIS, T. W. TEASDALE, R. CHAKABORTY, W. J. SCHULL & F. SCHULSINGER. 1986. An adoption study of obesity. N. Engl. J. Med. **314:** 193–198.
21. SAHLINS, M. 1972. Stone Age Economics. Aldine. Chicago, IL.
22. WENKE, R. J. 1980. Patterns in Prehistory. Oxford. New York.
23. COHEN, M. N. & G. J. ARMELAGOS, Eds. 1984. Paleopathology at the Origins of Agriculture. Academic Press. New York.
24. TROWELL, H. 1975. Obesity in the western world. Plant Foods for Man **1:** 157–165.
25. GILBERT, R. I. & J. H. MIELKE, Eds. 1985. The Analysis of Prehistoric Diets. Academic Press. New York.
26. EATON, S. B. & M. KONNER. 1985. Paleolithic nutrition: a consideration of its nature and current implications. N. Eng. J. Med. **312:** 283–289.
27. WHITING, M. G. 1958. A cross-cultural nutrition survey. Doctoral Thesis. Harvard School of Public Health. Cambridge, MA.
28. KNOWLER, W. C., D. J. PETTITT, P. J. SAVAGE & P. H. BENNETT. 1981. Diabetes incidence in Pima Indians: contribution of obesity and parental diabetes. Am. J. Epidemiol. **113:** 144–156.
29. MINNIS, P. E. 1985. Social Adaptation to Food Stress: A Prehistoric Southwestern Example. University of Chicago Press. Chicago, IL.
30. TRUSWELL, A. S. & J. D. L. HANSEN. 1977. Diet and nutrition of hunter-gatherers. *In* Health and Disease in Tribal Societies. Ciba Foundation. Eds. 213–226. Elsevier. Amsterdam.
31. WILMSEN, E. 1978. Seasonal effects of dietary intake in the Kalahari San. Fed. Proc. Fed. Am. Soc. Exp. Bio. **37:** 65–71.
32. HUNTER, J. M. 1967. Seasonal hunger in a part of the west African savanna: a survey of body weights in Nangodi, north-east Ghana. Trans. Inst. Br. Geog. **41:** 167–85.

33. STEIN, Z. & M. SUSSER. 1975. The Dutch famine, 1944-1945, and the reproductive process. Pediatr. Res. **9:** 70-76.
34. SCOTT, E. C. & C. J. BAJEMA. 1982. Height, weight and fertility among participants of the third Harvard growth study. Hum. Biol. **54:** 501-516.
35. GARN, S. M., S. M. BAILEY & I. T. T. HIGGENS. 1980. Effects of socioeconomic status, family life, and living together on fatness and obesity. In Childhood Prevention of Atherosclerosis and Hypertension. R. Lauer & R. Skekelle, Eds. Raven Press. New York.
36. EASTMAN, N. J. & E. JACKSON. 1968. Weight relationships in pregnancy. Obstet. Gynecol. Surv. **23:** 1003-1025.
37. NAEYE, R. L. 1979. Weight gain and outcome of pregnancy. Am. J. Obstet. Gynecol. **135:** 3-9.
38. BLACKBURN, M. W. & D. H. CALLOWAY. 1976. Energy expenditure and consumption of mature, pregnant and lactating women. J. Am. Diet. Assoc. **69:** 29-37.
39. NAEYE, R. L. & E. C. PETERS. 1982. Working during pregnancy: effects on the fetus. Pediatrics **69:** 725-727.
40. THOMSON, A. M., F. E. HYTTEN & W. Z. BILLEWICZ. 1970. The energy cost of human lactation. Br. J. Nutr. **24:** 565-572.
41. BUTTE, N. F., C. GARZA, J. E. STUFF, E. O. SMITH & B. L. NICHOLS. 1984. Effect of maternal diet and body composition on lactational performance. Am. J. Clin. Nutr. **39:** 296-306.
42. PRENTICE, A. M., R. G. WHITEHEAD, M. WATKINSON, W. H. LAMB & T. J. COLE. 1983. Prenatal dietary supplementation of African women and birth-weight. Lancet **1:** 489-492.
43. DELGADO, H., A. LECHUG, C. YARBROUGH, R. MARTORELL, R. E. KLEIN & M. IRWIN. 1977. Maternal nutrition—its effect on infant growth and development and birth spacing. In Nutritional Impacts on Women. K. S. Moghissi & T. N. Evans, Eds. Harper & Row. Hagerstown, MD.
44. COLSON, E. 1979. In good years and bad: food strategies of self-reliant societies. J. Anthropol. Res. **35:** 18-29.
45. CAHNMAN, W. J. 1968. The stigma of obesity. Sociol. Q. **9:** 294-297.
46. GAMPEL, B. 1962. The "Hilltops" community. In Practice of Social Medicine. S. L. Kark & G. E. Steuart, Eds. E. & S. Livingstone. London.
47. EVREUX, Y. 1864. Voyage dans le Nord du Bresil Fait durant les Annees 1613 et 1614. F. Denis, Ed. A. Franch. Paris and Leipzig.
48. BOHANNAN, P. & L. BOHANNAN. 1969. A source notebook on Tiv religion (5 vol.). Human Relations Area Files. New Haven, CT.
49. RITENBAUGH, C. 1982. Obesity as a culture-bound syndrome. Cult. Med. Psychiatry **6:** 347-361.
50. Metropolitan Life Foundation. 1983. Height and Weight Tables. Metropolitan Life Insurance Company.
51. BURTON, B. T., W. R. FOSTER, J. HIRSCH & T. B. VAN ITALLIE. 1985. Health implications of obesity: an NIH consensus development conference. Intl. J. Obesity **9:** 155-169.
52. MALCOM, L. W. G. 1925. Note on the seclusion of girls among the Efik at Old Calabar. Man **25:** 113-114.
53. SMITHSON, C. L. 1959. The Havasupai Woman. U. Utah Press. Salt Lake City, UT.
54. BENNETT, W. C. & R. M. ZINGG. 1935. The Tarahumara: an Indian Tribe of Northern Mexico. U. Chicago Press. Chicago, IL.
55. MESSING, S. D. 1957. The Highland Plateau Amhara of Ethiopia. Doctoral Dissertation (Anthropology). U. Pennsylvania. Philadelphia, PA.
56. POWDERMAKER, H. 1960. An anthropological approach to the problem of obesity. Bull. N.Y. Acad. Sci. **36:** 286-295.
57. BRAIN, R. 1979. The Decorated Body. Harper & Row. New York.
58. AMNAR, H. 1954. Growing Up in an Egyptian Village. Routledge & Kegan Paul. London.
59. BEAGLEHOLE, E. & P. BEAGLEHOLE. 1938. Ethnology of Pukapuka. Bernice P. Bishop Museum. Honolulu, HA.

60. STRAHERN, A. 1971. The Rope of Moka. Cambridge University Press. New York.
61. GIFFORD, E. W. 1929. Tongan Society. Bernice P. Bishop Mus. Bull. 61. Honolulu, HA.
62. RICHARDS, A. I. 1939. Land, Labour and Diet in Northern Rhodesia: an Economic Study of the Bemba Tribe. Oxford University Press. London.
63. MASSARA, E. B. 1979. Que gordita! a study of weight among women in a Puerto Rican community. Ph.D. dissertation. Bryn Mawr College. Philadelphia, PA.
64. MASSARA, E. B. 1980. Obesity and cultural weight evaluations. Appetite 1: 291–298.
65. STYLES, M. H. 1980. Soul, black women and food. In A Woman's Conflict: The Special Relationship between Women and Food. J. R. Kaplan, Ed. Prentice Hall. Englewood Cliffs, N.J.
66. GARNER, D. M., P. E. GARFINKEL, D. SCHWARTZ & M. THOMPSON. 1980. Cultural expectations of thinness in women. Psychol. Rep. 47: 483–491.
67. FALLON, A. E. & P. ROZIN. 1985. Sex differences in perceptions of desirable body shape. J. Abnorm. Psychol. 94: 102–105.
68. Physician Task Force on Hunger in America. 1985. Hunger in America: the Growing Epidemic. Harvard University School of Public Health. Boston, MA.

Childhood Obesity[a]

WILLIAM H. DIETZ JR.

New England Medical Center
Boston, Massachusetts 02111

DEFINITION

Obesity is currently defined as a triceps skinfold in excess of the 85th percentile for children or adolescents of the same age and sex. Obviously, this definition represents a statistical rather than a pathological definition, and depends strongly on the correlation between the triceps skinfold and fatness.

Total body fat varies widely between male and female adolescents. In normal males, body fat accounts for approximately 13% of body weight, whereas in adolescent females, fat represents approximately 25% of body weight.[1] Likewise, in a normal 40 kg adolescent male, 5.2 kg of body weight will be fat, whereas a normal 60 kg adolescent male of the same size will have 50% more total body fat. A definition of obesity that relies on total body fat is therefore probably less reliable than one that reflects percentage body weight as fat.

The correlation coefficients among a variety of body indices and percentage weight as fat are shown in TABLE 1.[2] All of the correlation coefficients are highly significant (p < .001). The highest correlation coefficients for both sexes in both age groups are with triceps skinfold thickness. Because the sample sizes are relatively small, however, the confidence intervals overlap for the correlation coefficients for all the variables except weight. Therefore, all of the anthropometric measurements shown, except weight, are probably equally reliable in their prediction of percentage body weight as fat.

A major difficulty with the indices that incorporate stature is that they are confounded by frame size. Two sources of data support this assertion. The most commonly used index is the body mass index (BMI, weight in kg/height in meters²). As shown in TABLE 2, however, both bony chest breadth (a measure of frame size) and the triceps skinfold correlate equally well with BMI (S. Garn, personnel communication). In addition, the correlation coefficient of lean body mass with BMI approximates r = 0.65. Secondly, we have recently shown that frame size introduces a wide variation in the use of weight for height (W. H. Dietz and S. Gortmaker, unpublished observations). In samples of children controlled for age, sex, height, and triceps skinfold thickness, weight varied by 20% on either side of the mean for both boys and girls aged six to eleven years old.

These observations indicate that indices that incorporate both weight and stature do not provide accurate measures of fatness, but appear to measure both lean body mass and fatness with equal reliability. Furthermore, frame size appears to account for a variation of 20% in weight for children of the same age, sex, height, and fatness.

Although the correlation coefficient for the triceps skinfold with fat as a percentage of body weight may not differ significantly from indices that include both weight and stature, it appears more logical to determine obesity with a direct

[a] The author is the recipient of a Research Career Development Award #5K04HD00644 from the National Institute of Child Health and Human Development.

47

TABLE 1. Correlation Coefficients Among Common Indices of Weight and Percentage Body Weight as Fat (%BF)[2]

| | Ages 6–12.9 | | Ages 13–17.9 | |
Index	Boys (n = 68)	Girls (n = 49)	Boys (n = 63)	Girls (n = 81)
Weight	0.33	0.23	0.30	0.72
Relative weight	0.73	0.69	0.71	0.77
Weight/stature[2]	0.68	0.55	0.61	0.77
Weight/stature[3]	0.74	0.62	0.71	0.74
Triceps skinfold	0.84	0.83	0.78	0.83

measure of fatness, such as the triceps skinfold. The development of a pathologic diagnosis of obesity depends first on a reliable measure of fatness, and subsequently, a correlation of fatness with its pathologic consequences. Although the triceps skinfold provides a reliable measure of fatness to differentiate the obese from the nonobese, the lack of reproducibility of this measure in those identified as obese suggests that an alternative measure of the degree of obesity must be sought.

PREVALENCE

Reliable estimates of prevalence have been hampered by the selection of unrepresentative samples of the United States population, and by the use of varied criteria to define obesity. We have recently approached this problem[3] by defining obesity as a triceps skinfold greater than the 85th percentile for children or adolescents of the same age and sex sampled in cycles II and III of the National Health Examination Survey (NHES) in the mid-1960s. Each survey provided a sample of approximately 7000 subjects representative of the noninstitutionalized population of children and adolescents in the United States. The skinfold criteria were subsequently used to evaluate the changes in the national samples provided in the first and second Health and Nutrition Examination Surveys (HANES) performed during the early and late 1970s.

Over the 15-year period encompassed by these surveys, the prevalence of obesity increased by approximately 40% in both children and adolescents. Although the prevalence of obesity was greater in whites than in blacks in both NHES cycles, HANES I, and HANES II, more rapid increases in prevalence occurred among blacks than among whites.

TABLE 2. Correlation Coefficients Among Body Mass Index, Bony Chest Breadth, and the Triceps Skinfold[a]

Sex	Age	Bony Chest Breadth	Triceps Skinfold
Males	5–10	0.51	0.62
	11–15	0.65	0.72
	16–18	0.53	0.72
Females	5–10	0.52	0.60
	11–15	0.63	0.81
	16–18	0.55	0.74

[a] Garn, personal communication.

No further information is available regarding the prevalence, or changes in prevalence among other ethnic groups. Among adults, obesity appears to be more prevalent among recently arrived immigrant families, but resembles the prevalence among other U.S. groups by the third generation.[4] Variations in ethnicity may also help to explain the marked variations in regional prevalence that we have recently reported.

NATURAL HISTORY

The two most important determinants of the natural history of childhood obesity are age of onset and severity. As we have discussed elsewhere in detail,[5] crude incidence rates increase, and remission rates decrease, with advancing age. Current estimates suggest that obesity persists into adulthood in over 80% of obese adolescents.[6] Likewise, the likelihood of remission decreases as severity increases. Assuming that all excess weight is fat, approximately 1.5 years of weight maintenance is required for each 20% increment of weight in excess of ideal to achieve ideal body weight.[7] Although the effect of severity on the likelihood of persistence has rarely been studied, calculations from a cohort of obese seven-year old Swedish boys support this observation. In this group, approximately 30% of boys who were 120% of ideal body weight achieved ideal body weight within a seven-year period, whereas no boy whose weight was in excess of 160–170% of ideal achieved ideal body weight within this period of time.[8]

Obese adolescents who become obese adults may be more obese than obese adults who had onset of their obesity in adulthood. For example, over half of a large group of severely obese adult women had been obese as adolescents,[9] although obese adolescents account for only 30% of obese adults.[10] Mortality rates are markedly increased in obese men whose weights were in excess of 200% of ideal.[11] The majority of these men were likely obese as adolescents.

PHYSICAL, BIOCHEMICAL, AND BEHAVIORAL ABNORMALITIES

Childhood and adolescent obesity is accompanied by a variety of physical, biochemical, and behavioral abnormalities. Obese children tend to be taller at all ages than their nonobese counterparts.[12] Increased height provides a useful feature that differentiates exogenous obesity from most of the congenital and acquired causes of childhood obesity. The latter are frequently accompanied by short stature. Bone age is also advanced in childhood obesity, but whether bone age is disproportionate to height age has not been determined.

Lean body mass is also increased in childhood obesity. As we[13] and others[14] have shown elsewhere, these increases may account for as much as 50% of the excess weight associated with obesity. The source of the increase in lean body mass is not apparent, but may be due to muscle hypertrophy to support the increased mass associated with obesity, or may reflect the nuclear mass of adipocytes. Increased lean body mass has several important implications. First, the increases in lean body mass may confound the use of anthropometric indices that incorporate weight to define obesity. Second, the ideal weight used to define protein intake during hypocaloric diets must account for the increases in lean body mass. Third, the increase in lean body mass may by itself account for some of the pathological effects of obesity, such as hypertension.[15]

A variety of biochemical abnormalities consistent with an increased cardiovascular risk are also associated with obesity. Glucose intolerance is among the most frequent. Although studies of adults suggest that upper segment fatness is the principal determinant of the areas under the glucose and insulin curves in response to a glucose tolerance test,[16,17] such studies have rarely employed partial correlations to control for the effects of total body fat. In adolescents, both total body fat and the waist : hips ratio predict the glucose and insulin response to a glucose tolerance test, but when controlled for total body fat, the effect of the waist : hips ratio on the glucose and insulin responses is no longer significant.[18]

Hypertension also occurs with an increased prevalence among obese children and adolescents. Although sustained elevated blood pressures occur in only a small percentage of children and adolescents,[19] over half of those with hypertension are obese.[20] The effect of lean body mass on blood pressure in children and adolescents has not been examined. The morbidity of hypertension associated with obesity is highly significant. Over 25% of obese, hypertensive adolescents had a significant morbid cerebro- or cardiovascular event within seven years of follow-up.[21]

A third important cardiovascular risk factor is hyperlipidemia.[22] Obese children tend to have an increased low density lipoprotein level and a decreased high density lipoprotein level. Hypertriglyceridemia also occurs, but may only reflect the hyperinsulinemia associated with obesity. Aerobic fitness minimally alters the association of these variables with fatness.[23]

Behaviorally, it is commonly assumed that obese children and adolescents have a marked imbalance between energy intake and expenditure. Several observations suggest that this is not the case. First multiple dietary histories from clinical patients fail to reveal substantial and consistent differences between either the frequency, pattern, or types of foods consumed by obese children and adolescents. Second, careful inspection of the growth charts of obese children suggests that even among the most obese, excess weight gains are rarely in excess of five to ten pounds per year. Weight gains of this magnitude can be explained by the ingestion of 50–100 extra kilocalories/day. In this context, excess energy ingested as fat may be more likely to produce obesity than excess energy ingested as carbohydrate, because approximately 25% of the energy contained in carbohydrate is consumed when carbohydrate is converted into fat.[24] No studies, however, have yet demonstrated that the obese overconsume fat.

In the steady state, energy expenditure can be basically divided into the energy costs of basal metabolic rate (BMR), the thermic effects of food, and the energy costs of activity. Because lean body mass is the principal determinant of BMR, BMRs are increased in adolescent obesity.

The thermic effect of food describes the rise in metabolic rate that follows a meal, and generally accounts for five to ten percent of the energy contained in the meal. We (L. Bandini and W. H. Dietz, unpublished observations) have been unable to detect any significant difference between the thermic effects of food in obese and nonobese adolescents, either in response to a weight maintenance diet, or when they are fed surfeit carbohydrate calories.

Although observed activity is decreased among obese adolescents,[25] the energy costs of activity for obese and nonobese adolescents have never been measured. Perhaps the most useful measure of this relationship is the expression of basal metabolic rate as a percentage of total daily energy expenditure. Preliminary data from studies currently in progress in our laboratory have failed to detect significant differences in this measure between obese and nonobese adolescents.

Although the observations with respect to energy balance suggest that differences between obese and nonobese adolescents have yet to be demonstrated, the magnitude of these differences indicates that they can only be detected with techniques more sensitive than those currently in use. An alternative approach to this problem is to examine the epidemiologic correlates of obesity, and to test the hypotheses these correlates suggest.

Obesity occurs with the highest prevalence in the Northeast, followed by the Midwest, South, and West.[26] It is more prevalent in the winter and spring, than it is in the summer and fall. Finally, it is more common in urban areas than it is in areas with a lower population density. The causal linkages that explain these associations are lacking, but on a population level, factors such as weather, activity, or the availability of inexpensive foods of low caloric density such as fruits and vegetables appear possible explanations.

A variety of family variables are also associated with obesity. The association of obesity in children with parental obesity has been well described.[27] Although this association has been cited as evidence of a genetic casualty, genetic factors do not account for the resemblance in fatness between unrelated spouses,[28] or pets and their owners.[29] The association of obesity in parents and children can be readily explained by environmental factors or familial practices, although genetic factors may affect susceptibility.

Obesity is directly related to socioeconomic class and level of parental education.[30] The relationship of obesity with family size is reciprocal; obesity occurs with the highest prevalence among single children, and decreases in prevalence as family size increases.[31]

Two types of behavioral analysis will probably be required to link these epidemiologic variables to the onset or persistence of childhood obesity. The first approach will be to examine the behaviors that are currently the focus of behavioral modification therapy. These include the frequency and types of foods consumed, the circumstances surrounding eating, and individual behaviors such as eating speed. The second approach will require a sophisticated analysis of family behavior that focuses on both the explicit and implicit messages regarding fatness, food consumption, and activity. Our understanding of family interactions and their measure is rudimentary, but a focus on these patterns has provided a useful therapeutic framework to develop and test hypotheses regarding the changes necessary within families to achieve weight loss.

At the present, the only behavior that has been causally linked to childhood obesity is television viewing.[31] Using data collected during NHES cycles II and III, we[32] have shown that time spent viewing television is directly and significantly related to the prevalence of obesity in both children and adolescents. Furthermore, time spent viewing television in children 6–11 years of age proved the most powerful predictor of the development of obesity during adolescence. The cross-sectional and longitudinal associations all persisted when they were controlled for other variables known to affect the prevalence of obesity such as season, region, population density, race, socioeconomic class, and family size.

These data fulfill the epidemiologic criteria for causality. The associations are consistent in several studies, highly significant, and temporally related. Furthermore, a logical mechanism exists to explain the associations. Time spent viewing television is time away from more energy-intensive activities. Snacking while watching television is directly related to the time spent watching television.[33] In addition, the more television that children view, the more likely they are to consume the foods advertised on television.[33] Foods advertised on television tend to be foods of higher caloric density.[34] Because childhood obesity appears to be a disease that results from a small daily caloric imbalance, the reduced activity or excess consumption of calorically dense foods may produce the disorder.

SYNDROMES ASSOCIATED WITH OBESITY

The recognizable syndromes associated with childhood obesity are rare, and can be grouped into congenital, endocrine, and oncologic categories. The two most frequent congenital syndromes associated with obesity are myelodysplasia and Prader-Labhart-Willi syndrome. Myelodysplasia occurs in approximately one per thousand live births. Atrophy of the large muscles of the lower extremities is associated with a decreased metabolic rate, and probably a reduction in energy expended during activity. Preliminary data from our studies suggest that the relationship between lean body mass and BMR in this population does not differ significantly from the correlation observed in normal or obese populations matched for age and sex. In our experience, obesity appears to result from a failure on the part of caretakers to recognize the low energy requirements associated with the syndrome.

Prader-Labhart-Willi syndrome[35] is associated with small deletions of chromosome 15.[36] In approximately half of all clinical cases, the deletion cannot be recognized. Those patients without the deletion resemble those with the deletion in virtually every respect. Characteristically, affected children are born with hypotonia and feed poorly in early infancy. At several years of age, a ravenous appetite develops. Patients frequently eat garbage, and a pathognomonic sign is a lock on the refrigerator. Hypogonadism, mild to moderate mental retardation, and short stature invariably accompany this disease. Temper tantrums and extremely resourceful food seeking behaviors are commonplace.

As in myelodysplasia, changes in body composition and energy expenditure occur, but do not readily account for the disease. In contrast to exogenous obesity, lean body mass is reduced, so that even when weight for height is normal, patients are obese by triceps skinfold criteria. Basal metabolic rate is reduced, but comparable to normal subjects when expressed per kg of lean body mass (D. A. Schoeller, L. Bandini, and W. H. Dietz, unpublished observations). Although anecdotal observations suggest excessive carbohydrate ingestion, and the characteristics of the syndrome support a hypothalamic origin, treatment with fenfluramine has failed to produce either weight loss or changes in behavior. Furthermore, sucrose ingestion has failed to produce behavior changes.[37]

The major endocrine abnormality associated with obesity is Cushing's syndrome. This syndrome is rare and is readily differentiated from childhood obesity; short stature and violaceous striae accompany the disease. A buffalo hump or hypertension occur in exogenous obesity and is not a useful differentiating feature. Obesity appears to result from the action of steroids; lean body mass is reduced and fat is increased. The prevalence of hypothyroidism among the obese probably does not exceed its prevalence in the general pediatric population.

Finally, although hypothalamic tumors are associated with hyperphagia and obesity, they are exceedingly rare. Craniopharyngiomas are among the most frequent of such tumors, and are typically accompanied by volatile moods. Like Prader-Willi syndrome, the behaviors are so reproducible that they suggest a neurologic basis.

The absence of clearly reproducible behavioral patterns and the altered body composition that accompanies exogenous obesity suggests that a central basis for this disorder is unlikely. Furthermore, the absence of differences in the relationship of BMR to lean body mass in the Prader-Labhart-Willi syndrome suggests that the fundamental problem is one of the central regulation of energy balance.

ACKNOWLEDGMENTS

The assistance of Sandy Smith in the preparation of this manuscript is gratefully acknowledged.

REFERENCES

1. CHEEK, D. B. Human Growth. Philadelphia. Lea and Febiger Company.
2. ROCHE, A. F., R. M. SIERVOGEL, W. C. CHUMLEA & P. WEBB. 1981. Grading fatness from limited anthropometric data. Am. J. Clin. Nutr. **34**: 2831–38.
3. DIETZ, W. H., S. L. GORTMAKER & A. M. SOBOL. 1985. Trends in the prevalence of childhood and adolescent obesity in the United States. Pediatr. Res. **19**: 198A.
4. DIETZ JR., W. H. 1981. Obesity in infants, children and adolescents in the United States. I. Identification, natural history and aftereffects. Nutr. Res. **1**: 117–137.
5. GOLDBLATT, P. B., M. E. MOORE & A. J. STANKARD. 1965. Social factors in obesity. J. Am. Med. Assoc. **192**: 97–100.
6. LLOYD, J. L., O. H. WOLFF & W. S. WHELAN. 1961. Childhood obesity. Br. Med. J. **2**: 145–148.
7. DIETZ, W. H. 1983. Childhood obesity. Susceptibility, cause and management. J. Pediatr. **103**: 676–686.
8. BORJESON, M. 1962. Overweight children. Acta Pediatr. Scand. **51**: Suppl 132.
9. RIMM, I. J. & A. A. RIMM. 1976. Association between juvenile onset obesity and severe adult obesity in 73,532 women. Am. J. Public Health **66**: 479–481.
10. ABRAHAM S. & M. NORDSIECK. 1960. Relationship of excess weight in children and adults. Public Health Rep. **75**: 263–73.
11. DRENICK, E. J., G. S. BOLE, F. SELTZER & D. G. JOHNSON. 1980. Excessive mortality and causes of death in morbidly obese men. J. Am. Med. Assoc. **243**: 443–445.
12. FORBES, G. B. 1977. Nutrition and growth. J. Pediatr. **91**: 40.
13. DIETZ, W. H. & D. A. SCHOELLER. 1982. Optimal dietary therapy for obese adolescents: comparison of protein plus glucose and protein plus fat. J. Pediatr. **100**: 638–44.
14. FORBES, G. B. 1964. Lean body mass and fat in obese children. Pediatrics **34**: 308–314.
15. WIENSIER, R. L., D. J. NORRIS, R. BORCH, R. S. BERNSTEIN, J. WANG, M.-U. YANG, R. N. PIERSON JR. & T. B. VAN ITALLIE. 1985. Obesity and hypertension. Hypertension **7**: 578–85.
16. KISSEBAH, A. H., N. VYDELINGUM, R. MURRAY, D. J. EVANS, A. J. HARTZ, R. K. KALKHOFF & P. W. ADAMS. 1982. Relation of body fat distribution to metabolic complications of obesity. J. Clin. Endocrinol. Metab. **54**: 254–60.
17. EVANS, D. J., R. G. HOFFMAN, R. K. KALKHOFF & A. H. KISSEBAH. 1984. Relationship of body fat topography to insulin sensitivity and metabolic profits in premenopausal women. Metab. Clin. Exp. **33**: 68–75.
18. BANDINI, L., W. H. DIETZ & D. A. SCHOELLER. 1986. Total body fat, fat distribution, and glucose tolerance in adolescents. Am. J. Clin. Nutr. **42**: 696.
19. LAUER, R. M., W. E. CONNOR, M. A. REITER & W. R. CLARKE. 1975. Coronary heart disease risk factors in school children: the Muscatine Study. J. Pediatr. **86**: 697–706.
20. RAMES, L. K., W. R. CLARKE, W. E. CONNOR, M. A. REITER & R. M. TAUER. 1978. Normal blood pressures and the evaluation of sustained blood pressure elevation in childhood: the Muscatine Study. Pediatrics **61**: 245–251.
21. HEYDEN, S., A. G. BERTEL, C. G. HAMES & J. R. McDONOUGH. 1969. Elevated blood pressure levels in adolescents, Evans County, Georgia. J. Am. Med. Assoc. **209**: 1683–1698.

22. VOORS, A. W., D. W. HARSHA, L. S. WEBBER, B. RADHAKRISHNAMURTHY, S. R. SIMAVASAN & G. S. BERENSON. 1982. Clustering of anthropometric parameters, glucose tolerance, and serum lipids in children with high and low B- and pre-B-lipoproteins. Atherosclerosis 2: 346–355.

23. FRIPP, R. R., J. L. HODGSON, P. O. KWITEROVICH, J. C. WERNER, H. G. SCUSLER & V. WHITMAN. 1985. Aerobic capacity, obesity, and arteriosclerotic risk factors in male adolescents. Pediatrics 75: 813–8.

24. FLATT, J. P. 1978. The biochemistry of energy expenditure. In Recent Advances in Obesity Research: II. G. Bray, Ed: 211–228. Newman Publishing. London.

25. JOHNSON, M. L., B. S. BURKE & J. MAYER. 1956. Relative importance of inactivity and overeating in the energy balance of obese high school girls. Am. J. Clin. Nutr. 4: 37–44.

26. DIETZ, W. H. & S. L. GORTMAKER. 1984. Factors within the physical environment associated with childhood obesity. Am. J. Clin. Nutr. 39: 619–624.

27. GARN, S. M. & D. C. CLARK. 1976. Trends in fitness and the origins of obesity. Pediatrics 57: 443–456.

28. GARN, S. M., S. M. BAILEY & P. E. COLE. 1979. Synchronous fatness changes in husbands and wives. Am. J. Clin. Nutr. 32: 2375–2377.

29. MASON, E. 1970. Obesity in pet dogs. Vet. Rec. 86: 612–616.

30. GARN, S. M., S. M. BAILEY, P. E. COLE & I. T. T. HIGGINS. 1976. Level of education, level of income, and level of fatness in adults. Am. J. Clin. Nutr. 30: 721–7.

31. RAVELLI, G. P. & L. BELMONT. 1979. Obesity in nineteen-year-old men: family size and birth order associations. Am. J. Epidemiol. 109: 66–70.

32. DIETZ, W. H. & S. L. GORTMAKER. 1985. Do we fatten our children at the TV set? Television viewing and obesity in children and adolescents. Pediatrics 75: 807–12.

33. DUSSERE, S. A. 1976. The effects of television advertising on children's eating habits. Masters Thesis. Amherst, University of Massachusetts.

34. DIETZ, W. H. & P. A. CURATALO. 1983. Energy per serving of sugared and nonsugared cereals. J. Nutr. Ed. 15: 84.

35. BRAY, G. A., W. T. DAHMS, R. S. SWERDLOFF, R. H. FISER, R. L. ATKINSON & R. E. CARREL. 1983. The Prader-Willi syndrome: a study of 40 patients and a review of the literature. Medicine (Baltimore) 62: 59–80.

36. LEDBETTER, D. H., V. M. RICCARDI, S. D. AIRHART, R. J. STROBEL, B. S. KEENAN & J. D. CRAWFORD. 1981. Deletions of chromosome 15 as a cause of the Prader-Willi syndrome. N. Engl. J. Med. 304: 325–29.

37. OTTO, P. L., S. I. SULZBACHER & B. S. WORTHINGTON-ROBERTS. 1982. Sucrose-induced behavior changes of persons with Prader-Willi syndrome. Am. J. Ment. Def. 86: 335–41.

Psychopathology and Obesity[a]

THOMAS A. WADDEN AND ALBERT J. STUNKARD

Department of Psychiatry
University of Pennsylvania School of Medicine
Philadelphia, Pennsylvania 19104-3246

Obesity has historically been linked to emotional factors by clinicians and the lay public alike. Early psychiatric studies reinforced the popular perception that psychopathology is common among the overweight and plays an important role in the development of obesity. This notion has been challenged by recent investigations which suggest that psychological disturbances are more likely to be the consequences than the causes of obesity.[1] Emotional difficulties faced by the obese may be largely attributable to an entrenched cultural contempt for the obese and a pervasive preoccupation with thinness.

PSYCHOPATHOLOGY AMONG THE OBESE

General Populations

The long-standing belief that obese persons suffer disproportionately from severe emotional disturbances appears to be incorrect. This belief was first challenged by Moore and colleagues[2] in a study of 1660 people in midtown Manhattan. They found that obese persons scored significantly higher than nonobese persons on only three of nine measures of psychological functioning: immaturity, suspiciousness, and rigidity. Even on these measures, moreover, differences between groups were too small to be judged clinically significant.[1] Similarly, in a study of 344 British persons by Silverstone,[3] "the prevalence of neuroticism and psychiatric disturbance among obese patients was found to be no greater than among normals, even when any possible influence of age and social class had been controlled for."

Five other large European studies (each of at least 500 subjects) have supported the conclusion that emotional disturbance is no more common among the obese than among normal-weighted persons.[4-8] Indeed, some studies have suggested that the obese exhibit less psychopathology than do their nonobese counterparts. For example, Crisp and McGuiness[9] studied 739 British citizens and found significantly less anxiety and depression among overweight persons than among their normal-weight peers. Similar results were obtained by Stewart and Brook[10] in a study of 5817 people, although differences between groups in this study were small.

Studies of obese children are consistent with those of adults. In the two largest American studies of nonclinical samples, obese children and adolescents showed

___
[a] This work was supported in part by a Grant from the National Institute of Child Health and Human Development to T. A. Wadden, by a Career Scientist Award from the National Institute of Mental Health to A. J. Stunkard, and by a Grant from the MacArthur Foundation.

levels of self-esteem similar to those of their nonobese peers, with all scores falling well within normal limits.[11,12] Sallade[11] observed no significant differences between obese and nonobese children on measures of personality functioning.

Clinical Populations

In contrast to studies of the obese population as a whole, there have been several reports of increased psychopathology among severely overweight persons seeking dietary or surgical treatment. These studies have typically used the Minnesota Multiphasic Personality Inventory (MMPI)[13] to assess psychopathology.

Ten studies[14-23] found at least mild elevations in depression, as defined by a T score of 60 (one standard deviation above the mean). Mild to moderate elevations have also been observed on scales measuring hypochondriasis, hysteria, and impulsivity,[14-25] leading investigators such as Hutzler and colleagues[25] to conclude that severely obese patients have "fairly high levels of psychopathology."

By failing to include appropriate control groups, many of these reports may overstate the magnitude of psychopathology in obese patients. Thus, patients seeking treatment for any disorder may exhibit elevated levels of psychopathology. Swenson and colleagues[26] have reported MMPI scores for 18,328 women between the ages of 20 and 60 seen at the Mayo Clinic for general medical and surgical procedures. Scores for this sample on the hypochondriasis, depression, and hysteria scales were at least one standard deviation above the mean—the criterion for psychopathology in the studies of obese patients. Moreover, the T scores on each of these scales, for approximately 15% of the Mayo Clinic patients, reached 70, which is two standard deviations above the mean and indicative of clinically significant psychopathology.

Apparently, then, the degree of psychopathology evident in obese patients is no greater than that of other patients presenting for medical and surgical treatment. Carefully controlled studies using either the MMPI[23,27] or other objective measures of psychological adjustment[28,29] support this conclusion. When significant differences have been found, they have been small,[14,30] and no single psychopathological profile has been consistently found to characterize obese patients.[14,31]

Several studies have relied on the psychiatric interview rather than paper and pencil tests to assess psychological adjustment. Four such studies of severely obese persons obtained contradictory results: two studies showed extensive evidence of psychopathology,[32,33] whereas the other two found little evidence.[34,35] The validity of these reports is difficult to evaluate because all four were uncontrolled studies of small samples, and diagnostic criteria were not clearly stated.

In the largest study to date, Halmi and colleagues[36] assessed 86 morbidly obese persons using criteria of the Diagnostic and Statistical Manual of Mental Disorders (DSM-III).[37] The lifetime prevalence of an axis I clinical psychiatric diagnosis was 47.5%, with depressive disorders occurring at 28.7 percent. This lifetime prevalence of depression is similar to the 24.7 percent observed by Weissman and Meyers[38] in an epidemiologic survey that used research diagnostic criteria[39] similar to those of the DSM-III. Halmi and associates[36] concluded that "there is no evidence of an increased prevalence of major psychiatric disorders in obese persons when strictly defined diagnostic criteria are used."

We have seen that epidemiological and clinical studies refute the popular notion that overweight persons as a group are emotionally disturbed. This does not mean, however, as McReynolds[40] reported, that all obese persons are free of psychological problems. Like their normal-weight counterparts, some overweight adults, adolescents, and children suffer from severe depression and anxiety and require professional attention.[31,32,41–43] Furthermore, many overweight persons may experience emotional difficulties that are not measured by standard psychological tests. Such difficulties are likely to involve weight specific issues such as a sense of isolation due to the failure of family and friends to understand the frustration of a weight problem. These kinds of issues may engender emotional disturbances that are an unfortunate consequence of being obese.

PSYCHOPATHOLOGY AS A CONSEQUENCE OF OBESITY

The Pain of Obesity

The finding that overweight persons on the whole are not significantly more emotionally disturbed than normal-weight persons is rather remarkable given the unique psychological stresses they must face. America's contempt for the obese and its preoccupation with thinness are everywhere evident. Research has shown that there is a strong prejudice against the obese that cuts across age, sex, race, and socioeconomic status.[41,44]

Children as young as six years describe silhouettes of an obese child as lazy, dirty, stupid, ugly, cheats, and liars.[45] When shown black and white line drawings of a normal weight child, an obese child, and children with various handicaps, including missing hands and facial disfigurement, children and adults rate the obese child as the least likable.[46–48] Not only is this prejudice relatively uniform among blacks and whites and persons from rural and urban settings, but it is also, sadly, seen among obese persons themselves.[45,48]

The obese must also contend with discrimination, the behavioral enactment of prejudice. Numerous reports have documented the stigmatization of obese persons in various spheres of social functioning. Canning and Meyer[49] found lower acceptance rates into prestigious colleges for obese high school students compared to normal-weight students, even though the two groups did not differ in high school performance, academic qualifications, or application rates to colleges. In a similar study, Pargaman[50] found that obese persons were underrepresented in a private college in the Northeast.

Several reports indicate that the obese face discrimination in seeking employment and on the job.[51] Employers rate overweight individuals as less desirable employees than normal-weight individuals, even when they believe the two groups have the same abilities.[52] Roe and Eickwort[53] found that 16% of employers surveyed said they would not hire obese women under any condition, and an additional 44% would not hire them under certain circumstances. One survey of executives found discrimination against the overweight manifested in earning potential.[54] Only 9% of executives surveyed with salaries of $25,000 to $50,000 were more than 10 pounds overweight, whereas 39% of those earning only $10,000 to $20,000 were comparably overweight. The authors estimated that each pound of fat could cost an executive $1,000 a year.

The full extent of job-related discrimination against the obese is impossible to ascertain because of the reluctance of employers to discuss their biases.[41,51] The armed services and police and fire departments will not enlist severely overweight persons and often reprimand or discharge persons who fail to maintain an acceptable weight.[41] Even obese persons holding physically nondemanding jobs may experience weight-related discrimination. Recently, some obese Americans have initiated organized responses to such discrimination in the form of advocacy groups (most notably, the National Association to Aid Fat Americans) and an increasing number of weight-discrimination lawsuits.[41]

Weight-related discrimination may extend to other social institutions, including marriage. Few studies have examined whether obese persons are less likely to marry than are nonobese persons.[55] For women of lower socioeconomic status, however, physical attractiveness is an important predictor of marrying men of a higher socioeconomic status.[56] One study[57] found that only 12% of women who moved into a higher social class were obese, whereas 22% who moved to a lower class were overweight.

Psychopathology Specific to the Obese

The stigma attached to being overweight does take its toll on the emotional health of some obese persons. Although they show no greater disturbance on conventional measures of psychopathology, many overweight persons suffer from psychological problems specific to the obese. One important example of such problems is disparagement of body image.

Obese persons characteristically view their own bodies as grotesque and loathsome and believe that others view them with hostility and contempt.[58,59] Individuals with body image disturbance are completely preoccupied with their obesity and related feelings of self-loathing. The disorder is an internalization of parental and peer criticism and persists in the absence of continued deprecation.

Given the prevalence of weight-related prejudice described above, one might expect all obese persons to despise their own physical appearance, but such is not the case. Emotionally healthy obese persons have no body-image disturbance. The disturbance is most often seen in young women of middle and upper-middle socioeconomic status, groups in which obesity is less prevalent and for which the sanctions against it are stronger. The disturbance is generally confined to persons who have been obese since childhood, who have a generalized neurotic disturbance, and whose parents and friends have chided them for their overweight. Adolescence appears to be the period of greatest risk for the development of the disorder.[60]

EMOTIONAL DISTURBANCE AS A CONSEQUENCE OF DIETING

Social sanctions against the overweight and a prevailing obsession with thinness have engendered a widespread fear of obesity.[61] This fear, even more than a recognition of the health risks of obesity, may be the most powerful incentive for many overweight persons to undertake reducing diets. Unfortunately, dieting itself may be a source of psychological disturbance.

Untoward Emotional Responses

The incidence of emotional disturbance secondary to dieting was first reported in 1957 by Stunkard,[62] who found that more than half of the respondents who had dieted had experienced depression, nervousness, weakness and/or irritability in response to dieting. Subsequently, a dieting depression and other adverse emotional reactions have been observed in a variety of reducing regimens.[63-68] Psychological disturbance was seen in outpatients consuming diets of 400[65,66] or 1000 kcal,[62,63] and in inpatients who fasted.[15,64,67]

The adverse emotional responses of obese persons who diet resemble those reported by Keys and associates[69] in their study of normal-weight male volunteers on semistarvation diets. In the course of losing one-quarter of their body weight, these men experienced depression, apathy, diminished libido and a profound preoccupation with food. These symptoms have been attributed to a reduction of body weight below a biological set point. The same biological pressures may account for the negative emotions experienced by obese persons who diet and attempt to maintain a reduced body weight.[1]

Weight reduction does not always entail adverse psychological consequences, however. Two relatively recent advances in the treatment of obesity appear to avoid the negative emotional reactions associated with older dietary treatments. The first of these, behavior modification for weight control, may mediate the emotional response to dieting. In combination with diets providing as little as 400 kcal[70] or as much as 1000 kcal,[71] behavior therapy is associated with decreased anxiety and depression, or, at least, with no worsening of these affects.[72] Although these findings would suggest that behavior therapy should always accompany dieting, the precise mechanisms for this improvement are poorly understood.[73] It should also be recognized that the nature of emotional changes observed during weight reduction depends on the method used to assess mood and that some of the favorable results of behavior therapy may be due to the way in which they were measured.[74,75]

Like behavior modification, surgery for obesity has been associated with improvements in affect, even though the weight losses it produces are far greater. In 1974, Solow and associates[21] reported dramatic improvements in mood, self-esteem, interpersonal and vocational effectiveness, body image, and activity levels in severely obese patients following jejunoileal bypass surgery. Subsequent studies corroborated the improved psychological functioning associated with this operation.[76,77] Because of the high incidence of serious physical complications following jejunoileal bypass, the operation has been largely replaced by gastric restriction procedures. These operations produce similar improvements in mood, body image, and social functioning with fewer physical complications.[78-80]

Bulimia

Apart from its potential to provoke untoward emotional reactions, prolonged dieting may be a precipitating factor in the development of bulimia. This eating disorder has recently become widely known and is thought to be so common that *Newsweek* called 1981 "the year of the binge-purge syndrome".[81]

Bulimia, which unlike obesity is now a psychiatric diagnosis in the Diagnostic and Statistical Manual of the American Psychiatric Association,[37] is characterized by episodes of binge eating, followed by depressed mood and self-deprecating thoughts.[1,37] The disorder occurs in persons of all weights, and its has been estimated that 5% of all obese persons are bulimic. Unlike their nonobese counterparts, however, obese bulimics do not typically vomit after binge eating, so they must cope with increased weight in addition to the burden of a distressing pattern of behavior.[1]

The role of dieting in the onset of bulimia has been suggested by both clinical reports and epidemiologic surveys, which indicate that the disorder usually begins during a period of severe dietary restriction. For example, 83% of subjects reported by Fairburn and Cooper[82] and 88% reported by Pyle and associates[83] were dieting at the time of their initial binge-purge episode, despite the fact that most subjects were not overweight. Ironically, the role of dieting has not been closely examined in obese persons because it is viewed as appropriate.[84] Nonetheless, severe dietary restriction appears to have the same negative behavioral consequences in obese persons as it does in both normal-weight and underweight persons.

The desperation and compulsiveness with which many persons seek to lose weight reflect a prevailing climate of fear and intolerance with respect to obesity. This climate is surely a factor in the alarming incidence of bulimia and anorexia nervosa. At heart, both disorders represent an intense fear of becoming overweight and thus becoming the object of scorn and ridicule that obese persons face. Both disorders provide eloquent testimony of *The Pain of Obesity*.[85]

GROUPS AT INCREASED RISK

Adolescent Girls

The subjective importance of physical appearance is particularly great among girls in their teens. Survey studies reveal that adolescent girls are especially dissatisfied with their body weights. Half of the 10th, 11th, and 12th-grade girls in one study believed that they were overweight, and nearly two-thirds wanted to lose weight. By contrast, most of the boys surveyed were either satisfied with their weight or believed they were too thin. Significantly, the prevalence of overweight was identical (25%) in the two groups.

Adolescence is the period of greatest risk for the development of body image disturbance, and girls seem to be particularly vulnerable. Self-conscious and embarassed about the physical changes that accompany puberty, they are often desperately anxious about any failure to conform to popular ideals of feminine beauty. Several reports have shown that most teenage girls are uncomfortable with their physical appearance. One study[87] found that 11- to 19-year-old girls reported less satisfaction with their bodies than did boys. Girls expressed the least satisfaction with their weight, legs, waist, and hips. In another study,[88] 59% of normal-weight female college students rated themselves low on satisfaction with their "figure."

Women

As they progress into adulthood, adolescent girls face continuing social pressure to maintain a lean physical appearance. They are clearly the victims of a weight-related double standard that condemns obesity in women while forgiving it in men.[52,89,90] Although there is no great sex difference in the prevalence of obesity, women are overrepresented in both research and clinical programs for the treatment of obesity. As a consequence, research on the social and psychological hazards of obesity has been confined almost exclusively to obese women. Seeking to escape the powerful stigma directed against female obesity, women outnumber men nine to one in diet clinics and contribute a disproportionate amount to the $20 billion-a-year diet and exercise industry.[52]

The heightened emotional stresses facing overweight women may well increase their vulnerability to psychological disturbance, including obsessive dieting and an irrational fear of obesity. Even in a nonclinical program, conducted at a worksite, more women (55%) enrolled in the program than considered themselves to be overweight (45%) (R. Y. Cohen, A. J. Stunkard and M. R. J. Felix, unpublished observations). Not surprisingly, the prevalence of bulimia in women far exceeds that in men.

Severely Obese

Severely obese persons (100% or more overweight) are members of a true minority. The prevalence of severe obesity may be as low as 0.1%, making population studies of this group impossible.[91] As a result, most of our information about severe obesity has been derived from clinical experience.

Although they are the smallest of the groups at increased risk, the severely obese face the greatest psychological burden because of their overweight. The prejudice and discrimination directed against them is far more pervasive and damaging than that directed against less overweight persons.[51] Unlike other overweight persons, most severely obese persons suffer from body image disparagement. It is not clear whether this greater prevalence of body image disparagement is due primarily to a greater severity of overweight or to the childhood onset of obesity, an apparently necessary condition for the development of the disorder.

The severely obese are also more vulnerable to the adverse psychological consequences of dieting.[78] Because they diet more frequently and lose and regain greater amounts of weight than do less obese persons, the severely obese are at greater risk of the negative emotional reactions and binge eating that may be precipitated by prolonged dietary restriction.

A variety of physical and environmental difficulties also add stress to the lives of the severely obese. The physical handicaps associated with morbid obesity may make participation in work or recreational activities extremely difficult. In addition, severely obese persons must constantly contend with environmental limitations due to their physical size. Often, the result is frustration and humiliation. Many cannot fit through turnstiles and revolving doors; access to public transportation is limited. The environment may be so constraining, that many severely obese persons may become confined to their homes. In almost every aspect of living, the severely obese person ". . .is made to feel different and is made aware of the fact that he or she really doesn't fit."[92]

IMPLICATIONS FOR TREATMENT

An understanding of the social and psychological consequences of obesity may provide an important perspective for those who treat the obese. At lesser degrees of overweight, the problems associated with the psychological hazards of obesity may exceed those associated with its physical hazards. In particular, it is important to address the needs of those groups at greatest risk for the negative psychological sequelae of obesity. For example, creative responses are needed to the problems of adolescent girls, in whom unnecessary dieting and weight consciousness may contribute to body image disparagement, bulimia, and anorexia nervosa.

Health-care professionals have a unique potential to either alleviate or exacerbate the emotional pain borne by many obese persons. Unfortunately, studies indicate that health-care providers are likely to share the prevailing contempt for the obese. In one study,[93] a group of 77 physicians described their obese patients as weak-willed, ugly, and awkward. Keys[94] has suggested that the physician's antipathy to the obese is based on the belief that the overweight are self-indulgent, "hence at least faintly immoral and inviting retribution." Needless to say, there is no evidence that moral condemnation offers any therapeutic benefit to the obese patient.

It is our hope that this description of the suffering undergone by obese persons will help health-care professionals to understand better what their patients have endured and that this understanding will awake in them a measure of compassion for those who have suffered so much.

ACKNOWLEDGMENTS

The authors thank Jordan W. Smoller for his assistance in preparing this manuscript.

REFERENCES

1. STUNKARD, A. J. OBESITY. 1985. *In* Comprehensive textbook of psychiatry. H. I. Kaplan, A. M. Freedman & B. J. Sadock, Eds.: 1133–1142. Williams & Wilkins. Baltimore.
2. MOORE, M. E., A. J. STUNKARD & L. SROLE. 1962. Obesity, social class and mental illness. J. Am. Med. Assoc. **181:** 962–966.
3. SILVERSTONE, J. T. 1968. Psychosocial aspects of obesity. Proc. R. Soc. Med. **61:** 371–375.
4. HALLSTROM, T. & H. NOPPA. 1981. Obesity in women in relation to mental illness, social factors and personality traits. J. Psychosom. Res. **25:** 75–82.
5. HALLBERG, L., A-M. HOGDAHL, L. NILSSON & G. RYBO. 1966. Fetma hos kvinnor: Sociala data, symtom och fynd. Lakartidn **63:** 621.
6. FLODERUS, B. 1974. Psycho-social factors in relation to coronary heart disease and associated risk factors. Nord. Hyg. Tidskr. Suppl 6.
7. KITTEL, F., R. M. RUSTIN, M. DRAMAIX, G. DE BACKER & M. KORNITZER. 1978. Psychosocio-biological correlates of moderate overweight in an industrial population. J. Psychosom. Res. **22:** 145.
8. LARSSON, B. 1978. A population study of men, with special reference to the development and consequences for health. Doctoral Dissertation. University of Göteborg, Gotab, Kunglav, Sweden.
9. CRISP, A. H. & B. McGUINESS. 1976. Jolly fat: Relation between obesity and psychoneurosis in general population. Br. Med. J. **3:** 7–9.
10. STEWART, A. L. & R. H. BROOK. 1983. Effects of being overweight. Am. J. Public Health **73:** 171–178.
11. SALLADE, J. 1973. A comparison of the psychological adjustment of obese vs. nonobese children. J. Psychosom. Res. **17:** 89–96.
12. WADDEN, T. A., G. D. FOSTER, K. D. BROWNELL & E. FINLEY. 1984. Self-concept in obese and normal-weight children. J. Consult. Clin. Psychol. **52:** 1104–1105.
13. HATHAWAY, S. R. & J. C. McKINNLEY. 1982. Minnesota Multiphasic Personality Inventory. University of Minnesota. Minneapolis.
14. JOHNSON, S. F., W. M. SWENSON & C. F. GASTINEAU. 1976. Personality characteristics in obesity: Relation of MMPI profile and age of onset of obesity to success in weight reduction. Am. J. Clin. Nutr. **29:** 626–632.
15. KOLLAR, E. J., R. M. ATKINSON & D. L. ALBIN. 1968. The effectiveness of fasting in the treatment of superobesity. Psychosomatics **10:** 125–135.
16. LAUER, J. B., R. S. WAMPLER, J. B. LANTZ & C. J. ROMINE. 1979. Psychosocial aspects of extremely obese women joining a diet group. Int. J. Obesity **3:** 153–161.

17. LEON, G. R., E. D. ECKERT, D. TEED & H. BUCHWALD. 1979. Changes in body image and other psychological factors after intestinal bypass surgery for massive obesity. J. Behav. Med. **2:** 39–55.
18. MCCALL, R. J. 1973. MMPI factors that differentiate remediably from irremediably obese women. J. Commun. Psychol. **1:** 34–36.
19. POMERANTZ, A. S., S. GREENBERG & G. L. BLACKBURN. 1977. MMPI profiles of obese men and women. Psychol. Rep. **41:** 731–734.
20. ROSEN, L. W. & A. S. ANISKIEWICZ. 1973. Psychosocial functioning of two groups of morbidly obese patients. Int. J. Obesity **7:** 53–59.
21. SOLOW, C., P. M. SILBERFARB & K. SWIFT. 1974. Psychosocial effects of intestinal bypass surgery for severe obesity. N. Engl. J. Med. **290:** 300–4.
22. SVANUM, S., J. B. LANTZ, J. B. LAUER, R. S. WAMPLER & J. A. MADURA. 1981. Correspondence of the MMPI and the MMPI-168 with intestinal bypass surgery patients. J. Clin. Psychol. **37:** 137–141.
23. WEBB, W. W., R. PHARES, H. S. ABRAM, S. A. MEIXEL, H. W. SCOTT & J. T. GERDES. 1976. Jejunoileal bypass procedures in morbid obesity: Preoperative psychological findings. J. Clin. Psychol. **32:** 82–5.
24. CASTELNUOVO-TEDESCO, P. & D. SCHIEBEL. 1975. Studies of superobesity I: Psychological characteristics of superobese patients. Int. J. Psychiatry **6:** 465–480.
25. HUTZLER, J. C., J. KEEN, V. MOLINARI & L. CAREY. 1981. Super-obesity: A psychiatric profile of patients electing gastric stapling for the treatment of morbid obesity. J. Clin. Psychiatry **42:** 458–461.
26. SWENSON, W. M., J. S. PEARSON & D. OSBORNE. 1973. An MMPI Source Book. University of Minnesota Press. Minneapolis.
27. CRUMPTON, E., D. B. WINE & H. GROOT. 1966. MMPI profiles of obese men and six other diagnostic categories. Psychol. Rep. **19:** 1110–1115.
28. MENDELSON, M., N. WEINBERG & A. J. STUNKARD. 1961. Obesity in men: A clinical study of twenty-five cases. Ann. Intern. Med. **54:** 660–671.
29. HOLLAND, J., J. MASLING & D. COPLEY. 1970. Mental illness in lower class normal, obese and hyperobese women. Psychosom. Med. **32:** 351–357.
30. LEON, G. R., R. KOLOTKIN & G. KORGESKI. 1979. MacAndrew Addiction Scale and other MMPI characteristics associated with obesity, anorexia and smoking behavior. Addictive Behav. **4:** 401–407.
31. DUCKRO, P. N., J. N. LEAVITT, D. G. BEAL & A. F. CHANG. 1983. Psychological status among female candidates for surgical treatment. Int. J. Obesity **7:** 477–486.
32. ATKINSON, R. M. & E. L. RINGUETTE. 1967. A survey of biographical and psychological features in extraordinary fatness. Psychosom. Med. **29:** 121–133.
33. FINK, G., H. GOTTESFELD & L. GLICKMAN. 1962. The superobese patient. J. Hillsdale Hospital **11:** 97–119.
34. WISE, T. & F. FERNANDEZ. 1979. Psychological profiles of candidates seeking surgical correction for obesity. Obesity/Bariatric Med. **8:** 83–86.
35. CASTELNUEVO-TEDESCO, P. & D. SCHIEBEL. 1976. Studies of superobesity: II. Psychiatric appraisal of surgery for superobesity. Am. J. Psychiatry **133:** 26–31.
36. HALMI, K. A., M. LONG & A. J. STUNKARD. 1980. Psychiatric diagnosis of morbidly obese gastric bypass patients. Am. J. Psychiatry **137:** 470–472.
37. Diagnostic and Statistical Manual of Mental Disorders (DSM-III). 1980. American Psychiatric Association.
38. WEISSMAN, M. & J. MYERS. 1978. Affective disorders in a US urban community. Arch. Gen. Psychiatry **35:** 1304–1311.
39. SPITZER, R. L., J. ENDICOTT & E. ROBBINS. 1975. Research diagnostic criteria (RDC) for a selected group of functional disorders, 2nd ed. Biometrics Research. New York State Psychiatric Institute. New York.
40. MCREYNOLDS, W. T. 1982. Toward a psychology of obesity: Review of research on the role of personality and level of adjustment. Int. J. Eating Disorders **2:** 37–57.
41. ALLON, N. 1975. The stigma of overweight in everyday life. *In* Obesity in perspective. G. Bray, Ed. Washington, D.C.: DHEW, U.S. Government Printing Office.
42. DWYER, J. & J. MAYER. 1975. The dismal condition: Problems faced by obese adolescent girls in American society. *In* Obesity in perspective. G. Bray, Ed. Washington, D.C.: DHEW, United States Government Printing Office.

43. WERKMAN, S. L. & E. S. GREENBERG. 1967. Personality and interest patterns in obese girls. Psychosom. Med. **29:** 72–80.
44. ALLON, N. 1979. Self-perceptions of the stigma of overweight in relationship to weight-losing patterns. Am. J. Clin. Nutr. **32:** 470–480.
45. STAFFIERI, J. R. 1967. A study of social stereotype of body image in children. J. Pers. Soc. Psychol. **7:** 101–104.
46. RICHARDSON, S. A., N. GOODMAN, A. H. HASTORF & S. M. DORNBUSCH. 1961. Cultural uniformity in reaction to physical disabilities. Am. Sociol Rev. **26:** 241–247.
47. GOODMAN, N., S. M. DORNBUSCH, S. A. RICHARDSON & A. H. HASTORF. 1963. Variant reactions to physical disabilities. Am. Sociol Rev. **28:** 429–435.
48. MADDOX, G. L., K. BACK & V. LIEDERMAN. 1968. Overweight as social deviance and disability. J. Health Soc. Behav. **9:** 287–298.
49. CANNING, H. & J. MAYER. 1966. Obesity—its possible effects on college admissions. N. Engl. J. Med. **275:** 1172–1174.
50. PARGAMAN, D. 1969. The incidence of obesity among college students. J. Sch. Health **29:** 621–625.
51. ALLON, N. 1982. The stigma of overweight in everyday life. *In* Psychological aspects of obesity: A handbook. B. Wolman, Ed. 130–174. Van Nostrand Reinhold Co., New York.
52. LARKIN, J. E. & H. A. PINES. 1979. No fat persons need apply. Sociology of Work and Occupations. **6:** 312–327.
53. ROE, D. A. & K. R. EICKWORT. 1976. Relationships between obesity and associated health factors with unemployment among low income women. J. Am. Med. Women's Assoc. **31:** 193–194, 198–199, 203–204.
54. Fat execs get slimmer paychecks. 1974. Industry Week. **180:** 21, 24.
55. SOBALL, J. 1984. Marriage, obesity and dieting. Marriage Fam. Rev. **7:** 115–139.
56. ELDER, G. H. 1969. Appearance and education in marriage mobility. Am. Sociol Rev. **34:** 519–527.
57. GOLDBLATT, P. B., M. E. MOORE & A. J. STUNKARD. 1962. Obesity, social class, and mental illness. J. Am. Med. Assoc. **192:** 1039–1044.
58. STUNKARD, A. J. & M. MENDELSON. 1961. Disturbances in body image of some obese persons. J. Am. Dietet. Assoc. **38:** 328–331.
59. STUNKARD, A. J. & M. MENDELSON. 1967. Obesity and the body image: I. Characteristics of disturbances in the body image of some obese persons. Am. J. Psychiatry **123:** 1296–1300.
60. STUNKARD, A. J. & V. BURT. 1967. Obesity and the body image: II. Age at onset of disturbances in the body image. Am. J. Psychiatry **123:** 1443–7.
61. BENNETT, W. & J. GURIN. 1982. The dieter's dilemma: Eating less and weighing more. Basic Books. New York.
62. STUNKARD, A. J. 1957. The dieting depression: untoward responses to weight reduction. Am. J. Med. **23:** 77–86.
63. SWANSON, D. W. & F. A. DINELLO. 1970. Follow-up of patients starved for obesity. Psychosom. Med. **32:** 209–214.
64. SWANSON, D. W. & F. A. DINELLO. 1970. Severe obesity as a habituation syndrome. Arch. Gen. Psychiatry **22:** 120–7.
65. CRISP, A. H. & E. STONEHILL. 1970. Treatment of obesity with special reference to seven severely obese patients. J. Psychosom. Res. **14:** 327–345.
66. GLUCKSMAN, M. L. & J. HIRSCH. 1968. The response of obese patients to weight reduction: a clinical evaluation of behavior. Psychosom. Med. **30:** 1–11.
67. ROWLAND, C. V. 1968. Psychotherapy of six hyperobese adults during total starvation. Arch. Gen. Psychiatry **18:** 541–548.
68. STUNKARD, A. J. & J. RUSH. 1974. Dieting and depression reexamined: A critical review of reports of untoward responses during weight reduction for obesity. Ann. Intern. Med. **81:** 526–533.
69. KEYS, A., J. BROZEK, A. HENSCHEL, O. MICKELSON & H. L. TAYLOR, Eds. 1950. The biology of human starvation, vol. II. University of Minnesota. Minneapolis.

70. WADDEN, T. A. & A. J. STUNKARD. 1986. A controlled trial of very-low-calorie diet, behavior therapy, and their combination in the treatment of obesity. J. Consult. Clin. Psychol. **54:** 482–488.
71. CRAIGHEAD, L. W., A. J. STUNKARD & R. M. O'BRIEN. 1981. Behavior therapy and pharmacotherapy for obesity. Arch. Gen. Psychiatry **38:** 763–768.
72. WING, R. R., L. H. EPSTEIN, M. D. MARCUS & D. J. KUPFER. 1984. Mood changes in behavioral weight loss programs. J. Psychosom. Res. **28:** 189–196.
73. WADDEN, T. A. 1984. Communication to the editor. J. Psychosom. Res. **28:** 345–346.
74. WADDEN, T. A., A. J. STUNKARD & J. W. SMOLLER. 1986. Dieting and depression: A methodological study. J. Consult. Clin. Psychol. **54:** 869–871.
75. SMOLLER, J. W., T. A. WADDEN & A. J. STUNKARD. Dieting and depression: A critical review of the literature. J. Psychosom. Res. In press.
76. CRISP, A. J., R. S. KALUCY, T. R. E. PILKINGTON & J-C. GAZET. 1977. Some psychological consequences of ileojejunal bypass surgery. Am. J. Clin. Nutr. **30:** 109–120.
77. KULDAU, J. M. & C. S. W. RAND. 1980. Jejunoileal bypass for obesity: general and psychiatric outcome after one year. Psychosomatics **21:** 534–539.
78. HALMI, K. A., A. J. STUNKARD & E. E. MASON. 1980. Emotional responses to weight reduction by three methods: diet, jejunoileal bypass and gastric bypass. Am. J. Clin. Nutr. **33:** 351–357.
79. SALZSTEIN, E.C. & M. C. GUTMANN. 1980. Gastric bypass for morbid obesity. Arch. Surg. **115:** 21–28.
80. GENTRY, K., J. D. HALVERSON & S. HEISLER. 1984. Psychological assessment of morbidly obese patients undergoing gastric bypass: A comparison of preoperative and postoperative adjustments. Surgery **95:** 218–220.
81. Looking back at 1981. 1982. Newsweek. Jan. 4:26–29.
82. FAIRBURN, C. G. & P. J. COOPER. 1982. Self-induced vomiting and bulimia nervosa: An undetected problem. Br. Med. J. **284:** 1153–1155.
83. PYLE, R. L., J. E. MITCHELL & E. D. ECKERT. 1981. Bulimia: A report of 34 cases. J. Clin. Psychiatry **42:**(2): 60–64.
84. WARDLE, J. & H. BEINHART. 1981. Binge eating—a theoretical review. Br. J. Clin. Psychology **20**(2): 97–111.
85. STUNKARD, A. J. 1976. The pain of obesity. Bull Publishing. Palo Alto.
86. HUENEMANN, R. L., L. R. SHAPIRO, M. C. HAMPTON & B. W. MITCHELL. 1966. A longitudinal study of gross body composition and body confirmation and their association with food and activity in a teen-age population. Am. J. Clin. Nutr. **18:** 325–338.
87. CLIFFORD, E. 1971. Body satisfaction in adolescence. Percept. Mot. Skills. **33:** 119–125.
88. DOUTY, H. I., J. B. MOORE & D. HARTFORD. 1974. Body characteristics in relation to life adjustment, body-image, and attitudes of college females. Percept. Mot. Skills **39:** 499–521.
89. WOOLEY, S. C. & O. W. WOOLEY. 1979. Obesity and women—I. A closer look at the facts. Women's Studies Int. Quart. **2:** 69–79.
90. WOOLEY, S. C., O. W. WOOLEY & S. R. DYRENFORTH. 1979. Obesity and women—II. A neglected feminist topic. Women's Studies Int. Quart. **2:** 81–92.
91. Obese and overweight adults in the United States. Rockville, Maryland: National Center for Health Statistics, 1983; DHHS publication no. (PHS) 82-1680. (Vital and health statistics; series 2; no. 230).
92. STRAUS, R. 1966. Public attitudes regarding problem drinking and problem eating. Ann. N.Y. Acad. Sci. **133:** 792–802.
93. MADDOX, G. L. & V. LIEDERMAN. 1969. Overweight as a social disability with medical implications. J. Med. Educ. **44:** 214–220.
94. KEYS, A. 1955. Editorial: Obesity and heart disease. J. Chronic Dis. **1:** 456–460.

Fat Cell Distribution and Metabolism

PER BJÖRNTORP

*Department of Medicine I
Sahlgren's Hospital
University of Göteborg
Göteborg, Sweden*

Obesity is the condition where the lipid store of the body, adipose tissue, is enlarged. The main, functional unit of adipose tissue is the adipocyte. Enlargement of the storage capacity of adipose tissue is accomplished first by enlargement of the adipocyte contents of storage fat, triglyceride, and later on, when available adipocytes are filled to full capacity, by the formation of new fat cells. It should be emphasized, that adipocytes have a unique ability to change their capacity for triglyceride storage. An essentially triglyceride-free adipocyte has a diameter of about 15 μm, which can be expanded by increased triglyceride contents about tenfold. This means a theoretical flexibility of volume by a factor of about one-thousand. It is clear then that limited variations in the size of adipose tissue can be obtained simply by variations in the amount of fat in each of the available adipocytes. It is only when excess obesity is present that new fat cells are needed to further reinforce the capacity of adipose tissue to store excess triglyceride.

Adipose tissue is spread out over the body in a subcutaneous layer, and there are also visceral fat deposits. It is well-known that the distribution of fat among these different fat deposits is different between sexes and that there are also large individual variations. Recent work has now demonstrated that this is due to a regulation that includes genetic, nervous, endocrine, and metabolic factors. These factors exert their regulating functions at different points in the process of accumulating circulating energy substrate in the adipocytes of the various fat depots.

After a meal, circulating fat in the form of chylomicra and very low density lipoprotein particles is caught in the capillary network surrounding the adipocytes. Available evidence suggests that the lipid transport particles are caught by glucoseaminoglucans, located at the surface of the endothelial cells. The triglyceride is then hydrolyzed here by lipoprotein lipase, synthetized in the adjacent adipocytes, and transported to the endothelial cell surface system for triglyceride hydrolysis.[1] It seems likely that the regional activity of lipoprotein lipase is an early regulatory factor determining in which region circulating triglycerides will be primarily taken up and stored. There are, however, other probable regulatory steps here, including other parts of the local capture-hydrolysis process, blood flow, and availability of capillary surface area. Genetic factors play a role also. This is not well-defined either, but seems to be by way of regulation of metabolic factors such as lipoprotein lipase.[2]

Recent work has revealed the role of steroid hormones in the regulation of lipoprotein lipase activity in different adipose tissue regions of humans. This problem can be studied by examining activity in relation to known exposure of these hormones alone or in combination. In normal, nonobese women with intact ovarian and adrenal functions, there is a marked variation in lipoprotein lipase activity in different adipose tissue regions. Of particular interest here is the relative increase of activity in the femoral-gluteal subcutaneous adipose tissue region.[3] The activity does not seem to vary in the menstrual cycle, but the preponderance of the femoral activity is further accentuated during the early phases of pregnancy. During lactation, the specific increase of activity in the femoral region has disappeared.[3] This chain of events is suggesting regulation by sex steroid hormones, which vary widely in concentration in the conditions mentioned. This assumption is strengthened by the fact that the specific activity increase of femoral-gluteal adipocytes is vanishing with menopause and can be brought back with substitution by estrogen plus gestagen in postmenopausal women.[4,5]

These descriptive data suggest that female sex hormones stimulate the lipoprotein lipase activity specifically in the gluteal-femoral adipocytes. It is of interest that this seems to be a unique feature for this region; other regions such as subcutaneous abdominal, various intraabdominal, and mammary adipose tissues do not show these characteristics.[5] It is of interest in this connection that the femoral-gluteal subcutaneous adipose tissue seems to be a fat depot that is typically found in women, and seldom in nonobese men. The presence of fat in this region in women is, of course, due to the presence of adipocytes here, but is more marked because of the enlargement of the adipocytes in this region, a phenomenon parallel to the increased activity of lipoprotein lipase activity.[3,4,6] This regional fat accumulation is probably further accentuated by the low capacity to mobilize fat from these adipocytes, as will be seen below.

It is not known from human studies which of the female sex hormones is the most important for the induction of lipoprotein lipase activity in the femoral region. Rat studies have shown, however, that progesterone seems to exert the effect in question.[7] Estrogen is needed, however, as a prerequisite for the progesterone effect, apparently by being necessary for the formation of specific progesterone receptors mediating the transport of hormone to its active site in the cell nucleus.[8] It is suggested that similar mechanisms are responsible for the phenomena observed in women, and that these effects are specific for the gluteal-femoral region.

As stated above, the storage capacity of the adipocyte is considerable. When, however, this capacity tends to be fully utilized, new adipocytes appear.[9] This process is also subjected to regulation at several points, mechanisms that are only partially known. An important step here, however, is probably where the adipocyte precursor cell is differentiated to express its full adipocyte phenotype.

Recent studies suggest that this differentiation is also regulated by sex steroid hormones, where estrogen and progesterone, as well as androgens play a role. Progesterone seems to stimulate differentiation at physiological concentrations in studies *in vitro* with adipose precursor cells,[10] whereas androgens, particularly dihydrotestosterone, are markedly inhibitory (unpublished results). The dual role of progesterone, suggested by the studies referred to, both to induce lipoprotein lipase activity to facilitate lipid accumulation in adipocytes, as well as to stimulate the formation of new fat cells, seems to be a most useful mechanism to promote triglyceride accumulation. In women, this then seems to occur specifically in the gluteal-femoral subcutaneous depot. In addition to other known functions of progesterone to protect the developing fetus, this specific fat accumulating property is also useful for this purpose, because, as will be seen below, there is evidence to suggest that the specific accumulation of lipid energy in the gluteal-femoral region may serve a specific purpose—to furnish energy for the development of the fetus and newborn child, by being useful primarily during the last part of pregnancy and during lactation.[3]

Accumulation of triglyceride in adipocytes is the end result of the balance between triglyceride uptake and release. Therefore, obviously, lipid mobilization is of importance for the regional distribution of adipose tissue. Also, this process is probably regulated by steroid hormones, although this picture seems less clear than the regulation by sex steroid hormones of lipoprotein lipase activity. In women with intact ovarian function, lipolysis, stimulated by norepinephrine, is higher in the abdominal region than in the femoral region. This difference seems to disappear with menopause, due to a decrease of abdominal lipolysis, which seems roughly proportional to remaining circulating estrogen.[4,5] In the rat 17-β-estradiol increases lipolytic sensitivity to norepinephrine, an effect that varies in different regions, and that does not require corticosteroid hormones.[11] Although available evidence suggests that estrogen is stimulating lipolytic sensitivity specifically in the abdominal region in women, the evidence is not conclusive. Direct hormone substitution experiments with postmenopausal women are needed.

It is remarkable that the femoral adipocytes have a specifically low sensitivity to the lipolytic response of norepinephrine.[3–5,12,13] It seems that this is not sex specific; femoral adipocytes from men are also insensitive to lipolytic stimulation. It is only in women during the late pregnancy and during lactation that femoral lipolysis has been found to be as sensitive to norepinephrine as abdominal adipocytes.[3] The direct cause to this is not known. It does not seem to be an effect of prolactin, because women with elevated plasma prolactin levels do not have increased lipolysis in femoral adipocytes (Rebuffé-Scrive, personal communication). The biological significance of an increased lipolysis in the femoral region during late pregnancy and lactation is interesting, suggesting that the depot fat, presumably deposited here specifically by gestagen effects, is available for the needs of the fetus during late pregnancy, when much energy is needed for the formation of fetal tissue, as well as during lactation, providing the newborn child with energy.

It should be emphasized that the picture of the regional-specific metabolism of adipocytes is based almost entirely on in vitro studies of adipose tissue. Recent studies have examined some of these problems in vivo in humans. This has been possible by following the half-life of labeled glucose, incorporated into adipose tissue triglyceride-glycerol. The half-life is about 12 months in the abdominal and 19 months in the femoral adipocytes, suggesting a higher lipolytic activity in the abdominal as compared with femoral adipocytes, in excellent agreement with the in vitro studies (Mårin et al. unpublished).

The effects of testosterone are not clear. It is also likely that testosterone exerts regionally specific metabolic effects, because administration of testosterone to castrated rats results in regional changes in adipocyte size, the end result of metabolic regulation of adipocytes. It has been suggested that the effects of testosterone on adipocyte metabolism might be induced by estrogen, formed by way of aromatization of testosterone.[14]

Corticosteroid hormone effects are also not clear in their details. Empirically, we have known for a long time that excess cortisol production results in redistribution of adipose tissue from peripheral to central depots. This seems to correspond to a decrease of gluteal adipocyte size in women,[15] suggesting either inhibition of lipoprotein lipase activity, or stimulation of lipolysis. Direct studies of this problem have shown that abdominal and femoral lipolysis increases after short-term administration of low doses of corticosteroids (Rebuffé-Scrive, personal communication). This may well be different after long-term, high-dose administration, however. Specific binding of corticosteroid hormone occurs in human adipocytes, and this is also a regionally specific effect.[16] Clearly, more studies are needed in this area.

In summary, the physiological regulation of deposition and mobilization of depot fat results in a specific female depot of fat in the femoral-gluteal adipose tissue regions. Clearly then, steroid hormones play an important role for metabolic regulation, and perhaps also for the formation of new fat cells. In this way, sex steroid hormones help to develop secondary sex characteristics in adipose tissue in an analogous way as in other tissues such as muscle and hair. Control by nervous and circulatory factors is not known, but may be expected to play roles also. Finally, as mentioned above, there is evidence of genetic factors of importance seen, for example, in the similarity of adipose tissue distribution between monozygotic twins.

The gluteal-femoral region of adipose tissue is thus typically seen in women. Both sexes have intra- and extraabdominal adipose tissue as well as some other adipose tissue regions of minor quantitative importance. In obesity, the excess depot fat is presumably accumulated in the available depots and directed to these depots by principally the same regulatory mechanisms as in the physiological nonobese state. Women that are capable of accumulating fat in the femoral-gluteal region will primarily accumulate excess fat in this area. This then is the typical female type of obesity. Occasionally this is also seen in obese men, although an isolated increase of these depots, as seen frequently in women, is very rarely found in men. Men instead have, typically, enlarged abdominal tissue stores. This might be due to the simple fact that these are the main adipose depots present in men. Excess adipose tissue in the abdominal regions is frequently seen in obese women, particularly in severely obese women. It is not unusual that women have an excess of abdominal fat without much adipose tissue in the gluteal-femoral region.[17] These women with the android type adipose tissue distribution are those who are prone to develop various metabolic derangements, and are therefore a clinically important group. Women with an exaggeration of the typical normal female distribution of adipose tissue, gynoid obesity, on the other hand, are rarely affected by these conditions.[17,18] Information on the distribution of adipocytes in these different regions in different forms of obesity is useful knowledge, because with different distribution, the risk for a number of diseases, as well as premature mortality, clearly varies.[19,20] Thus, obese men and women with android obesity need particular attention paid to complicating disorders; they should, therefore, be treated more intensively than gynoid obese women. Women and men with specific enlargement of the abdominal adipose tissue regions, even without an excess of total adipose tissue, seem to have an increased risk for myocardial infarction.[19,20]

Moderate obesity with gynoid distribution is then probably a benign condition from the viewpoint of risking development of insulin resistance, diabetes mellitus, hyperlipidemia, and hypertension. It seems likely that this condition is mainly a slight exaggeration of the physiological accumulation of fat. It is a common experience that female obesity begins and is exaggerated with pregnancy. With the background of physiological regulation, summarized above, it may be suspected that this would mainly be obesity of the gynoid type. Epidemiological evidence for this suggestion, is, however, lacking. Furthermore, from functional aspects, it might be suspected that the moderate weight increase often seen at menopause would be due to accumulation of excess fat primarily in abdominal regions, because the specific sex hormone effects leading to accumulation of fat in the femoral-gluteal regions, as well as the potential lipolysis stimulating effect of estrogen in the abdominal region, have both vanished. Direct epidemiological evidence for this possibility is also lacking. This is of potential interest, because after menopause, the risk for ischemic heart disease is rapidly increasing in women, and abdominal obesity is known to be a risk factor for ischemic heart disease in women.[20]

Although there is reason to suspect that gynoid obesity in women is just an exaggeration of a physiological condition, it is not known why certain obese women have an android adipose tissue distribution. It might be speculated that genetic factors are important, because this is known for adipose tissue distribution in general. It is important to realize that these android obese women also have a number of other male characteristics, not confined to adipose tissue.

First, muscle tissue has a number of android features, including an increased mass, fiber composition with less slow twitch fiber, and a response to physical training with a further increase of muscle mass.[21] Furthermore, these women often have menstrual irregularities, hirsutism, increased plasma-free testosterone, and decreased sex-hormone–binding globulin concentrations.[22] Some of these features may also have a genetic background, such as muscle fiber composition.[23] The pathogenesis of this condition is, however, not known.

THERAPEUTIC ASPECTS

Although the description and risks of different distribution of excess adipose tissue in obesity are now fairly well established, potential differences in the success of therapy is less well documented. In general, severe obesity is difficult to treat with remaining success.[24] Adipose tissue characteristics have been used previously as a prognostic instrument in studies, suggesting that an increased number of adipocytes is associated with a poor treatment prognosis, particularly as far as maintenance of the lower weight after treatment is concerned.[25] Although not examined in the report by Krotkiewski et al.,[25] it seems likely that the treated hyperplastic subjects (mainly women) were gynoid obese, because this type of obesity has an extra fat depot, the femoral-gluteal depot, which is not so apparent in male or android female obesity. It is an attractive possibility, therefore, that gynoid obesity is more difficult to treat than android obesity. This suggestion is supported by other observations. It is known that obesity in men have a somewhat better treatment prognosis than obesity in women.[26] Furthermore, the fact that the femoral-gluteal depot, the gynoid characteristic, is less readily mobilized than the abdominal fat means that it is more difficult to treat gynoid obesity, particularly because the difficulty of mobilizing this fat is exaggerated during at least the early phases of weight loss.[27] A recent study suggests that there is no difference in the diet treatment prognosis of android and gynoid obesity,[28] but this question needs further study.

The alternate treatment of obesity is exercise. A recent study examining this question has shown that men and android obese women, who were subjected to a controlled, long-term exercise program, eating ad libitum, did indeed decrease in body fatness, while muscle mass increased. By contrast, obese women, particularly those with gynoid adipose tissue distribution, increased their body fat mass during the training program.[21] These findings indicate that gynoid obesity is indeed more difficult to treat by exercise. The interesting observation in this study where body fat actually increased shows that these women were on a positive caloric balance during the training program. This observation might indicate fundamental differences in gynoid and android obesity in energy expenditure and/or energy intake regulation. The work intensity and duration was identical in android and gynoid obese women in this study, making it unlikely that energy expenditure in the training program was different in these two groups. There is currently little evidence that defect thermogenetic mechanisms play an important role in the pathogenesis of human obesity.[29] Therefore, it seems more attractive to speculate that the positive caloric balance of the gynoid obese women was due to a defect regulation of food intake in response to the increased need in the training program. Maybe food intake was not adjusted finely enough and resulted in overeating. Such a mechanism has been observed in female rats subjected to exercise, whereas male rats are more efficient in this regard.[30] It is a remaining possibility that such an "overshoot" of energy intake after exercise is characteristic of women rather than specifically of gynoid obese women. The importance of progesterone for energy intake regulation in quantitative terms is known from rat studies.[7] The regulatory role of progesterone on adipocyte lipid storage capacity has been discussed above. Whether progesterone effects on adipocyte metabolism, and on food intake regulation are parallel phenomena, or the adipocyte metabolism modifications precede the effects of progesterone on energy intake regulation,[7] is not yet definitely known. Other studies also suggest a regulatory role of adipocytes on energy intake regulation both in rat[31] and human.[32] This area remains inconclusive, however, until a potential signal from adipocytes to energy intake regulation has been identified.

REFERENCES

1. OLIVECRONA, T., G. BENGTSSON, S. E. MARKLUND, U. LINDAHL & M. HÖÖK. 1977. Fed. Proc. Fed. Am. Soc. Exp. Biol. 36: 60–65.
2. BOUCHARD, C. 1985. In Metabolic Complications to Human Obesities. J. Vague et al., Eds.: 87–96. Excerpta Medica. Amsterdam.
3. REBUFFÉ-SCRIVE, M., L. ENK, N. CRONA, P. LÖNNROTH, L. ABRAHAMSSON, U. SMITH & P. BJÖRNTORP. 1985. J. Clin. Invest 75: 1973–1976.
4. REBUFFÉ-SCRIVE, M., P. LÖNNROTH, P. MÅRIN, C. WESSLAU, P. BJÖRNTORP & U. SMITH. 1986. Int. J. Obesity. In press.
5. REBUFFÉ-SCRIVE, M., J. ELDH, L. O. HAFSTRÖM & P. BJÖRNTORP. 1986. Metab. Clin. Exp. 35: 792–797.
6. WADE, G. N. & J. M. GRAY. Cytoplasmic 17 β- (^{3}H) estradiol binding in rat adipose tissues. 1975. Endocrinology 103: 1695–1701.
7. STEINGRIMSDOTTIR, L., J. BRASEL & M. R. S. GREENWOOD. 1980. Hormonal modulation on adipose tissue lipoprotein lipase may alter food intake in rats. Am. J. Physiol. 239: (Endocrinol. Metab.), E 167–180.
8. WADE, G. N. 1976. Sex hormones, regulatory behaviors, and body weight. In Advances in the study of behavior. 6: 201–279. J. S. Rosenblatt, R. A. Hinde, E. Shaw & C. G. Beer, Eds. Academic Press. New York.
9. FAUST, I. M., P. R. JOHNSON, J. S. STERN & J. HIRSCH. 1978. Am. J. Physiol. 235: E 279–E 286.
10. XUE FAN, X. & P. BJÖRNTORP. 1986. Submitted for publication.
11. REBUFFË-SCRIVE, M. 1986. Acta Physiol. Scand. In press.
12. SMITH, U. J. P. HAMMERSTEN. P. BJÖRNTORP & J. KRAL. 1979. Regional differences and effect of weight reduction on human fat cell metabolism. Eur. J. Clin. Invest. 9: 327–332.
13. LA FONTAN, M., L. DANG-TRAN & M. BERLAN. 1979. Alpha-adrenergic antilipolytic effect of adrenaline in human fat cells of the thigh: comparison with adrenaline responsiveness of different fat deposits. Eur. J. Clin. Invest. 9: 261–266.

14. WADE, G. N. & J. M. GRAY. 1979. Gonadal effects on food intake and adiposity: A metabolic hypothesis. Physiol. Behav. 22: 583–593.
15. KROTKIEWSKI, M., G. BLOHMÉ, N. LINDHOLM & P. BJÖRNTORP. 1976. The effects of adrenal corticosteroids on regional adipocyte size in man. J. Clin. Endocrinol. Metab. 42: 91–97.
16. REBUFFÉ-SCRIVE, M., K. LUNDHOLM & P. BJÖRNTORP. 1985. Glucocorticoid hormone binding to human adipose tissue. Eur. J. Clin. Invest. 15: 267–271.
17. VAGUE, J., P. VAGUE, J-M., MEIGNEN, J. JUBELIN & M. TRAMONI. 1985. In Metabolic Complications to Human Obesities. J. Vague et al., Eds.: 3–12. Excerpta Medica. Amsterdam.
18. KROTKIEWSKI, M., P. BJÖRNTORP, L. SJÖSTRÖM & U. SMITH. 1983. Impact of obesity on metabolism in men and women. Importance of regional adipose tissue distribution. J. Clin. Invest. 72: 1150–1162.
19. LARSSON, B., K. SVÄRDSUDD, L. WELIN, L. WILHELMSEN, P. BJÖRNTORP & G. TIBBLIN. 1984. Abdominal adipose tissue distribution, obesity and risk of cardiovascular disease and death: 13 year follow up of participants in the study of men born in 1913. Br. Med. J. 288: 1401–1404.
20. LAPIDUS, L., C. BENGTSSON, B. LARSSON, B. K. PENNERT, E. RYBO & L. SJÖSTRÖM. 1984. Distribution of adipose tissue and risk of cardiovascular disease and death: a 12 year follow up of participants in the population study of women in Gothenburg, Sweden. Br. Med. J. 289: 1257–1261.
21. KROTKIEWSKI, M. & P. BJÖRNTORP. 1986. Int. J. Obesity. 10: 331–341.
22. EVANS, D. J., R. G. HOFFMAN, R. K. KALKHOFF & A. KISSEBAH. 1983. J. Clin. Endocrinol. Metab. 57: 304–310.
23. SALTIN, B., J. HENRIKSSON, E. NYGAARD, P. ANDERSEN & E. JANSSON. 1977. Ann. N.Y. Acad. Sci. 301: 3–29.
24. STUNKARD, A. J. & M. McLAREN-HUME. Arch. Intern. Med. 103: 79–86.
25. KROTKIEWSKI, M., L. SJÖSTRÖM, P. BJÖRNTORP, G. CARLGREN, G. GARRELICK & U. SMITH. 1977. Int. J. Obesity 1: 395–416.
26. BRAY, G. A. 1970. Am. J. Clin. Nutr. 23: 1141–1151.
27. ÖSTMAN, J., P. ARNER, P. ENGFELDT & L. KAGER. 1979. Regional differences in the control of lipolysis in human adipose tissue. Metab. Clin. Exp. 12: 1198–1205.
28. LANSKA, D. J., M. J. LANSKA, A. J. HARTZ, R. K. KALKHOFF, D. RUPLEY & A. A. RIMM. 1985. Int. J. Obesity 9: 241–246.
29. SJÖSTRÖM, L. 1985. Int. J. Obesity Suppl. 2: 123–129.
30. NANCE, D. M., B. BROMLEY, R. J. BARNARD & R. A. GORSKI. 1977. Physiol. Behav. 19: 155–158.
31. FAUST, I. M., P. R. JOHNSON & J. HIRSCH. 1976. Am. J. Physiol. 231: 538–544.
32. BJÖRNTORP, P., G. CARLGREN, B. ISAKSSON, M. KROTKIEWSKI, B. LARSSON & L. SJÖSTRÖM. 1975. Am. J. Clin. Nutr. 28: 445–452.

Energy Utilization in Human Obesity

ERIC JÉQUIER

Institute of Physiology
University of Lausanne
1005 Lausanne, Switzerland

INTRODUCTION

Obesity is the consequence of a chronic imbalance between nutrient intake and energy expenditure. In spite of the large number of published studies, it is not yet clearly established whether the main abnormality that is responsible for the development of obesity is a chronic excess of energy intake, or whether a defect in energy expenditure may also be involved. Everyone agrees, however, that during weight gain, energy intake exceeds energy expenditure: there is either a lack of adjustment of intake to the level of expenditure, or energy expenditure does not rise sufficiently to match the fluctuations in intake. The major difficulty of any study on the regulation of energy balance in humans is the necessity of measuring small differences between energy intake and output. In an adult man, if energy intake was to exceed energy output by 5% each day during one year, a daily gain of approximately 125 kcal/day (*i.e.* 46 625 kcal in one year) would result, which corresponds to a weight gain of about 7 kg over one year. This example illustrates the need to use very precise methods in order to assess small changes in energy balance.

It is likely that conventional crude methods that have been previously used to measure oxygen consumption in humans for periods of several hours have been inadequate to show subtle differences in metabolic rate. For instance, the use of the Douglas bag technique to collect gas samples through a mouthpiece to assess the changes in metabolic rate during several hours following a meal cannot produce reliable results because of the discomfort of the subject and the risk of air leaks. Continuous measurements of metabolic rate using the ventilated hood system or the respiration chamber has allowed reassessment of the control of energy turnover in obese men and women with greater accuracy than before. Several recent reviews on the regulation of energy balance in humans[1-4] and animals[5] have been recently published. This presentation will not review the vast literature of experimental aspects of energy metabolism in animals, because different mechanisms may apply to small rodents and humans. In particular, the role of brown adipose tissue as an energy dissipative mechanism in young rodents is well established.[6,7] In the adult human, however, there is no conclusive evidence that this tissue plays a role in the regulation of energy balance. Instead of duplicating the excellent reviews on energy expenditure in obesity,[1-5] this presentation will be limited to the discussion of a few important questions that have recently received much attention.

HOW MUCH ENERGY DO OBESE SUBJECTS EXPEND?

Total Energy Expenditure (TEE)

In sedentary subjects who spend 24 hours in a respiration chamber, TEE in absolute terms, was found to be more elevated in obese than in lean subjects;[8–10] a linear correlation has been obtained between body weight and TEE measured under the sedentary conditions of a respiration chamber.[8] The observation of an elevated TEE in obese subjects is a consistent finding among the various groups using respiration chambers[8,10] or direct calorimeters.[9] This has the important implication that most obese individuals must have a greater daily energy intake than lean sedentary subjects to maintain their body weight and body composition. If the results of TEE are expressed per kg of fat-free mass (FFM), the values obtained in lean and obese subjects are found to be similar.[8,10] This illustrates the fact that the greater TEE in obese subjects is mainly related to their larger FFM than that of lean individuals. This also explains why the basal metabolic rate is more elevated in obese than in lean subjects.[8,11,12] In summary, the answer to the question mentioned above is clear: obese subjects expend more energy than lean sedentary controls.

WHAT IS THE RELATIVE IMPORTANCE OF THE COMPONENTS OF ENERGY EXPENDITURE IN OBESE AND LEAN SUBJECTS?

The TEE can be divided into three main components, that is, basal metabolic rate (BMR), thermogenesis, and physical activity.

Basal Metabolic Rate (BMR)

The BMR depends on the mass of active cells, that is, the body cell mass (BCM). The BCM is the best reference point for BMR, and there is an excellent correlation between these two terms.[13] The BCM is usually estimated from total exchangeable potassium (K_e) using regression equations developed by Moore et al.[14] In most studies on the body composition of obese subjects, however, BCM has not been measured, but the lean body mass was derived from ^{40}K assays,[12,15] or the fat free mass was calculated from body density,[8,16] or more indirectly from regression equations between skinfold measurements and the body fat mass.[8] The BMR was found to be better correlated with FFM than with body weight or body surface area.[8,12] It was concluded that the elevated BMR of obese subjects depends mostly on their excess FFM.[8,12] The latter includes an increased BCM (which is due to muscular hypertrophy, and enlarged cytoplasm of adipose cells[2]) and a large extracellular mass (ECM). It is only the BCM that consumes energy, whereas ECM represents a liquid space for transport of ions and nutriments, which does not perform any work. It is important to emphasize that in addition to the enlarged fat mass, which characterizes obesity, obese patients also have a larger mass of metabolically active tissues than sedentary lean controls,[15] which accounts for their elevated BMR.[8,11,12] Because BMR represents 65 to 75% of TEE in most sedentary individuals,[2,8,10] it's value has a major influence on TEE.

Thermogenesis

Thermogenesis refers to the conditions that increase the metabolic rate at rest, the most important of which is dietary thermogenesis. Cold exposure, ingestion of caffeine, and smoking, however, are also conditions that stimulate resting metabolic rate.

Dietary thermogenesis includes two components. The first is obligatory thermogenesis, which depends upon the energy cost of digesting, absorbing and processing, or storing the nutrient. The second component is facultative thermogenesis, which represents an additional energy expenditure that is not accounted for by the known energy costs of obligatory thermogenesis.[17] Recent studies in animals show that the sympathetic nervous system plays a role in modulating facultative thermogenesis. Carbohydrate ingestion activates norepinephrine turnover in rat heart,[18] liver, and pancreas.[19] In humans, glucose administration promotes a rise in plasma norepinephrine levels, whereas fat or protein consumption does not have the same effect.[20] Furthermore, the administration of the beta-receptor antagonist propranolol[21,22] suppresses most of the facultative thermogenesis in humans. This suggests that in humans, as in experimental animals, activation of β-adrenergic receptors mediates a part of the glucose-induced thermogenesis. Because propranolol inhibits most of the facultative thermogenesis, other mechanisms, such as sodium pumping[23] and increased protein turnover,[24] are less likely to be responsible for this phenomenon.

While sympathetic-mediated activation of brown adipose tissue metabolism is of major importance in rats on a cafeteria diet,[5,6] there is no convincing evidence that this tissue is functional in adult humans. It is not known, however, in which tissue(s) carbohydrate-induced facultative thermogenesis takes place in humans. Astrup et al.[25,26] have recently shown that the major part of thermogenesis elicited by exogenous β-agonists occurs in skeletal muscle and not in brown adipose tissue.[26] In addition, an oral glucose load elicits an early component of skeletal muscle thermogenesis coinciding with the muscular uptake of glucose, followed by a late facultative thermogenesis that seems to be mediated by a sustained rise in arterial concentration of epinephrine and perhaps also of norepinephrine.[27]

The thermogenic response to a meal or to a single nutrient has been studied by many authors. TABLE 1 summarizes the main results: on 16 studies, 10 report a decreased thermogenic response to meal (or to a single nutrient) ingestion in obese subjects, whereas 6 studies show similar responses in lean and obese individuals. The reasons for these conflicting results are still unclear: differences in test meal composition, in the duration of the measurements, and in the technique used to measure energy expenditure may account for some of the discrepant results. Furthermore, recent evidence suggests that there may be subgroups of obese individuals with a thermogenic defect, whereas other obese individuals have a normal thermogenic response to food ingestion.[4] Obese individuals with a marked insulin resistance have a low thermogenic response to glucose ingestion, whereas obese individuals with moderate insulin resistance do not have a significant decrease in glucose-induced thermogenesis.[33]

Physical Activity

The total daily energy expenditure depends upon the degree of physical activity in everyday life. It is evident that people involved in heavy physical activity expend more energy than less active subjects. When comparing the energy expenditure of physical activity of sedentary lean and obese people, the weight-bearing activity, such as walking and ascending stairs, costs more energy in obese individuals. Yet we have found no significant difference in the energy expenditure due to physical activity when comparing lean and obese women who spent 24 hours in a respiration chamber with ad libitum physical activity.[40]

In answer to the question about the relative importance of the components of energy expenditure in obese and lean subjects, it can be concluded that the basal metabolic rate expressed in absolute terms is more elevated in obese subjects. The diet-induced thermogenesis appears to be decreased in several groups of obese individuals. Other thermogenic stimuli such as cold exposure,[39] caffeine ingestion,[43] or smoking have either a similar effect on energy expenditure or a slightly smaller effect in obese individuals when compared with lean subjects.[39,43] Physical activity is variable, but obese subjects may spend more energy than lean individuals in weight-bearing activities.[10]

TABLE 1. Studies on the Thermogenic Responses to Meals or to Single Nutrients in Obesity

Authors	No. of Obese Studied	Meal or Nutrient	Thermogenesis	Duration of Measurement	Reference No.
Kaplan and Leveille	4	meal	decreased	5 h	28
Pittet et al.	11	glucose	decreased	2.5 h	29
Shetty et al.	5	meal	decreased	2.5 h	30
Danforth et al.	6	meal	decreased	3 h	31
Sharief and McDonald	5	glucose (sucrose)	similar	3 h	32
Golay et al.	55	glucose	decreased	3 h	33
Welle and Campbell	13	glucose	similar	3 h	34
Felig et al.	10	meal	similar	3 h	35
Segal and Gutin	10	meal	similar	4 h	36
Schwarz et al.	6	meal	decreased	2 h	37
Bessard et al.	6	meal	decreased	6 h	38
Blaza and Garrow	5	meal	similar	24 h	39
Schutz et al.	20	meal	decreased	24 h	40
Swaminathan et al.	11	meal	decreased	2 h	41
Segal et al.	8	meal	decreased	3 h	16
Anton-Kuchly et al.	10	protein	similar	5 h	42

WHAT MECHANISMS ACCOUNT FOR THE LOW DIET-INDUCED THERMOGENESIS (DIT) OBSERVED IN SOME SUBGROUPS OF OBESE PATIENTS?

Several mechanisms explain a low DIT in obese subjects. They include insulin resistance,[33,44–46] a blunted thermogenic response to norepinephrine,[47] and/or a blunted responsiveness of the sympathetic nervous system to changes in energy balance.[48,49]

Insulin Resistance

Obese patients with a large hyperinsulinemic response to an oral glucose load have a lower thermogenic response to glucose ingestion than obese patients, with an unaltered insulin response, or control subjects.[33] These results suggest that insulin resistance in obese subjects contributes to a lower thermic effect of glucose. Ravussin et al.[44] have shown that the thermic effect of infused glucose and insulin was decreased in obesity and noninsulin-dependent diabetes: with increased insulin resistance, the lower thermic effect of infused glucose-insulin was a consequence of lower carbohydrate storage rates and possibly a greater inhibition of gluconeogenesis. When the impairment of glucose uptake due to insulin resistance in obese subjects is overcome by infusing an extra amount of insulin, the thermogenic response to glucose becomes similar to that observed in lean individuals.[46] Thus the impaired rate of glucose uptake in obese individuals with insulin resistance is related to the low thermogenic response to glucose-insulin infusions. In lean non-insulin-resistant subjects, the high rate of glucose uptake, after an oral glucose load or during intravenous glucose-insulin infusion, favors glucose storage as muscle glycogen,[50] an energy requiring process, whereas in insulin-resistant subjects, a low rate of uptake allows "on-line" oxidation of glucose with less storage in glycogen, and an economy of energy expenditure.[46]

Thermogenic Response to Norepinephrine Infusion and Turnover of Norepinephrine in Lean and Obese Subjects

In order to mimic situations that occur when the sympathetic nervous system is stimulated (such as nonshivering thermogenesis and glucose administration), norepinephrine was infused into lean and obese subjects. Jung et al.[47] observed a lower thermogenic response to norepinephrine infusion in two groups of patients (obese and postobese women) than in lean subjects. Subsequent studies by Katzeff et al.[51] in obese women have failed to confirm this observation; the reasons for these discrepant results are not clear. The marked degree of obesity, which was very likely mainly due to hyperphagia, in the obese subjects studied by Katzeff et al.,[51] may have induced maximal stimulation of any thermogenic mechanism,[2] whereas this may not have been the case in moderately obese or postobese patients with restrained eating habits.[47]

Changes in energy balance through overeating or undereating lead, respectively, to increased or decreased turnover of tissue or plasma norepinephrine in rats[52] and in humans.[49] Bazelmans et al.,[48] however, showed in six obese men that the norepinephrine turnover failed to change in response to ten-day periods of overeating or undereating. These results suggest that the sympathetic nervous system responsiveness to the energy state is blunted in the obese. The role of the sympathetic nervous system in modulating energy expenditure in relationship to changes in energy intake needs to be further evaluated in lean and obese individuals.

WHAT IS THE INFLUENCE OF A LOW THERMOGENIC RESPONSE TO FOOD INGESTION ON BODY WEIGHT?

The overall energy expenditure of obese individuals is usually found to be higher than that of lean controls, even in situations in which a thermogenic defect may be present, that is, after a meal or during cold exposure.[8-11] The conclusion that has been drawn from these data is that the lower thermogenic responses to various stimuli cannot have any important role in causing obesity.[53] Whereas the energy-saving mechanism due to low DIT in people with established obesity is offset by a larger BMR and an increased energy cost of physical activity,[10] it cannot be ruled out that an impaired thermogenesis may have contributed to the development of obesity. The factors that are involved in the dynamic phase of weight gain are still poorly understood, because it is impossible to predict who are the individuals who are prone to become obese later on. Furthermore, a small daily energy gain that is very difficult to measure if integrated during several months or years can lead to severe obesity. Instead of studying preobese subjects, it is possible to measure the overall energy expenditure of obese individuals before and after a substantial weight loss; by studying postobese individuals it is possible to assess whether energy-saving mechanisms are still present after weight loss, or in other words, whether the thermogenic defect is a consequence or a possible cause of obesity.

In our group, Bessard et al.[38] showed that the reduced thermogenic response to a meal observed in six obese women was not normalized after a mean weight loss of 12 kg; Schutz et al.[54] reached the same conclusion in three groups of obese subjects, with various degrees of insulin resistance, when studying the glucose-induced thermogenesis before and after weight loss. In these studies, the postobese subjects had not reached a normal body weight, and they expended slightly more energy than lean controls in the postprandial state due to their elevated BMR. Recently, 12 obese subjects were studied before (mean body weight 83 ± 2 kg) and after weight loss (mean body weight 68 ± 2 kg) (Golay, personal communication). The glucose-induced thermogenesis was significantly reduced in the obese subjects before and after weight loss as compared with that of lean controls. The BMR of the obese was greater than that of controls before weight loss, but it was similar, after weight loss. As a result of the low thermogenic response to glucose ingestion, the postprandial energy expenditure was significantly lower in the postobese subjects (FIG. 1). Thus blunted DIT in postobese individuals explains the relapse of weight gain, if their energy intake is not reduced accordingly. In addition, these studies show that the thermogenic defect is not normalized after weight loss. This suggests that the impaired thermogenic response to meal ingestion is not a consequence of obesity, but it could be a constitutive factor of genetic origin that predisposes the subject to obesity. Other investigators have, however, reported a partial restoration of the thermic effect of glucose by weight loss in obese subjects.[44,55]

We have proposed that a certain weight gain must occur in an individual with a thermogenic defect in order to compensate for it.[4]

Studies in the respiration chamber show a linear relationship between excess body weight and total energy expenditure.[8] The slope of this regression line is about 16 kcal/kg body weight per day, which means that for each kilogram of excess body weight, the overall energy expenditure is increased by 16 kcal per day. Using a respiration chamber, we reported that the thermic response induced by three meals over 14 hours was 14.8 ± 1.1% (of the ingested energy) in lean subjects and 8.7 ± 0.5% in a group of 20 obese women with a childhood history of obesity.[40] The difference of 6% between these responses represents an economy of 150 kcal/day for an energy intake of 2500 kcal/day. If two subjects were to eat the same amount of food energy, that is, 2500 kcal/day, one with a DIT of 15%, and the other a DIT of 9%, the economy of energy (i.e. 150 kcal/day in the latter) would favor weight gain. The body weight gain that is needed to compensate for reduced DIT would be 9.4 kilograms. DIT of 9% represents the mean value for the obese group; in this study, however, two obese subjects had DIT of 3.5%, that is, a difference of 11.5% with the mean value of 15% in the controls. This lower thermogenic response corresponds to an economy of energy of about 300 kcal per day, which could be compensated by a weight gain of approximately 18 kg. These calculations are made on the presuppositions that the preobese subjects have the same defective thermogenic response as the obese, and that they have the same caloric intake as a control subject who maintains energy balance. Furthermore, it is possible that the value of 16 kcal/kg excess body weight, which was measured in a respiration chamber, underestimates the true energy expenditure due to excess body weight in everyday life.[10] It is not known whether physical activity could be used to compensate for an abnormally low DIT. By taking into account all these reservations, low DIT in preobese subjects can account for an increase in body weight of 10 to 15 kg; a greater increase in body weight cannot be explained solely on this basis, and increased energy intake must also occur.

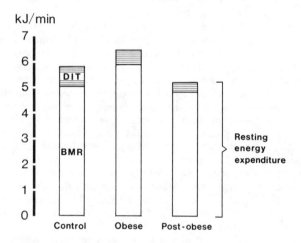

FIGURE 1. Basal metabolic rate (open columns) and DIT (hatched columns) in a group of 17 control subjects (body weight 63 ± 2 kg) and a group of 12 obese subjects (body weight 83 ± 2 kg). The same obese individuals were studied after a mean weight loss of 15 ± 2 kg consecutive to a 17 ± 3 week hypocaloric diet followed by 4 weeks of a maintenance diet (*i.e.*, postobese). DIT was measured during three hours following a 100 g oral glucose load. The resting energy expenditure (BMR + DIT) was greater in the obese than in the control subjects, but it was lower in the postobese group than in the control group (Golay, personal communication).

WHAT PROPORTION OF OBESE INDIVIDUALS HAVE AN IMPAIRED THERMOGENIC RESPONSE TO FOOD INGESTION?

The discrepant results on DIT in obese subjects reported in the literature suggest that obese patients represent a heterogenous group. In a recent study,[4] we measured the DIT response to three meals over 24 hours in a respiration chamber in 35 obese women from the outpatient clinic of the hospital and 17 age-matched controls. The only criteria for the selection of the obese was a body fat mass greater than 35 percent of body weight. A third of the obese women had reduced DIT (lower than 10.5%), whereas only one control woman had a low thermogenic response (the latter was a typical restrained eater).[5,6] The majority of the obese women had unaltered DIT.

These results show that less than half of an unselected obese population present a thermogenic defect. Further studies are needed to better identify who are the obese with reduced DIT. Recently, Molnar et al.[57] showed that food-induced thermogenesis was reduced in the early phase of childhood obesity but increased in the later phase. Griffiths and Payne[58] reported a lower daily energy expenditure in children of obese parents than in children of normal weight parents; the former also had a lower energy intake than the latter. The low energy expenditure of children of obese parents may contribute to weight gain if energy intake is not maintained at a reduced level.

WHAT IS THE CONTRIBUTION OF GENETIC FACTORS AND OF THE FAMILY ENVIRONMENT TO HUMAN OBESITY?

In a recent study, Stunkard et al.[59] examined the contribution of genetic factors and the family environment to obesity in 540 adult Danish adoptees. They found a strong relation between the weight class of the adoptees and the body mass index of their biologic parents, but there was no relation between the weight class of the adoptees and the body mass index of their adoptive parents. They concluded that genetic influences have an important role in determining human fatness in adults, whereas the family environment alone has no apparent effect.

It is clear that environment has a permissive effect on the development of obesity; for instance, famine could prevent the expression of a genetic tendency towards obesity. The availability of food above the famine level might permit expression of the strongest genetic tendency.[59] The data of Stunkard et al.[59] do not tell us whether the genetic trait towards obesity is expressed as an excessive food intake or a low energy expenditure. The genetic influence may be expressed as an inability to adapt energy expenditure to a variable intake, or conversely, it may determine a defective control of food intake that does not adapt energy intake to changes in energy expenditure. Poehlman et al.[60] recently reported a similarity of the thermic effect of a meal within twin pairs, which supports the concept of a genetic dependency for the thermic effect of a meal.

Future research in human obesity should be aimed at obtaining a better understanding of the determinants of this condition. If the genetic determinants are more important than the environment, it would be of great interest to identify genetic markers that are involved in the control of the efficiency of energy utilization and in the control of food intake.

REFERENCES

1. WOO, R., R. DANIEL-KUSH & E. S. HORTON. 1985. Regulation of energy balance. Annu. Rev. Nutr. **5:** 411–433.
2. JAMES, W. P. T. 1985. Is there a thermogenic abnormality in obesity? In Substrate and Energy Metabolism. J. S. Garrow & D. Halliday, Eds.: 108–118. John Libbey. London.
3. SJÖSTRÖM, L. 1985. A review of weight maintenance and weight changes in relation to energy metabolism and body composition. In Recent Advances in Obesity Research: IV. J. Hirsch & T. B. Van Itallie, Eds.: 82–94. John Libbey. London.
4. JÉQUIER, E. 1984. Energy expenditure in obesity. Clin. Endocrinol. Metab. **13:** 563–580.
5. ROTHWELL, N. J. & M. J. STOCK. 1981. Regulation of energy balance. Annu. Rev. Nutr. **1:** 235–256.

6. ROTHWELL, N. J. & M. J. STOCK. 1979. A role for brown adipose tissue in diet-induced thermogenesis. Nature (London) **281:** 31–35.
7. ROTHWELL, N. J. & M. J. STOCK. 1984. Brown adipose tissue. Recent Adv. Physiol. **10:** 349–384.
8. RAVUSSIN, E., B. BURNAND, Y. SCHUTZ & E. JÉQUIER. 1982. Twenty-four-hour energy expenditure and resting metabolic rate in obese, moderately obese, and control subjects. Am. J. Clin. Nutr. **35:** 566–573.
9. BLAZA, S. & J. S. GARROW. 1983. Thermogenic response to temperature, exercise and food stimuli in lean and obese women, studied by 24 h direct calorimetry. Br. J. Nutr. **49:** 171–180.
10. PRENTICE, A. M., A. E. BLACK, W. A. COWARD, H. L. DAVIES, G. R. GOLDBERG, P. R. MURGARTROYD, J. ASHFORD, M. SWAYER & R. G. WHITEHEAD. 1986. High-levels of energy expenditure in obese women. Br. J. Med. **292:** 983–987.
11. JAMES, W. P. T., H. L. DAVIES, J. BAILIES & M. J. DAUNCEY. 1978. Elevated metabolic rates in obesity. Lancet **1:** 1122–1125.
12. HALLIDAY, D., R. HESP, S. F. STALLEY, P. WARWICK, D. G. ALTMAN & J. S. GARROW. 1979. Resting metabolic rate, weight, surface area and body composition in obese women. Int. J. Obesity **3:** 1–6.
13. ROZA, A. M. & H. M. SHIZGAL. 1984. The Harris Benedict equation reevaluated: resting energy requirements and the body cell mass. Am. J. Clin. Nutr. **40:** 168–182.
14. MOORE, F. D., K. H. OLESON, J. D. MCMURPHY, H. V. PARKER, M. R. BELL & C. M. BOYDEN. 1963. The body cell mass and its supporting environment. *In* Body Composition in Health and Disease. W. B. Saunders & Co. Philadelphia, PA.
15. FORBES, G. B. & S. L. WELLE. 1983. Lean body mass in obesity. Int. J. Obesity **7:** 99–107.
16. SEGAL, K. R., B. GUTIN, A. M. NYMAN & F. X. PI-SUNYER. 1985. Thermic effect of food at rest, during exercise, and after exercise in lean and obese men of similar body weight. J. Clin. Invest. **76:** 1107–1112.
17. ACHESON, K. J., E. RAVUSSIN, J. WAHREN & E. JÉQUIER. 1984. Thermic effect of glucose in man. Obligatory and facultative thermogenesis. J. Clin. Invest. **74:** 1572–1580.
18. YOUNG, J. B. & L. LANDSBERG. 1977. Stimulation of the sympathetic nervous system during sucrose feeding. Nature (London) **269:** 615–617.
19. YOUNG, J. B. & L. LANDSBERG. 1979. Effect of diet and cold exposure on norepinephrine turnover in pancreas and liver. Am. J. Physiol. **236:** E524–E533.
20. WELLE, S., U. LILAVIVAT & R. G. CAMPBELL. 1981. Thermic effect of feeding in man: increased norepinephrine levels following glucose but not protein or fat consumption. Metab. Clin. Exp. **30:** 953–958.
21. ACHESON, K., E. JÉQUIER & J. WAHREN. 1983. Influence of beta-adrenergic blockade on glucose-induced thermogenesis in man. J. Clin. Invest. **72:** 981–986.
22. DEFRONZO, R. A., D. THORIN, J. P. FELBER, D. C. SIMONSON, D. THIÉBAUD, E. JÉQUIER & A. GOLAY. 1984. Effect of beta and alpha-adrenergic blockade on glucose-induced thermogenesis in man. J. Clin. Invest. **73:** 633–639.
23. GUERNSEY, D. L. & W. K. MORISHIGE. 1979. Na^+ pump activity and nuclear T_3 receptors in tissues of genetically obese (ob/ob) mice. Metab. Clin. Exp. **28:** 629–632.
24. MILLER, B. G., W. R. OTTO, R. F. GRIMBLE *et al.* 1979. The relationship between protein turnover and energy balance in lean and genetically obese (ob/ob) mice. Br. J. Nutr. **42:** 185–199.
25. ASTRUP, A., J. BULOW, J. MADSEN & N. J. CHRISTENSEN. 1985. Contribution of BAT and skeletal muscle to thermogenesis induced by ephedrine in man. Am. J. Physiol. **248:** E507–E515.
26. ASTRUP, A., J. BULOW, N. J. CHRISTENSEN & J. MADSEN. 1984. Ephedrine-induced thermogenesis in man: no role for interscapular brown adipose tissue. Clin. Sci. **66:** 179–186.
27. ASTRUP, A., J. BULOW, N. J. CHRISTENSEN, J. MADSEN & F. QUAADE. 1986. Facultative thermogenesis induced by carbohydrate: a skeletal muscle component mediated by epinephrine. Am. J. Physiol. **250:** E226–E229.

28. KAPLAN, M. L. & G. A. LEVEILLE. 1976. Calorigenic response in obese and non-obese women. Am. J. Clin. Nutr. **23:** 1108–1113.
29. PITTET, P., P. CHAPPUIS, K. J. ACHESON, F. DE TECHTERMANN & E. JÉQUIER. 1976. Thermic effect of glucose in obese subjects studied by direct and indirect calorimetry. Br. J. Nutr. **35:** 281–289.
30. SHETTY, P. S., R. T. JUNG, W. P. T. JAMES, M. A. BARRAND & B. A. CALLINGHAM. 1981. Postprandial thermogenesis in obesity. Clin. Sci. (London) **60:** 519–525.
31. DANFORTH JR., E., R. J. DANIELS, H. L. KATZEFF, E. RAVUSSIN & J. S. GARROW. 1981. Thermogenic responsiveness in Pima Indians. Clin. Res. **29:** 663A.
32. SHARIEF, N. N. & I. MACDONALD. 1982. Differences dietary induced thermogenesis with various carbohydrates in normal and overweight men. Am. J. Clin. Nutr. **35:** 267–272.
33. GOLAY, A., Y. SCHUTZ, H. U. MEYER, D. THIÉBAUD, B. CURCHOD, E. MAEDER, J. P. FELBER & E. JÉQUIER. 1982. Glucose-induced thermogenesis in nondiabetic and diabetic obese subjects. Diabetes **31:** 1023–1028.
34. WELLE, S. L. & R. G. CAMPBELL. 1983. Normal thermic effect of glucose in obese women. Am. J. Clin. Nutr. **37:** 87–92.
35. FELIG, P., J. CUNNINGHAM, M. LEVITT, R. HENDLER & E. NADEL. 1983. Energy expenditure in obesity in fasting and postprandial state. Am. J. Physiol. **244:** E45–E51.
36. SEGAL, K. R. & B. GUTIN. 1983. Thermic effects of food and exercise in lean and obese women. Metab. Clin. Exp. **32:** 581–589.
37. SCHWARTZ, R. S., E. RAVUSSIN, M. MASSARI, M. O'CONNELL & D. C. ROBBINS. 1983. The thermic effect of carbohydrate versus fat feeding in man. Metab. Clin. Exp. **32:** 581–589.
38. BESSARD, T., Y. SCHUTZ & E. JÉQUIER. 1983. Energy expenditure and postprandial thermogenesis in obese women before and after weight loss. Am. J. Clin. Nutr. **38:** 680–693.
39. BLAZA, S. & J. S. GARROW. 1983. Thermogenic response to temperature, exercise and food stimuli in lean and obese women, studied by 24 h direct calorimetry. Br. J. Nutr. **49:** 171–180.
40. SCHUTZ, Y., T. BESSARD & E. JÉQUIER. 1984. Diet induced thermogenesis measured over a whole day in obese and nonobese women. Am. J. Clin. Nutr. **40:** 542–552.
41. SWAMINATHAN, R., R. F. G. J. KING, J. HOLMFIELD, R. A. SIWEK, M. BAKER & J. K. WALES. 1985. Thermic effect of feeding carbohydrate, fat, protein and mixed meal in lean and obese subjects. Am. J. Clin. Nutr. **42:** 177–181.
42. ANTON-KUCHLY, B., M. LAVAL, M.-L. CHOUKROUN, G. MANCIET, P. ROGER & P. VARENE. 1985. Postprandial thermogenesis and hormonal release in lean and obese subjects. J. Physiol. (Paris) **80:** 321–329.
43. ACHESON, K. J., B. ZAHORSKA-MARKIEWICZ, PH. PITTET & E. JÉQUIER. 1980. Caffeine and coffee: their influence on metabolic rate and substrate utilization in normal weight and obese individuals. Am. J. Clin. Nutr. **33:** 989–997.
44. RAVUSSIN, E., C. BOGARDUS, R. S. SCHWARTZ, D. C. ROBBINS, R. R. WOLFE, E. S. HORTON, E. DANFORTH JR., E. A. H. SIMS. 1983. Thermic effect of infused glucose and insulin in man. Decreased response with increased insulin resistance in obesity and noninsulin-dependent diabetes mellitus. J. Clin. Invest. **72:** 893–902.
45. FELIG, P. 1984. Insulin is the mediator of feeding-related thermogenesis: insulin resistance and/or deficiency results in a thermogenic defect which contributes to the pathogenesis of obesity. Clin. Physio. **4:** 267–273.
46. RAVUSSIN, E., K. J. ACHESON, O. VERNET, E. DANFORTH & E. JÉQUIER. 1985. Evidence that insulin resistance is responsible for the decreased thermic effect of glucose in human obesity. J. Clin. Invest. **76:** 1268–1273.
47. JUNG, R. T., P. S. SHETTY, W. P. T. JAMES, M. BARRAND & B. A. CALLINGHAM. 1979. Reduced thermogenesis in obesity. Nature (London) **279:** 322–323.
48. BAZELMANS, J., P. J. NESTEL, K. O'DEA & M. D. ESLER. 1985. Blunted norepinephrine responsiveness to changing energy states in obese subjects. Metab. Clin. Exp. **34:** 154–160.

49. O'DEA, K., M. D. ESLER, P. LEONARD, J. R. STOCKIGT & P. NESTEL. 1982. Noradrenaline turnover during under- and overeating in normal weight subjects. Metab. Clin. Exp. **31:** 896–899.
50. JACOT, E., R. A. DEFRONZO, E. JÉQUIER, E. MAEDER & J. P. FELBER. 1982. The effect of hyperglycemia, hyperinsulinemia and route of glucose administration on glucose oxidation and glucose storage. Metab. Clin. Exp. **31:** 922–930.
51. KATZEFF, H. L., M. O'CONNELL, E. S. HORTON, E. DANFORTH JR., J. B. YOUNG & L. LANDSBERG. 1986. Metabolic studies in human obesity during overnutrition and undernutrition: thermogenesis and hormonal responses to norepinephrine. Metab. Clin. Exp. **35:** 166–175.
52. YOUNG, J. R., E. SAVILLE, N. J. ROTHWELL *et al.* 1982. Effect of diet and cold exposure on norepinephrine turnover in brown adipose tissue of the rat. J. Clin. Invest. **69:** 1061–1071.
53. GARROW, J. S. 1981. Thermogenesis and obesity in man. *In* Recent Advances in Obesity Research III. P. Björntorp, M. Cairella & A. N. Howard, Eds.: 208–215. John Libbey. London.
54. SCHUTZ, Y., A., GOLAY, J. P. FELBER & E. JÉQUIER. 1984. Decreased glucose-induced thermogenesis after weight loss in obese subjects: a predisposing factor for relapse of obesity? Am. J. Clin. Nutr. **39:** 380–387.
55. SCHWARTZ, R. S., J. B. HALTER & E. BIERMAN. 1983. Reduced thermic effect of feeding in obesity: role of norepinephrine. Metab. Clin. Exp. **32:** 114–117.
56. STUNKARD, A. J. 1981. "Restrained eating": What it is and a new scale to measure it. *In* The Body weight regulatory system: Normal and disturbed mechanisms. L. A. Cioffy, W. P. T. James & T. B. Van Itallie, Eds.: 243–251. Raven Press. New York.
57. MOLNAR, D., P. VARGA, I. RUBECZ, A. HAMAR & J. MESTYAN. 1985. Food-induced thermogenesis in obese children. Eur. J. Pediatr. **144:** 27–31.
58. GRIFFITHS, M. & P. R. PAYNE. 1976. Energy expenditure in small children of obese and non-obese parents. Nature (London) **260:** 698–700.
59. STUNKARD, A. J., T. I. A. SORENSEN, C. HANIS, T. W. TEASDALE, R. CHAKRABORTY, W. J. SCHULL & F. SCHULSIGER. 1986. An adoption study of human obesity. N. Engl. J. Med. **314:** 193–198.
60. POEHLMAN, E. T., A. TREMBLAY, E. FONTAINE, J. P. DESPRÉS, A. NADEAU, J. DUSSAULT & C. BOUCHARD. 1986. Genotype dependency of the thermic effect of a meal and associated hormonal changes following short-term overfeeding. Metab. Clin. Exp. **35:** 30–36.

Insulin Resistance and Amino Acid Metabolism in Obesity

BENJAMIN CABALLERO

Department of Applied Biological Sciences
and
The Clinical Research Center
Massachusetts Institute of Technology
Cambridge, Massachusetts 02142

The association of obesity with high plasma insulin levels has been known for over 20 years.[1] This hyperinsulinemia appears to be a compensatory response to a decreased tissue sensitivity to insulin's action on glucose metabolism in the obese, and is manifested by a decreased peripheral glucose uptake, excessive hepatic glucose production in the basal state, and inadequate suppression of hepatic glucose output by exogenous insulin.[2] Most moderately obese persons have a normal oral glucose tolerance test (OGTT), but they exhibit an excessive insulin rise in response to glucose intake, consistent with the lower tissue responsiveness to insulin. Thus, obese persons may be exposed for long periods of time to abnormally high plasma insulin levels, which may, in fact, be necessary to sustain a normal glycemia; but because the responsiveness to insulin may be different for other insulin-dependent metabolic functions, this hyperinsulinemia may be either excessive or insufficient for these processes.

Systemic insulin concentration results from the balance between pancreatic B-cell production and hepatic removal, and an impairment in either one of these processes has been proposed to explain the hyperinsulinemia of obesity. Some studies found that exogenous insulin is unable to completely suppress pancreatic insulin production, as estimated by the plasma C peptide level and the C peptide: insulin molar ratio (C : I);[3,4] others, however, found normal C peptide levels and a low C : I ratio in obese individuals.[5-7] The few studies that measured portal vein insulin concentrations directly found values similar to those in the systemic circulation.[8,9] Because these results reflect the response of a heterogeneous population of obese subjects, it is possible that overproduction or decreased removal of insulin is predominant in different types of obesity. Misbin[10] suggested that overproduction is predominant in obese with moderate hyperinsulinemia and normal glucose tolerance, whereas decreased insulin degradation plays the principal role in those with very high plasma insulin concentrations and impaired glucose tolerance.

The decreased tissue sensitivity to insulin of obesity involves receptor and postreceptor defects. Studies in obese humans and in animal models of obesity have shown a decreased number of insulin receptors in a variety of tissues: skeletal muscle,[11,12] adipocytes,[13] thymic lymphocytes,[14] hepatocytes[15,16] and circulating monocytes.[17] Studies in humans have also demonstrated a correlation between the number of receptors in circulating monocytes and insulin sensitivity measured by the insulin clamp technique.[18] Regional perfusion studies in obese humans show that insulin resistance is present in muscle (quantitatively the most important),[19] adipose tissue, liver,[2] and the splanchnic bed.[20,21] Because under normal conditions only a small number of receptors must be active to exert insulin

84

actions, most obese subjects exhibit a normal maximal insulin-stimulated glucose disposal rate when sufficient insulin is administered.[22] On the other hand, some obese persons cannot reach the maximum glucose output even when receiving very high amounts of insulin, presumably reaching receptor saturation without exhibiting an insulin effect.[23,24] These obese persons are characterized as having postreceptor defects, and in some studies the magnitude of this defect is correlated with fasting plasma insulin concentrations.[24]

EFFECTS OF INSULIN ON AMINO ACID METABOLISM

Insulin is an anabolic hormone that regulates protein synthesis at the transcriptional, translational, and posttranslational processing steps.[25,26] It can also indirectly modulate protein synthesis by controlling the rate of amino acid uptake into the cell. Insulin promotes the incorporation of branched chain amino acids into muscle, inhibits leucine oxidation,[27] and decreases protein degradation.[28] In 1928, Luck et al.[29] were the first to demonstrate that the injection of insulin into humans produces a significant decrease in total amino N in plasma. An inverse correlation between plasma insulin and branched chain amino acid concentrations over a wide range of insulin levels has been reported, from very low, such as in diabetes, to very high, as in functioning insulinoma.[30] A dose of 0.1 U/kg of insulin in an adult causes a significant fall in branched chain amino acids 20 minutes after injection;[31] carbohydrate intake produces a similar effect.[32] This insulin effect is most likely due to a stimulation of peripheral amino acid uptake, particularly into muscle tissue.[33] In a recent study, Fukagawa et al.[34] used the euglycemic clamp technique to quantify the sensitivity of the branched chain amino acids, tyrosine and phenylalanine, to insulin in normal men. They reported that insulin levels for half-maximal amino acid decrease are within the range of half-maximal glucose disposal.

INSULIN AND AMINO ACID METABOLISM IN OBESITY

Several years ago, Felig et al. and others[35,36] demonstrated that the insulin-dependent fall in plasma branched chain amino acids (BCAA) was impaired in obese subjects; in their study, obese subjects showed significantly higher fasting plasma levels of valine, leucine, isoleucine, tyrosine, and phenylalanine. After intravenous (i.v.) administration of 0.5 g/kg of glucose, the percent fall in neutral amino acids was significantly lower in obese, although the absolute fall for each of these amino acids was similar in lean and obese. Felig et al. suggested that this hyperaminoacidemia could constitute a feedback signal to increase insulin production in the face of the lower insulin sensitivity, given the known ability of most amino acids to stimulate pancreatic beta-cell output.[37] An alternative interpretation is that these elevated plasma amino acid levels result from the accumulation of amino acids within the plasma compartment, secondary to a decrease in their insulin-mediated uptake into peripheral tissues. This interpretation assumes that insulin resistance affects similarly glucose and amino acid metabolism. Although in normal humans the plasma insulin level for half-maximal glucose metabolic rate and half-maximal decrease in plasma amino acid levels is similar,[34] it is not known if this is the case in insulin-resistant states. Indeed, it has been shown that there is a dissociation between the responsiveness to insulin of glucose and of potassium and free fatty acids.[38] Insight into the mechanism of insulin resistance obtained from the study of other diseases also suggests that the responsiveness of glucose and amino acid uptake to insulin may not necessarily be parallel (TABLE 1). For example, the insulin resistance of uremia is associated with a decreased metabolic rate for glucose, but amino acid uptake is normal, to the point that the high plasma insulin response frequently produces a markedly low plasma level of branched chain amino acids.[39,40] Likewise, aging is associated with a progressive decline in the glucose metabolic response to insulin, whereas the amino acid response is preserved.[41] In obesity, results from other studies show that the hyperaminoacidemia is not a constant feature of insulin resistance.[42,43] In contrast to Felig *et al.,* studies by Forlani *et al.*[42] and Heraief *et al.*[43] found normal fasting plasma levels of branched chain amino acids in obese individuals, which were unrelated to plasma insulin concentrations. A study that compared the rate of disappearance from plasma of an i.v. valine dose in lean and obese adults, found that the metabolic clearance rate of the amino acid was the same in both groups, and that the obese adults actually had lower valine levels during the first 90 minutes of the study.[44] Conversely, Forlani *et al.*[42] found a reduced fall in plasma branched chain amino acid in the obese individuals during an euglycemic insulin clamp. These

TABLE 1. Insulin Action in Obesity, Uremia, and Type I Diabetes

	Obesity	Uremia	Diabetes
Glucose			
Plasma level	N[a]	↑	↑
Oral GTT	N	I[b]	I
Metabolism rate	↓	↓	↓
Insulin			
Plasma level	↑	↑	↑
Sensitivity	↓	↓	N, ↓
Amino Acids (BCAA)			
Plasma levels	↑	↓	↑
Uptake	↓	↑	↓

[a] N = normal
[b] I = impaired

investigators used a nonprimed insulin infusion and assumed a steady state condition after only 30 minutes, factors that may have complicated the interpretation of results.

Kinetic Studies

The high plasma amino acid concentrations associated with obesity could be due, theoretically, to impaired peripheral amino acid uptake, decreased protein synthesis, excessive protein breakdown, or a combination thereof. If the degree of hyperinsulinemia of an obese person is insufficient to support a normal amino acid metabolism, this person would be in a situation of relative insulin deficiency, similar to that of the insulin-deprived type I diabetic. In such a condition, there is an increase in the plasma concentration of BCAA, as well as in the rate of leucine flux and oxidation.[45] Studies on amino acid kinetics in obesity have focused on the effects of different weight reduction diets, to establish the optimum dietary energy and protein combination to spare body proteins while reducing body fat. This approach does not directly address the effects of hyperinsulinemia on amino acid metabolism, because dietary treatment and weight loss produce changes in the plasma levels of other substrates that also affect amino acid kinetics, such as ketone bodies.[46] Nevertheless, data from some of these studies, obtained prior to the initiation of dietary treatment, can offer some insight on the changes in amino acid kinetics associated with obesity. Vazquez et al.[47] studied leucine kinetics in a group of obese persons using a primed, 3-hour [^{14}C]leucine infusion, and reported a mean leucine flux (Q) of 8.7 mmoles/hour. A similar result (8.44 mmoles/hour) was found by Clugston et al.[48] in 10 obese women infused with [^{14}C]leucine for 24 hours. Using a constant 10-hour infusion of the same tracer, Garlick et al.[49] found a mean Q of 10.2 mmoles/hour (97.3 μmoles/kg/hour) in five obese adults. These values are substantially higher than those found by Fukagawa et al.[28] in five lean adults using [^{13}C]leucine and a similar kinetic model: 5.7 mmoles/hour (76.8 μmoles/kg/hour). Comparisons, however, between different studies should be made with caution, because differences in methods and/or theoretical assumptions in the kinetic parameters may produce differences unrelated to the physiological state of the subjects. Ideally, data from obese subjects should be compared only with a carefully matched group of lean subjects studied under the same conditions. Furthermore, as with other values of substrate concentrations in obese individuals, results can vary dramatically depending on whether they are expressed per kg of body weight, or lean body mass or surface area, and most studies on amino acid kinetics do not assess body composition. Likewise, the assessment of tissue and liver sensitivity to insulin is necessary to establish the relationship between insulin resistance and changes in whole body protein metabolism.

EFFECTS OF BODY COMPOSITION

The simple fact that weight reduction improves insulin sensitivity[50] suggests a relationship between body composition and insulin action. One proposed mechanism for this interaction is that the increase in fat cell mass and fat cell size may have as a consequence a decrease in the number of insulin receptors per cell, and thus decrease the response to insulin. Bjorntorp et al.[51] found a significant correlation between fasting insulin levels and fat cell diameter in obese persons, and the correlation of fasting insulin with body fat and with percent excess of ideal body weight (IBW) has also been reported by other investigators.[52,53] Measuring insulin sensitivity with the euglycemic clamp technique, Yki-Jarvinen and Koivisto[54] reported a significant negative correlation between percent body fat (estimated by skinfold thickness measurements) and insulin sensitivity. Bogardus et al.[55] also reported a nonlinear correlation between insulin sensitivity and fat mass measured by underwater weighing, with a cutoff point at approximately 28% of body fat. Using the steady state plasma glucose approach, Nagulesparan et al.[56] found a significant negative correlation between body mass index and insulin response. On the other hand, Reaven et al.[57] have shown that in obese subjects with normal OGTT, only plasma insulin response is correlated with degree of obesity, and not insulin-stimulated glucose disposal.

Muscle mass appears also to be an important determinant of insulin sensitivity, as evidenced by the decrease in basal plasma insulin after physical training, even when associated with slight increases in body fat mass.[58]

Body composition can also affect amino acid responses to insulin. Because branched chain amino acid metabolism takes place mainly in lean tissue, changes in the size of this compartment may conceivably affect blood levels of BCAA.

Obesity is usually associated with an increase in lean body mass that may comprise as much as 40% of the excess weight.[59] One study showed a significant correlation among plasma amino acids, insulin levels, and the ponderal index of obesity.[60] In another study in obese subjects before and after a 6-week period of physical training, a significant positive correlation was found between lean body mass (measured by [40]K) and the sum of branched chain amino acids, tyrosine, and phenylalanine, both before and after the training[61] (FIGURE 1). Other studies have also reported good correlations between percent fat mass and insulin sensitivity.[54]

INSULIN RESISTANCE AND BRAIN SEROTONIN SYNTHESIS

High plasma levels of large neutral amino acids (LNAA)—of which the branched chain comprise a large fraction—may affect the regulation of food intake and other behavioral and neuroendocrine processes involving the neurotransmitter serotonin. The synthesis of serotonin in the brain is dependent on the availability of its precursor amino acid tryptophan (Trp), which enters the brain at a rate determined by its plasma concentration relative to the other LNAA: valine, leucine, isoleucine, tyrosine, phenylalanine, and methionine.[62] This plasma Trp/LNAA ratio, therefore, predicts the availability of tryptophan to the brain,[63] which in turn determines its serotonin output in animals, and presumably in humans.[64,65] The insulin resistance of an obese person, by diminishing the insulin-mediated fall in plasma LNAA, would block the normal rise in the Trp/LNAA ratio produced by carbohydrate ingestion. Thus, less tryptophan would be available to the brain, and less serotonin would be released after a carbohydrate meal. Hence, insulin resistance for amino acid metabolism may play a role in sustaining an excessive food intake in obesity. Moderately obese persons exhibit a blunted fall in plasma branched chain amino acids after eating a 30 g carbohydrate snack,[66] in spite of their significantly higher insulin response, which completely suppresses the rise in the plasma Trp/LNAA ratio normally occurring in lean persons after

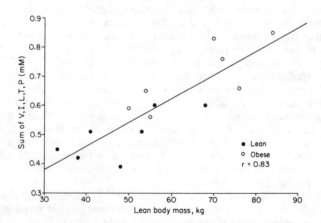

FIGURE 1. Correlation between lean body mass and the sum of plasma concentrations of valine, leucine, isoleucine, tyrosine, and phenylalanine in obese and control subjects.[6]

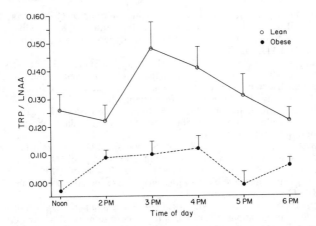

FIGURE 2. Changes in the plasma Trp/LNAA ratio in lean and obese subjects after ingestion of a 400 kcal meal at noon and a 30 g carbohydrate snack at 2:00 P.M.[66]

eating carbohydrates (FIGURE 2). Furthermore, absolute values of plasma tryptophan concentrations may be significantly lower in the obese hyperinsulinemic
than in lean subjects,[67] which produces even lower Trp/LNAA ratios. Along these
lines, the carbohydrate craving described in some obese persons[68] may be teleo-
logically interpreted as the failure of the brain to produce enough serotonin to
suppress carbohydrate intake. In fact, serotonin agonists have been shown to
selectively decrease carbohydrate intake in obese carbohydrate cravers,[68] and
tryptophan administration decreases overall energy intake in normal humans.[69,70]

CONCLUSIONS

Most obese persons can sustain a normal plasma glucose concentration, but
this requires abnormally high circulating levels of insulin. Even under this hyperinsulinemic condition, several insulin-mediated functions may be deficient,
such as glucose metabolic rate and maintaining normal plasma amino acid levels.
Chronic hyperinsulinemia has also been linked to complications similar to those
seen in long-standing obesity,[71,72] and as discussed above, insulin resistance may
also affect the physiological control of food intake by decreasing the availability of
precursor amino acids to the brain. Our understanding of the role of insulin
resistance on the pathophysiology of obesity may thus provide the rationale for
complementary therapeutic approaches to this condition.

REFERENCES

1. KARAM, J. H., G. M. GRODSKY & P. H. FORSHAM. 1963. Excessive insulin response to
   glucose in obese subjects measured by immunochemical assay. Diabetes **12:** 197–
   204.
2. DEFRONZO, R. A. 1982. Insulin secretion, insulin resistance, and obesity. Int. J. Obesity **6:** 73–82.

3. ELAHI, D., M. NAGULESPARAN, R. J. HERSCHCOPF, D. C. MULLER, J. D. TOBIN, P. M. BLIX, A. H. RUBENSTEIN & R. H. UNGER. 1982. Feedback inhibition of insulin secretion by insulin: relation to the hyperinsulinemia of obesity. N. Engl. J. Med. **306:** 1196–1202.

4. SAVAGE, P. J., E. V. FLOCK, M. E. MAKO, P. M. BLIX, A. H. RUBENSTEIN & P. H. BENNET. 1979. C-peptide and insulin secretion in Pima Indians and Caucasians: constant fractional hepatic extraction over a wide range of insulin concentrations and in obesity. J. Clin. Endocrinol. Metab. **48:** 594–598.

5. FABER, O.K., K. CHRISTENSEN, H. KEHLET, S. MADSBAD & C. BINDER. 1981. Decreased insulin removal contributes to hyperinsulinemia in obesity. J. Clin. Endocrinol. Metab. **53:** 618–621.

6. MEISTAS, M. T., S. MARGOLIS & A. A. KOWARSKI. 1983. Hypersinsulinemia of obesity is due to decreased clearance of insulin. Am. J. Physiol. **245:** E155.

7. BONORA, E., I. ZAVARONI, C. COSCELLI & U. BUTTURINI. 1984. Decreased hepatic insulin extraction in subjects with mild glucose intolerance. Metab. Clin. Exp. **32:** 438–446.

8. BLACKARD, W. G. & N. C. NELSON. 1970. Portal and peripheral vein immunoreactive insulin concentrations before and after glucose infusion. Diabetes **19:** 302–306.

9. WALTER, R. M., E. M. GOLD, C. A. MICHAS & J. W. ENSNICK. 1980. Portal and peripheral vein concentrations of insulin and glucagon after arginine infusion in morbidly obese subjects. Metab. Clin. Exp. **29:** 1037–1040.

10. MISBIN, R. I. 1985. Hyperinsulinemia in obesity: overproduction of insulin or decreased insulin clearance? Curr. Topics Nutr. Dis. **14:** 19–31.

11. FORGUE, M. E. & P. FREYCHET. 1975. Insulin receptors in the heart muscle. Demonstration of specific binding sites and impairment of insulin binding in the plasma membranes of the obese hyperglycemic mouse. Diabetes **24:** 715–723.

12. OLEFSKY, J., V. C. BACON & S. BAUR. 1976. Insulin receptors of skeletal muscle: specific insulin binding sites and demonstration of decreased number of sites in obese rats. Metab. Clin. Exp. **25:** 179–191.

13. OLEFSKY, J. M. 1976. Decreased insulin binding to adipocytes and circulating monocytes in obesity. J. Clin. Invest. **57:** 1165–1172.

14. SOLL, A. H., R. KAHN, D. M. NEVILLE & J. ROTH. 1975. Insulin receptor deficiency in genetic and acquired obesity. J. Clin. Invest. **56:** 769–780.

15. ARNER, P., K. EINARSSON, L. BACKMAN, K. NILSELL, K. M. LEREA & J. N. LIVINGSTON. 1983. Studies of liver insulin receptors in non-obese and obese human subjects. J. Clin. Invest. **72:** 1729–1736.

16. SOLL, A. H., C. R. KAHN & D. M. NEVILLE. 1975. Insulin binding to liver plasma membranes in the obese hyperglycemic (ob/ob) mouse. Demonstration of a decreased number of functionally normal receptors. J. Biol. Chem. **250:** 4702–4707.

17. ARCHER, J. A., P. GOLDEN, J. R. GAVIN, M. LESNIAK & J. ROTH. 1973. Insulin receptors in human circulating lymphocytes: application to the study of insulin resistance in man. J. Clin. Endocrinol. Metab. **36:** 627–633.

18. DEFRONZO, R. A., V. SOMAN, R. S. SHERWIN, R. S. HENDLER & P. FELIG. 1978. Insulin binding to monocytes and insulin action in human obesity, starvation and refeeding. J. Clin. Invest. **62:** 204–213.

19. RABINOWITZ, D. & K. L. ZIERLER. 1962. Forearm metabolism in obesity and its response to intraarterial insulin. Characterization of insulin resistance and evidence for adaptive hyperinsulinism. J. Clin. Invest. **41:** 2173–2181.

20. FELIG, P., J. WAHREN, R. HENDLER & T. BRUNDIN. 1974. Splanchnic glucose and amino acid metabolism in obesity. J. Clin. Invest. **53:** 582–590.

21. DEFRONZO, R. A., E. FERRANNINI, R. HENDLER, P. FELIG & J. WAHREN. 1983. Regulation of splanchnic and peripheral glucose uptake by insulin and hyperglycemia in man. Diabetes **32:** 35–45.

22. KOLTERMAN, O. G., G. M. REAVEN & J. M. OLEFSKY. 1976. Relationship between *in vivo* insulin resistance and decreased insulin receptors in obese man. J. Clin. Endocrinol. Metab. **48:** 487–494.

23. BOGARDUS, C., S. LILLIOJA, D. MOTT, G. R. REAVEN, A. KASHIWAGI & J. E. FOLEY.

1984. Relationship between obesity and maximal insulin-stimulated glucose uptake *in vivo* and *in vitro* in Pima Indians. J. Clin. Invest. **73:** 800–805.

24. KOLTERMAN, O. G., J. INSEL, M. SAEKOW & J. M. OLEFSKY. 1980. Mechanisms of insulin resistance in human obesity. Evidence for receptor and postreceptor defects. J. Clin. Invest. **65:** 1272–1284.

25. SALTER, J. & C. H. BEST. 1953. Insulin as a growth hormone. Br. Med. J. **2:** 353–356.

26. ROY, A. K., B. CHATTERJEE, M. S. K. PRASAD & N. J. UNAKAR. 1980. Role of insulin in the regulation of the hepatic messenger RNA for alpha-2u-globulin in diabetic rats. J. Biol. Chem. **255:** 11614–11618.

27. HUTSON, S. M., T. C. CREE & A. E. HARPER. 1978. Regulation of leucine and alpha-ketoisocaproate metabolism in skeletal muscle. J. Biol. Chem. **253:** 8126–8133.

28. FUKAGAWA, N. K., K. L. MINAKER, J. W. ROWE, M. N. GOODMAN, D. E. MATTHEWS, D. M. BIER & V. R. YOUNG. 1985. Insulin-mediated reduction of whole body protein breakdown. Dose-response effects on leucine metabolism in postabsorptive men. J. Clin. Invest. **76:** 2306–2311.

29. LUCK, J. M., G. MORRISON & L. F. WILBUR. 1928. Effect of insulin on amino acid content of blood. J. Biol. Chem. **77:** 151–156.

30. BERGER, M., H. ZIMMERMAN-TELSCHOW, P. BERCHTOLD, H. DROST, W. A. MUELLER, F. A. GRIES & H. ZIMMERMANN. 1978. Blood amino acid levels in patients with insulin excess (functioning insulinoma) and insulin deficiency (diabetic ketosis). Metab. Clin. Exp. **27:** 793–799.

31. SCHAUDER, P., K. SCHEDER, D. MATTHAEI, H. V. HENNING & U. LANGENBECK. 1983. Influence of insulin on blood levels of branched chain keto and amino acids in man. Metab. Clin. Exp. **32:** 323–327.

32. MARTIN-DUPAN, R., C. MAURON, B. GLAESER & R. J. WURTMAN. 1982. Effect of various oral glucose doses on plasma neutral amino acid levels. Metab. Clin. Exp. **31:** 937–943.

33. AKEDO, H. & H. N. CHRISTENSEN. 1962. Nature of insulin action on amino acid uptake by the isolated diaphragm. J. Biol. Chem. **237:** 118–122.

34. FUKAGAWA, N. K., K. L. MINAKER, V. R. YOUNG & J. W. ROWE. 1986. Insulin dose-dependent reductions in plasma amino acids in man. Am. J. Physiol. **250:** E13–E17.

35. FELIG, P., E. MARLISS & G. F. CAHILL. 1969. Plasma amino acid levels and insulin secretion in obesity. N. Engl. J. Med. **281:** 811–816.

36. SWENDSEID, M. E., C. Y. UMEZAWA & E. DRENICK. 1969. Plasma amino acid levels in obese subjects before, during, and after starvation. Am. J. Clin. Nutr. **22:** 740–743.

37. FELIG, P., E. MARLISS & G. F. CAHILL. 1969. Hyperaminoacidemia: possible mechanism of hyperinsulinemia in obesity (Abstr). Clin. Res. **17:** 382.

38. ZIERLER, K. L. & D. RABINOWITZ. 1964. Effect of very small concentrations of insulin on forearm metabolism. Persistence of its action on potassium and free fatty acids without its effect on glucose. J. Clin. Invest. **43:** 950–962.

39. DEFRONZO, R. A., J. D. TOBIN & J. W. ROWE. 1978. Glucose intolerance in uremia. Quantification of pancreatic beta cell sensitivity to glucose and tissue sensitivity to insulin. J. Clin. Invest. **62:** 425–435.

40. DEFRONZO, R. A., & P. FELIG. 1980. Amino acid metabolism in uremia: insights gained from normal and diabetic man. Am. J. Clin. Nutr. **33:** 1378–1386.

41. FUKAGAWA, N. K. 1985. Insulin-amino acid interrelationships in aging man. Ph.D. Thesis, Dept. of Applied Biological Sciences, MIT. Cambridge, MA.

42. FORLANI, G., P. VANNINI, G. MARCHESINI, M. ZOLI, A. CIAVARLLA & E. PISI. 1984. Insulin-dependent metabolism of branched-chain amino acids in obesity. Metab. Clin. Exp. **33:** 147–150.

43. HERAIEF, E., P. BURCKARDT, C. MAURON, J. J. WURTMAN & R. J. WURTMAN. 1983. The treatment of obesity by carbohydrate deprivation suppresses plasma tryptophan and its ratio to other large neutral amino acids. J. Neural Transm. **57:** 187–195.

44. GLASS, A. R., R. BONGIOVANNI, C. E. SMITH & T. M. BOEHM. 1981. Normal valine disposal in obese subjects with impaired glucose disposal: evidence for selective insulin resistance. Metab. Clin. Exp. **30:** 578–582.

45. ROBERT, J. J., B. BEAUFRERE, J. KOZIET, J. F. DESJEUX, D. M. BIER, V. R. YOUNG & H. LESTRADET. 1985. Whole body *de novo* amino acid synthesis in type 1 (insulin-dependent) diabetes studied with stable isotope-labeled leucine, alanine and glycine. Diabetes **34:** 67–73.
46. PAUL, H. S. & S. A. ADIBI. 1978. Leucine oxidation in diabetes and starvation: effects of ketone bodies on branched-chain amino acid oxidation *in vitro*. Metab. Clin. Exp. **27:** 185–200.
47. VAZQUEZ, J. A., E. L. MORSE & S. A. ADIBI. 1985. Effect of dietary fat, carbohydrate, and protein on branched-chain amino acid catabolism during caloric restriction. J. Clin. Invest. **76:** 737–743.
48. CLUGSTON, G. A. & P. J. GARLICK. 1982. The response of protein and energy metabolism to food intake in lean and obese man. Hum. Nutr. Clin. Nutr. **36C:** 57–70.
49. GARLICK, P. J., G. A. CLUGSTON & J. C. WATERLOW. 1980. Influence of low-energy diets on whole body protein turnover in obese subjects. Am. J. Physiol. **238:** E235–E244.
50. OLEFSKY, J. M., G. M. REAVEN & J. W. FARQUHAR. 1974. Effects of weight reduction on obesity. Studies on carbohydrate and lipid metabolism. J. Clin. Invest. **53:** 64–76.
51. BJORNTORP, P., P. BERCHTOLD & G. TIBBLIN. 1971. Insulin secretion in relation to adipose tissue in men. Diabetes **20:** 65–70.
52. BAGDADE, J. A., E. L. BIERMAN & D. PORTE. 1967. The significance of basal insulin levels in the evaluation of the insulin response to glucose in diabetic and nondiabetic subjects. J. Clin. Invest. **46:** 1549–1557.
53. EL KODARY, A. Z., M. F. BALL, I. M. OWEISS & J. J. CANARY. 1972. Insulin secretion and body composition in obesity. Metab. Clin. Exp. **21:** 641–654.
54. YKI-JARVINEN, H. & V. A. KOIVISTO. 1983. Effects of body composition on insulin sensitivity. Diabetes **32:** 965–969.
55. BOGARDUS, C., S. LILLIOJA, D. M. MOTT, C. HOLLENBECK & G. REAVEN. 1985. Relationship between degree of obesity and *in vivo* insulin action in man. Am. J. Physiol. **248:** E286–E291.
56. NAGULESPARAN, M., P. J. SAVAGE, R. UNGER & P. H. BENNET. 1979. A simplified method using somatostatin to assess *in vivo* insulin resistance over a range of obesity. Diabetes **28:** 980–983.
57. REAVEN, G. M., J. MOORE & M. GREENFIELD. 1983. Quantification of insulin secretion and *in vivo* insulin action in nonobese and moderately obese individuals with normal glucose tolerance. Diabetes **32:** 600–604.
58. BJORNTORP, P., K. DEJOUNGE, L. SJOSTROM & L. SULLIVAN. 1970. The effects of physical training on insulin production in obesity. Metab. Clin. Exp. **19:** 631–638.
59. FORBES, G. B. & S. L. WELLE. 1983. Lean body mass in obesity. Int. J. Obesity. **7:** 99–107.
60. PENNETI, V., A. GALANTE, L. ZONTA-SGARAMELLA & S. D. JAYAKAR. 1982. Relation between obesity, insulinemia, and serum amino acid concentration in a sample of Italian adults. Clin. Chem. (N.Y.) **28:** 2219–2224.
61. HOLM, G., L. SULLIVAN, R. JAGENBURG & P. BJORNTORP. 1978. Effects of physical training and lean body mass on plasma amino acids in man. J. Appl. Physiol. **45:** 117–181.
62. PARDRIDGE, W. M. 1977. Regulation of amino acid availability to the brain. *In* Nutrition and the Brain. R. J. Wurtman and J. J. Wurtman, Eds.: 141–204. Raven Press. New York.
63. FERNSTROM, J. D. & D. V. FALLER. 1978. Neutral amino acids in the brain: changes in response to food ingestion. J. Neurochem. **30:** 1531–1538.
64. FERNSTROM, J. D. & R. J. WURTMAN. 1972. Brain serotonin content: physiological regulation by plasma neutral amino acids. Science **178:** 414–416.
65. WURTMAN, R. J., F. HEFTI & E. MELAMED. 1980. Precursor control of neurotransmitter synthesis. Pharmacol. Rev. **3:** 315–345.
66. CABALLERO, B., N. FINER & R. J. WURTMAN. 1986. Plasma amino acid responses to carbohydrate intake in obesity. Submitted for publication.

67. ASHLEY, D. V. M., M. O. FLEURY, A. GOLAY, E. MAEDER & P. D. LEATHWOOD. 1985. Evidence for diminished brain 5-hydroxytryptamine biosynthesis in obese diabetic and nondiabetic humans. Am. J. Clin. Nutr. 42: 1240–1245.

68. WURTMAN, J. J., R. J. WURTMAN, J. H. GROWDON, P. HENRY, M. A. LIPSCOMB & S. H. ZEISEL. 1981. Carbohydrate craving in obese people: suppression by treatments affecting serotoninergic neurotransmission. Int. J. Eating Disord. 1: 2–15.

69. HRBOTICKY, N., L. A. LEITER & G. H. ANDERSON. 1985. Effects of l-tryptophan on short term food intake in lean men. Nutr. Res. 5: 595–607.

70. BLUNDELL, J. E., V. MAVJEE, C. J. WILLIAMS & A. J. HILL. 1986. Interactive effects of tryptophan and macronutrients on hunger motivation and dietary preferences. J. Cell. Metab. (Suppl.) In press.

71. GARCIA-WEBB, P. 1983. Insulin resistance—a risk factor for coronary heart disease? Scand. J. Clin. Lab. Invest. 43: 677–685.

72. STANDL, E. 1985. High serum insulin concentrations in relation to other cardiovascular risk factors in macrovascular disease of type II diabetes. Horm. Metab. Res. (Suppl.) 15: 46–51.

Exercise Effects on Calorie Intake

F. XAVIER PI-SUNYER

Division of Endocrinology and Diabetes
and Obesity Research Center
St. Luke's-Roosevelt Hospital Center
Columbia University
New York, New York 10025

The promotion of exercise for the treatment of obesity has been based on the double premise that exercise generates special metabolic signals and that these reduce food intake. The decrease in intake coupled with the increase in expenditure leads to weight loss. Strong support for this premise comes primarily from animal studies, not from studies in humans. This arises in part because the premise is so difficult to prove in people. It ought to be a simple matter to exercise sedentary people and watch them eat less. In fact, the methodologic problems associated with measuring energy expenditure, voluntary changes in energy intake, and small shifts in body composition are great. As a result, there is a paucity of information in this area.

STUDIES IN ANIMALS

The animal studies are more enlightening, though to some extent confusing, because they are not consistent. There is a sexual dimorphism in the food intake response of rodents to exercise. Generally, male rats tend to decrease food intake and lose weight, whereas female rats tend to maintain or increase intake and thereby maintain or gain weight.

Crews et al.[1] ran male rats 2.24 to 3.72 km/day for 5 days/week and found that they decreased their intake in comparison to sedentary controls. Tsuji et al.[2] exercised rats on treadmills for 28 days, increasing the distance run from 1.2 to 3.5 km/day and also found a decreased food intake. Pitts and Bull[3] exercised rats on treadmills for 106 days, reaching a level on the last 20 days of 1.08 km/day at 14% grade. Again, food intake was lower than in sedentary controls. Dohm et al.[4] ran male rats on treadmills for 6 weeks, with increasing speed and grade to a final level of 1 hr/day at 35 m/min at 8% grade. Caloric intake was significantly lower than sedentary controls. Other studies have confirmed these findings.[5-9] On similar exercise programs, female rats usually do not change or increase their food intake and tend to maintain their body weight.[6,7]

In studies in which rats were run for some days and not for others, food intake was reduced during the activity day and approached control levels on rest days.[10,11] The net effect was weight reduction as compared to sedentary control animals.

If rats are made to undergo isolated bouts of exercise, food intake is inhibited, and the decrease is greatest for the longest exercise period. In addition, the closer the meal is given to the termination of the exercise bout, the greater the inhibitory effect.[11]

94

An assumption is often made that the effect of exercise on food intake is the same irrespective of the level of exercise imposed. That level involves both the intensity of the effort (kcal/min) and the amount of work done (total caloric expenditure). Although it is unwise to extrapolate the findings in rats obtained by Mayer et al.[12] directly to humans, their study does address this issue. They describe three different activity zones in which three different intake responses were elicited: a very inactive zone where intake exceeded expenditure, an active zone where a tight concordance between the two occurred, and an extremely active zone where discordance recurred. As animals fatigued in this third zone of activity, they ate less than they expended.

Also, Katch et al.,[13] varying the intensity of exercise in male rats while keeping energy expenditure constant, found that the reduction of food intake was highest in the high-intensity group, and that the effect lasted up to three days postexercise.

It is possible that humans have a similar pattern, and that the effect of exercise will differ with the intensity or amount of work done. It may be that only intense, glycogen-depleting exercise produces weight loss, whereas milder exercise does not. Alternatively, if the less intense exercise is done for a longer period, this too may have a weight-reducing effect. A trade-off between work intensity and work duration could exist. It would be important to have more information about this problem because the knowledge gained could be applied usefully in public health education and exercise prescriptions.

STUDIES IN HUMANS

In humans, there is little experimental evidence on the effect of exercise on food intake. Although epidemiological data suggest a positive relation between activity and leaness, one cannot establish whether overweight and increased body fat are a product of, exacerbated by, or lead to, inactivity. A great deal of anecdotal allusion has been made to the inhibitory properties of exercise on calorie consumption. But strong support for this comes largely from animal studies, not from studies in humans.

There are few studies of the effect of exercise on food intake that have actually measured food intake. Generally, protocols have either estimated food intake, or they have simply followed body weight and have interpreted weight loss as reflecting a hypophagic response and weight stability or weight gain as a hyperphagic response.

Most studies of normal weight individuals show insignificant changes in body weights with moderate exercise. This would suggest that in these individuals, the increased energy expenditure is compensated for by a hyperphagic response commensurate with the expenditure change, so that body weight equilibrium is maintained.[14]

By contrast, studies in obese volunteers have shown variable results. This suggests that in the obese person, intake is not tightly coupled to activity expenditure. Two studies, one exercising obese men and the other obese women, reported weight loss, but the weight loss can all be attributed to the expenditure side of the equation.[15,16] Though the investigators did not measure food intake carefully, food records suggested no increase in intake, and this fit well with their balance calculations.[15]

Studies in obese subjects by some observers have shown a decrease in weight with activity.[17-19] One of the troubles with such studies is that often only finishers are counted. If a study is long and arduous, such as Gwinup's[17] (120 minutes a day, 7 days a week for a year), only the very motivated will stick out all the exercise (11 of 34 in this study), and they may also become motivated to changing their diet (even though this is not prescribed). If so, then it may not be the exercise that causes the decrease in food intake, but rather a change in life style that may include changes in food and possibly tobacco use and alcohol intake, as well as the changes in activity.

Two studies of exercise matched to a free diet showed little effect on weight.[20,21] Thus, as expenditure energy was increased, it was presumably made up by intake, though intake was not measured. Leon et al. reported weight loss in individuals who spent 1100 kcal per day exercising.[22] This is very heavy exercise. By contrast, Krotkiewsky et al.,[21] using lighter exercise for 30 minutes per day, obtained no effect in obese women. Thus, heavy or sustained exercise may be required before much weight loss occurs.

In a number of studies, the food intake has been estimated from dietary history or dietary recall, continuously[23-26] or occasionally[22,26-29] in free-living subjects. Because only one of these studies attempted to validate the accuracy of the subject records, these reports are very unreliable.

Only a few studies have actually measured food intake directly in response to exercise. Three have been in a metabolic ward setting, with an exercise prescription but no dietary limits. All three were on lean subjects[30-32] and were very short-term. Edholm et al.[33] varied the expenditures of twelve lean young men over 14 days and measured their food intake. Even though the overall energy intake matched energy expenditure, there was no correlation between the mean expenditure on one day and the intake on that day, but there seemed to be some correlation with intake two days later. In studies by Campbell[32] and Warnold,[31] the volunteers underate in their sedentary periods and then ate more during the active exercising period. Because no cross-over designs were used, a period effect cannot be ruled out. Also, the treatment periods (sedentary and exercise) were very short (5–7 days), and it may be that regulatory mechanisms require longer to manifest themselves.[33-35]

METABOLIC WARD STUDIES IN LEAN AND OBESE SUBJECTS

We (Woo and Pi-Sunyer[14]) have recently completed a study to try to determine the effect of exercise on food intake in lean women. A number of lean women (mean weight 97% of ideal) spent three 19-day periods in a metabolic ward. A 5-day evaluation phase preceded three 19-day treatment periods. During the 5-day period, their sedentary 24-hr energy expenditure was calculated. This became the basis for calculating the extra exercise that they were asked to perform during their mild and moderate exercise periods. They spent each one of the periods at one of three levels of activity: sedentary (no exercise), mild exercise (110% of the sedentary activity), that is, exercise was prescribed to raise their 24-hour energy expenditure by 10%, or moderate (125% of sedentary activity). The exercise was done on a treadmill at a speed that was comfortable for the individual, which averaged 3.5 to 4.0 mph. Energy expenditure was measured by daily activity diaries[36] in which eight activities could be recorded. The energy cost of the activities was measured by indirect calorimetry twice a week. In the mild exercise period, they expended a mean of 378 kcal/day walking on the treadmill for 139 minutes, and in the moderate period a mean of 772 kcal/day while walking for 250 minutes. Food intake was covertly monitored by serving all meals and all snacks to each subject as separate items in multiple portions on large platters, from which she freely served herself. The items were covertly weighed before and after serving. The results are shown in FIGURE 1.

It may be seen in FIGURE 1 that we achieved our objective of making the volunteers increase their expenditure to about the 10% and the 25% level for the two exercise periods. It is also clear that there was a significant increase in intake with increased expenditure. As a result, the volunteers remained in energy balance during all three periods. The somewhat lessened intake increment between mild and moderate exercise as compared to between sedentary and mild is interesting. Although it could be an artifact of the few subjects studied, it could also reflect a fatigue effect, because the moderate exercise required these lean, and therefore efficient women, to be on the treadmill an average of 4 plus hours per

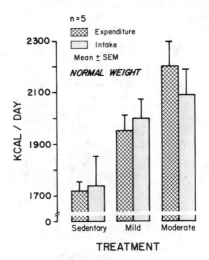

FIGURE 1. Mean energy expenditure and intake (in kcal/day) in five normal-weight women over three 19-day periods in which they were either sedentary or exercised on a treadmill at a mild (110% of sedentary daily activity) or moderate (125% of sedentary) degree. (R. Woo et al.[14] With permission from *Metabolism, Clinical and Experimental.*)

day. Such a fatigue effect has been described in exercising rats.[12] There were no changes in body weight, body fat, or lean body mass during the 57 days that this study was conducted.

In summary, over 19-day periods, lean women compensated for their increased intake by increasing their expenditure. There was no indication of an inhibitory effect of exercise on food intake, since at no time did the food intake fall below the sedentary intake when the lean subjects were exercising.

Having shown that lean individuals compensate by increasing food intake when expenditure is raised, we wished to test this in obese individuals who were sedentary (Woo, Garrow, and Pi-Sunyer[37]). The obese volunteers were six women between the ages of 22 and 61 years. Their ideal body weight ranged from 144 to 183% of ideal with a mean of 167 percent. They were studied on the metabolic ward for three consecutive 19-day periods. Each person was told that the study was to measure the effect of exercise on protein balance. They were also told that their weight might stay the same or actually go up. This was done to prevent individuals who were interested in losing weight from volunteering for the study.

The protocol was as described for the lean individuals. The three periods were sedentary, mild exercise (110% of sedentary expenditure), and moderate exercise (125% of sedentary expenditure). Subjects were assigned randomly to the three conditions in a Latin square design to control for period or time effect.

FIGURE 2 shows the daily energy expenditure for each activity during each of the three periods. Mean daily energy expenditures were 2221 + 71 kcal/day for sedentary, 2419 + 68 for mild, and 2714 + 119 for moderate exercise. The subjects expended about 200 extra calories during mild activity and 500 extra calories during moderate activity. To do this, they had to be on the treadmill an average of 39 min/day for mild and 96 min/day for moderate exercise.

FIGURE 2 demonstrates that energy intake did not increase as energy expendi-

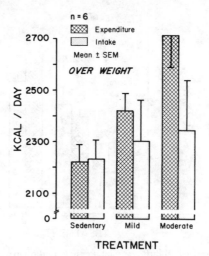

FIGURE 2. Mean energy expenditure and intake (in kcal/day) in six obese women over three 19-day periods in which they were either sedentary or exercised on a treadmill at a mild (110% of sedentary daily activity) or moderate (125% of sedentary) degree. (R. Woo *et al.*[14] With permission from *Metabolism, Clinical and Experimental*.)

ture increased. Mean daily intakes ranged between 2233–2345 kcal/day at all times. The intake seemed to be fixed and unchanged from treatment period to period. Also, the composition of the intake from period to period did not change. Because of the increase in expenditure and the lack of change of intake, caloric balance was negative in both the exercise periods.

These studies in obese women showed a dissociation between exercise and food intake. As exercise effort increased, food intake remained fixed, suggesting that exercise was not a variable in the determinants of food intake.

STUDIES FOR A LONGER TIME IN OBESE WOMEN

Inasmuch as we had shown a discrepancy between the effect of exercise on food intake in lean and obese women, suggesting that the obese exhibited a dissociation between exercise and food intake regulation, we felt it was important to see whether we could show this effect over a more extended period of time than a 19-day interval, which was the design of the initial studies. Although we felt that 19 days was significantly longer than any previous study of exercise effect on food intake, and should be enough time to give us information on long-term food intake regulation, we also felt that the studies would be bolstered if we showed similar behavior over a more extended period of time. As a result, we enlisted another group of women for a full 57-day period of moderate exercise (Woo, Garrow and Pi-Sunyer[38]). Three obese women, averaging 187% of ideal body weight, were volunteers. The initial protocol was identical to the previous two, which have been described. That is, they were admitted for an initial 5-day period where their sedentary energy intake and energy expenditure were measured. The volunteer obese women were then placed on a 57-day regimen of moderate exercise, which would raise their daily energy expenditure to 125% of the sedentary expenditure. Again, subjects could pick the treadmill speed that they considered comfortable, and then a time assignment was given to them to be done each 24 hours. The average expenditure, calculated at 125% of basal, was 2878, 2930, and 2839 kcal/day for the three 19-day periods making up the 57 days. The food intake per period was 1844, 1915, and 1950 kcal/day.

These women over the extended 57-day period maintained their food intake fixed. The intake did not correlate with their expenditure. Because of the difference between intake and expenditure, the obese volunteers lost a significant amount of weight over the period tested. As in the first study on obese women, food intake seemed to be determined by factors dissociated from the caloric expenditure.

FURTHER STUDIES IN OBESE MEN

Porikos et al.[39] who in our laboratory had provided obese persons with food in family-style platters and had taken great care to make the food tasty as well as plentiful, found that obese persons overate on such a regimen. With this in mind, we decided to do a pilot study in which we would serve the food in platters as previously but would take much greater care in making the food very tasty and variable: a gourmet cuisine.

For this study we enlisted four male volunteers (somewhat younger and less obese that the original group of six obese women) (Pi-Sunyer[40]). Their ages were 26–35 years. Their mean percent ideal body weight was 129% as calculated from the Metropolitan Life Tables. The protocol was different from the previous ones in a number of ways. The test periods were somewhat shorter at 10 days each. The subjects were not randomized for period, but all did the same sequence: sedentary, 120% of sedentary, 140% of sedentary, and back to sedentary. In this group, sedentary included some treadmill exercise because these men were younger and not as obese and gave us a history of greater daily activity in the free-living state. With the aid of pedometers that they wore for a week, we estimated their usual daily activity, so that in the sedentary period they were given treadmill assignments in order to emulate their normal 24-hour daily caloric expenditure. Treadmill exercise was then increased for the added 20% and 40% above the usual activity range. As a result, at the 40% range, these individuals were doing a great deal of treadmill walking, on an average, 3 hours and 16 minutes per day.

The results of this study are shown in FIGURE 3.[40] Caloric expenditure averaged 3000 + 92 kcal/day in the basal period. The activity goals were realized, with expenditure in the mild period being 122.5% of sedentary and in the moderate period 138.7 percent. Again, like the obese women, these obese men did not change their food intake. Values were not significantly different at 4488, 4248, 4128, and 3990 kcal/day for the four periods, so that as activity changed, caloric intake did not. Again, we saw a dissociation between food intake and energy expenditure.

It may be noted, however, that these individuals ate very much more than the obese women in the previous studies did. Why is this? We changed the protocol in this study to make the food presented to the individuals much more palatable. The foods were more gourmet including tastier desserts; greater effort was made to cook and present them in a very attractive fashion. Given this more gourmet presentation, the obese subjects took far more food that was the case with the sparer and less tasty hospital fare fed the obese women in the other studies. This, and the lack of correlation of the intake to the exercise, suggests that palatability and variety in the diet was more important in determining the amount of intake in

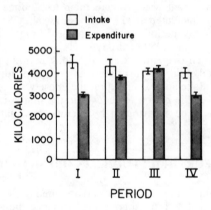

FIGURE 3. Mean energy intake and expenditure in four obese men over four 10-day periods (I to IV) in which they were at a basal level of activity (I and IV), or in which activity was increased by walking on a treadmill to a mild (110% of basal daily activity) (II), or a moderate (140% of basal) degree (III). (F. X. Pi-Sunyer.[39] With permission from John Libbey & Company Limited.)

the obese volunteers than was the particular caloric expenditure level they were maintaining.

SENSORY-SPECIFIC SATIETY

That the level of intake relates to the sensory aspects of the meals is in good agreement with data from Rolls et al.[41,42] They have suggested that satiety is sensory-specific, having shown that the intake of an individual can be changed by manipulating the sensory qualities of the foods presented. With greater variety of flavor, appearance, and taste, individuals eat more than if a more monotonous, less tasty fare is presented. Hence Rolls et al. hypothesize that satiety is not fixed but moves up or down according to the sensory qualities of the food available.

CONCLUSION

Our studies would suggest that the determinants of caloric intake in obese subjects may depend more on the sensory characteristics of the food presented than on any cues related to the energy expenditure. Subjects fixed on a particular caloric intake, which seemed to depend on the sensory qualities of the food presented, so that as pleasantness increased, intake went up. The fixity of caloric intake was not changed either up or down when caloric expenditure was increased to a very significant degree. Thus, we could find no evidence that the added exercise had any effect on the intake of calories.

We also found, however, that the lean individuals regulated intake very closely to expenditure. When expenditure was raised by increasing exercise, intake also went up.

It seems that obese individuals are not as sensitive to cues generated by exercise as are lean individuals. As a result, whereas lean persons tend to compensate for increasing exercise-induced expenditure with increased intake, the obese do not. It is possible that the insensitivity of the obese may be related to their increased adipose tissue stores. If so, at some point in a weight-loss curve, as adipose stores revert towards normal, it may be that obese individuals will become more responsive to exercise cues. It would be interesting to conduct studies in this regard; none have been done.

Nevertheless, inasmuch as exercise exerts neither a stimulatory nor an inhibitory effect on food intake in the obese individuals, a negative energy balance can be created by increasing caloric expenditure by exercise. This negative balance will be strictly equivalent to the increased expenditure. No specific inhibitory effect on food intake can be expected that would increase negative energy balance beyond the exercise calories expended. It is clear, therefore, that for a maximum effect on weight loss in an obese individual, a two-pronged approach is necessary. Not only must an emphasis be given to increasing expenditure, but strong emphasis must be placed on voluntarily decreasing dietary intake. The two seem to work relatively independently of each other, and stressing them both should lead to a maximum effect on weight loss.

REFERENCES

1. Crews III, E. L., K. W. Fuge, L. B. Oscai *et al.* 1969. Weight, food intake, and body composition: effects of exercise and protein deficiency. Am. J. Physiol. **216:** 275–287.
2. Tsuji, K., Y. Katayama & H. Koishi. 1975. Effects of dietary protein level on energy metabolism of rats during exercise. J. Nutr. Sci. Vitaminol. **21:** 437–449.
3. Pitts, G. C. & L. S. Bull. 1977. Exercise, dietary obesity, and growth in the rat. Am. J. Physiol. **232:** R38–R44.
4. Dohm, G. L., G. R. Beecher & T. P. Stephenson *et al.* 1977. Adaptations to endurance training at three intensities of exercise. J. Appl. Physiol. **42:** 753–757.
5. Oscai, L. B., P. A. Mole, B. Brei & J. O. Holloszy. 1971. Cardiac growth and respiratory enzyme levels in male rats subjected to a running program. Am. J. Physiol. **220:** 1238–1241.
6. Nance, D. M., B. Bromley, R. J. Barnard & R. A. Gorski. 1977. Sexually dimorphic effects of forced exercise on food intake and body weight in the rat. Physiol. Behav. **19:** 155–158.
7. Applegate, E. A., D. E. Upton & J. S. Stern. 1982. Food intake, body composition and blood lipids following treadmill exercise in male and female rats. Physiol. Behav. **28:** 917–920.

8. Oscai, L. B. & J. O. Holloszy. 1969. Effects of weight changes produced by exercise, food restriction, or over eating on body composition. J. Clin. Invest. **48:** 2124–2128.

9. Ahrens, R. 1972. Effects of age and dietary carbohydrate source on the response of rats to forced exercise. J. Nutr. **102:** 241–247.

10. Thomas, B. M. & A. T. Miller Jr. 1958. Adaptation to forced exercise in the rat. Am. J. Physiol. **193:** 350–354.

11. Stevenson, J. A. F., B. M. Box, V. Feleki & J. R. Beaton. 1966. Bouts of exercise and food intake in the rat. Appl. Physiol. **21:** 118–122.

12. Mayer, J., N. B. Marshall, J. J. Vitale *et al.* 1954. Exercise, food intake and body weight in normal rats and genetically obese adult mice. Am. J. Physiol. **177:** 544–548.

13. Katch, V. L., R. Martin & J. Martin. 1979. Effects of exercise intensity on food consumption in the male rat. Am. J. Clin. Nutr. **32:** 1401–1407.

14. Woo, R. & F. X. Pi-Sunyer. 1985. Effect of increased physical activity on voluntary intake in lean women. Metab. Clin. Exp. **34:** 836–841.

15. Dempsey, J. A. 1964. Anthropometrical observations on obese and non-obese young men undergoing a program of vigorous physical exercise. Res. Q. Am. Assoc. Health Phys. Educ. Recreat. **35:** 275–279.

16. Dudleston, A. K. & M. Bennion. 1970. Effect of diet and/or exercise on obese college women. J. Am. Diet Assoc. **56:** 126–129.

17. Gwinup, G. 1975. Effect of exercise alone on the weight of obese women. Arch. Intern. Med. **135:** 676–680.

18. Oscai, L. B. & B. T. Williams. 1968. Effect of exercise on overweight middle-aged males. J. Am. Geriatr. Soc. **16:** 794–797.

19. Boileau, R. A., E. R. Buskirk, D. H. Horstman *et al.* 1971. Body compositional changes in obese and lean men during physical conditioning. Med. Sci. Sports **3:** 183–189.

20. Weltman, A., S. Matter & B. A. Stamford. 1980. Caloric restriction and/or mild exercise: effects on serum lipids and body composition. Am. J. Clin. Nutr. **33:**1002–1009.

21. Krotkiewski, M., K. Mandroukas & L. Sjostrom *et al.* 1979. Effects of long-term physical training on body fat, metabolism and blood pressure in obesity. Metab. Clin. Exp. **28:** 650–658.

22. Leon, A. S., J. Conrad, D. B. Hunninghake & R. Serfass. 1979. Effects of a vigorous walking program on body composition and carbohydrate and lipid metabolism of obese young men. Am. J. Clin. Nutr. **33:** 1776–1787.

23. Bjorntorp, P., K. de Jounge & M. Krotkiewski *et al.* 1973. Physical training in human obesity. III. Effects of long-term physical training on body composition. Metab. Clin. Exp. **22:** 1467–1475.

24. O'Hara, W. J., C. Allen & R. J. Shepard. 1977. Treatment of obesity by exercise in the cold. Can. Med. Assoc. J. **117:** 773–786.

25. Parizkova, J. & O. Poupa. 1963. Some metabolic consequences of adaptation to muscular work. Br. J. Nutr. **17:** 341–345.

26. Skinner, J. S., J. O. Holloszy & T. K. Cureton. 1964. Effects of a program of endurance exercises on physical work. Am. J. Cardiol. **14:** 747–752.

27. Erkelens, D. W., J. J. Albers & W. R. Hazzard *et al.* 1979. HDL cholesterol in survivors of myocardial infarction. J. Am. Med. Assoc. **242:** 2185–2189.

28. Johnson, R. E., J. A. Mastropaolo & M. A. Wharton. 1972. Exercise, dietary intake, and body composition. J. Am. Diet. Assoc. **61:** 399–403.

29. Katch, F. I., E. D. Michael & E. M. Jones. 1969. Effects of physical training on the body composition and diet of females. Res. Q. Am. Assoc. Health Phys. Educ. Recreat. **40:** 99–104.

30. Passmore, R., J. G. Thomson & G. M. Warnock. 1952. A balance sheet of the estimation of energy intake and energy expenditure as measured by indirect calorimetry using the Kofranyi-Michaelis calorimeter. Br. J. Nutr. **6:** 253–264.

31. Warnold, J. & R. A. Lenner. 1977. Evaluation of the heart rate method to determine the daily energy expenditure in disease. A study in juvenile diabetics. Am. J. Clin. Nutr. **30:** 304–315.

32. CAMPBELL, R. G. & E. BECKER. April 1975. Effects of exercise on meal-taking in man. Presented at Eastern Psych. Assn. Meeting, Hartford, Conn.
33. EDHOLM, O. G. 1977. Energy balance in man-studies carried out by the Division of Human Physiology, National Institute of Medical Research. J. Hum. Nutr. **31:** 413–431.
34. DURNIN, J. V. G. A. 1961. 'Appetite' and the relationship between expenditure and intake of calories in man. J. Physiol. **156:** 294–306.
35. EDHOLM, O. G., J. M. ADAM & M. J. R. HEALY et al. 1970. Food intake and energy expenditure of army recruits. Br. J. Nutr. **24:** 1091–1107.
36. DURNIN, J. V. G. A. & J. M. BROCKWAY. 1959. Determination of the total daily energy expenditure in man by direct calorimetry: assessment of the accuracy of a modern technique. Br. J. Nutr. **13:** 41–53.
37. WOO, R., J. S. GARROW & F. X. PI-SUNYER. 1982. Effect of exercise on spontaneous calorie intake in obesity. Am. J. Clin. Nutr. **36:** 470–477.
38. WOO, R., J. S. GARROW & F. X. PI-SUNYER. 1982. Voluntary food intake during prolonged exercise in obese women. Am. J. Clin. Nutr. **36:** 478–484.
39. PORIKOS, K. P., G. BOOTH & T. B. VAN ITALLIE. 1977. Effect of covert nutritive dilution on the spontaneous food intake of obese individuals: a pilot study. Am. J. Clin. Nutr. **30:** 1638–1644.
40. PI-SUNYER, F. X. 1985. Effect of exercise on food intake. In Recent Advances in Obesity Research IV. J. Hirsch & T. B. Van Itallie, Eds.: 368–373. John Libbey. London.
41. ROLLS, B. J., E. T. ROWE & B. KINGSTON et al. 1981. Variety in a meal enhances food intake in man. Physiol. Behav. **26:** 215–221.
42. ROLLS, B. J., E. A. ROWE & E. T. ROLLS. 1982. How sensory properties of food affect human feeding behavior. Physiol. Behav. **29:** 409–417.

The Difference in the Storage Capacities for Carbohydrate and for Fat, and Its Implications in the Regulation of Body Weight[a]

J. P. FLATT

Department of Biochemistry
University of Massachusetts Medical School
Worcester, Massachusetts 01605

INTRODUCTION

Weight maintenance occurs when a situation is achieved in which energy intake and energy expenditure vary about the same mean value, and where protein balance, carbohydrate balance, and fat balance are all maintained as well. Because body weight is usually stable over prolonged periods, in spite of the appreciable deviations from exact balances that undoubtedly occur from day to day, it is evident that depletion or accumulation of body constituents must somehow elicit corrective responses. These may manifest themselves by influencing food intake, and/or by altering the rate of energy expenditure or the composition of the substrate mix used for energy generation. Thanks to these responses, the oxidative disposal of amino acids, glucose, and fatty acids can be made to occur at rates corresponding, in the average, to the relative proportions of protein, carbohydrate, and fat in the diet (with allowance for gluconeogenesis from amino acids and triglyceride-glycerol and the possible transformation of some carbohydrate into fat).

The need to properly adjust the composition of the fuel mix used for energy generation represents constraints beyond the mere need to achieve energy balance. The size of the body's protein pools, the state of repletion of its glycogen reserves, and the size of its adipose tissue mass influence the concentrations of circulating substrates and hormones, and thereby the rates of substrate utilization. Changes in body composition thus contribute to the adjustment of the composition of the fuel mix oxidized to the nutrient distribution in the diet. Therefore, one has to expect that a particular body composition must be reached by a given individual to permit the oxidation of a fuel mixture with an average composition equivalent to that provided by the diet consumed. By the same token, one is led to the realization that the composition of the diet is a factor in determining the body composition for which weight maintenance will be achieved.[1]

Adjustment of amino acid oxidation to protein intake is effectively achieved, as nitrogen balance (or a stable rate of protein accretion during growth) is achieved on high or low (but adequate) protein intakes, irrespective of the ratio of carbohydrate to fat in the diet and of the accuracy with which carbohydrate and fat balances are achieved. In view of this, and because carbohydrate and fat

[a] This work was supported by NIH Grant #AM 33214.

provide the bulk of the energy substrates used for adenosine triphosphate (ATP) generation, weight maintenance is determined primarily by events pertaining to the metabolism of carbohydrate and fat. Glucose and fatty acid oxidation provide together an amount of energy equal to the individuals' total energy expenditure, minus the energy provided by oxidation of amino acids, in amounts determined by protein intake. Carbohydrate and fat can both provide substrates for ATP generation, but the regulation of their metabolism is characterized by substantial differences.[1] As we will see, the origin of many of these differences can be attributed to the fact that the body's ability to store carbohydrate is two orders of magnitude less than its capacity for fat storage.[2] Biological evolution was therefore compelled to lead to the development of mechanisms (including hormonal responses) that give priority to the maintenance of the carbohydrate balance over that of the fat balance. The consequences that the very large difference in storage capability for carbohydrate and for fat can be expected to have on the body's ability to achieve a steady state can be appreciated by using a model.

DESCRIPTION OF THE MODEL

The basic operational conditions prevailing in a system that includes two reservoirs of very different capacities can be appreciated by considering an analogy with a hydraulic system (FIGURES 1 and 2). In this model, the two reservoirs provide the water needed to drive a turbine. The small reservoir (S for small and sugar) is meant to represent the body's limited capacity for storing glycogen, whereas the large reservoir (L for large and lipid) is analogous to the body's ability to store large amounts of fat. The model is assumed to have the following features: (a) The configuration of the turbine (A) is such that water will not be transferred from one compartment to the other, even when the hydrostatic pressures in the two compartments are different. (b) The total flow through the turbine is controlled so that it will generate a given amount of power, assumed to be proportional to the volume of water flowing through the turbine; (i.e. the power produced is not influenced by the hydrostatic pressures). (c) The flow of water contributed by the small and the large reservoirs to the turbine flux occurs in proportion to the hydrostatic pressures prevailing in S and L. (d) Replenishment of the reservoirs occurs when the water in the small reservoir has decreased to a particular level (S_1), which triggers the addition of a certain mass of water (M for mass of water or for meal). A portion of M is dumped into the large reservoir, whereas the other falls into the small reservoir. The fraction added to the large reservoir is F (for fraction of water or for the fat content of the diet). Thus L receives an amount equal to M × F, and S an amount equal to M × (1 − F), raising its level momentarily to a maximum height (S_2).

Given the large cross-sectional area of the large reservoir, the amount of water drained or added during one cycle will cause only an insignificant change in its water level. The cumulative effect, however, of repeated operation of the outflow-refilling cycle can lead to substantial changes in its content. Ultimately, the situation will be encountered in which the hydrostatic pressure in L will be just right for the outflow from L, during one cycle, to be equal to one water addition to it. Subsequently, water replenishments triggered at a frequency serving to maintain the content of S within its constant operating range (i.e. between S_1 and S_2) will cause no further accumulation or depletion in L. A steady state will then be reached. Thus, the water in the large reservoir will establish itself at a particular

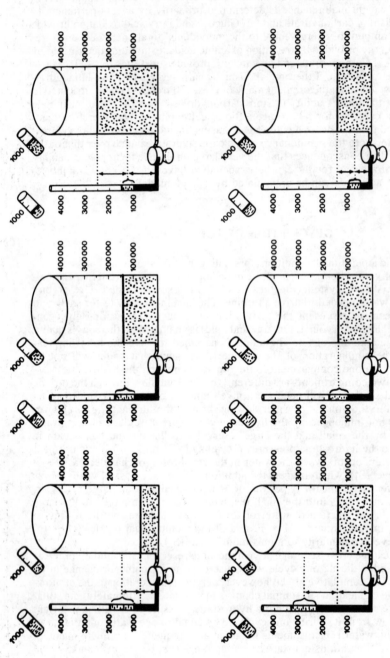

FIGURE 1. Hydraulic model of a turbine alimented by a small and a large reservoir. (Units were chosen to correspond approximately with the human body's glycogen and fat reserves, expressed in terms of kilocalories). It is assumed that the two reservoirs contribute to the turbine flux in proportion to the relative hydrostatic pressures prevailing in the ducts at any given time. Replenishment of the reservoirs is elicited when the water level in the small reservoir reaches a given minimal level (shown by the top of the black area in the small reservoir). Water is then added to the two reservoirs in proportions of 2 : 1 (left), 1 : 1 (middle), and 1 : 2 (right). Each scheme illustrates a particular steady state situation. (J. P. Flatt.[3] With permission from Wissenschaftliche Verlagsgesellschaft.)

level (L_s, for steady state level) without a sensor to measure its content, nor a regulatory mechanism that could drive the system toward some predetermined set-point value for its content.

As illustrated in FIGURE 1, changes in F cause a shift in the steady state level in L. For example, if one-third of the added water falls into L (*i.e.* F = 0.33), the level achieved in L corresponds to the situation where the hydrostatic pressure in the large reservoir is one-half of the average hydrostatic pressure prevailing in the small reservoir (left panel of FIG. 1). If F is 0.5, the level in the large reservoir rises until it is half way between S_1 and S_2 (middle panel). If F equals $\frac{2}{3}$, L_s must increase to twice the average hydrostatic pressure in S for the outflow from the large reservoir to be twice the outflow from the small reservoir (right panel). It is important to realize, however, that a constant level can be maintained in the large

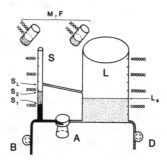

FIGURE 2. Hydraulic model used as an analogy for the body's acquisition, storage, and oxidation of carbohydrate and of fat. Turbine A is fed by the two reservoirs that contribute water in amounts proportional to the hydrostatic pressures prevailing in the two reservoirs. The power output from turbine A is variable (representative of physical activity changes). Turbine B is fed only from the small reservoirs and its outflow is constant (analogy with the brain's requirement for glucose). When the water level in the small reservoir declines to level S_1, a given mass of water M (meal) is added to the system, of which a fraction (F, corresponding to the fat content of the diet) falls into the large reservoir, the remainder being added to the small reservoir. When water accumulates to a sufficient height in the small reservoir (S_L), it can be transferred into the large reservoir (to mimic conversion of carbohydrate to fat); this transfer is not influenced by the level in the large reservoir. L_s indicates the level in the large reservoir when steady state conditions have become established. Turbine D is fed from the large reservoir only (analogy for diet-induced thermogenesis and the resulting high rates of fatty acid oxidation in brown adipose tissue).

reservoir as F increases (lower panels in FIG. 1), but this requires that the level that triggers water addition be adjusted to appropriately lower values in the small reservoir.

To provide a somewhat better analogy with flux and storage of sugar and lipid in the body, the following additional features can be incorporated into the model (FIG. 2), as summarized in TABLE 1: (e) A channel allows an overflow from the small into the large reservoir, should conditions be such that the small compartment overfills (*i.e.* when the water level in S reaches S_L). This transfer is assumed to be unaffected by the level in S; it is an analogy for the conversion of carbohydrate into fat. In adults consuming mixed diets *de novo*, lipogenesis appears to be of minor quantitative significance,[4] even in obese subjects.[5] This process becomes appreciable only when glycogen levels are raised to unusually high levels (*i.e.* > 8 g glycogen/kg body weight),[6] for example during total parenteral nutrition with

TABLE 1. Analogies Provided by the Model

Parameters in Model	Analogies
Geometry	Genetic (or fixed) traits
Diameters of large reservoirs	Number of adipocytes
Height of overflow from S into L (S_L)	Propensity toward lipogenesis
Size of ducts feeding turbine A	Balance between sympathetic and parasympathetic nervous system
Circumstantial Factor	Life-Style Factors
Height of S_1	Food availability
Height of S_2	Food palatability
Fraction added to L (F)	Fat content of diet
Ratio of $\dfrac{\text{Flux through B}}{\text{Total Flux}}$	Physical activity habits
Flow through D	Diet-induced thermogenesis in brown adipose tissue

hypertonic dextrose infusions,[6] or after deliberate ingestion of large excesses of carbohydrates during consecutive days.[7] (f) A second turbine can be driven only with water flowing out of the small reservoir. This additional turbine (B for brain) accounts for the constant requirement for glucose by the brain and other specialized cells that cannot use free fatty acids (FFA) for energy generation. The flux from S into B is, therefore, independent of the content of L. (g) The possibility exists to change the power demanded from the large turbine. This can mimic the effect of physical activity (turbine A for activity) or of other phenomena (such as cold exposure), which increase the body's overall rate of energy expenditure and substrate oxidation, while flux through B remains unaffected. (h) A small turbine is driven only by the outflow from L. This turbine (D for diet-induced thermogenesis) can be used to evaluate the effect of overfeeding-induced uncoupling of oxidative phosphorylation in brown adipose tissue (BAT), which primarily oxidizes fatty acids.[8] (This feature was used only in the computations used to generate FIG. 10).

RESPONSES OF THE MODEL

The rise in the steady state content of the large reservoir (L_s) as a function of increasing F (cf. upper half of FIG. 1 and dotted line in FIG. 3) is shifted upwards by increased drainage of the small reservoir through B. The full line in FIGURE 3 illustrates the situation where 20% of total outflow occurs through B (i.e. as the brain accounts for about 20% of basal metabolic expenditure[2]). An increase in total power output (increased physical activity) attenuates this effect; for example, the dashed line in FIGURE 3 could also be obtained by doubling total flux, thereby reducing the outflow through B to 10% of total flux. It is noteworthy that increases in total flux, in the absence of flow through turbine B, have no effect on the steady state content of L, as long as replenishment occurs whenever the content of S has decreased to a particular fixed level S_1. It is interesting, also, that an increase in flux through B, such as one would expect to occur during late pregnancy when the glucose requirements by the fetus augment, has the effect of elevating L_s.

In this and in many other ways, the model's "behavior" can help us to understand how various parameters contribute in determining to what extent the large compartment has to be filled for a steady state to become established. The content of L obviously depends on the particular geometry of the reservoirs and of the ducts alimenting turbine A, on the ratio of the diameters of the two reservoirs, on the height at which the overflow channel from S to L is placed (S_L), and on the dimensions of this conduit. These geometric properties are analogous to fixed or genetic traits, such as differences in the number of fat cells, or individual propensity toward converting sugar into lipid, or trends to metabolize at a relatively high or low respiratory quotient (RQ). The degree of filling of L is also influenced by circumstantial parameters that are akin to the influence of life-style variables on body weight. For instance, changes in the setting of S_1, which determines when replenishment is triggered, can be taken to reflect the leverage of food availability, whereas differences in S_2 can be seen as being related to food palatability and its influences on the degree of replenishment reached before further food intake is inhibited. As shown in FIGURE 4, the range within which the content of S is maintained (*i.e.* between S_1 and S_2) exerts a substantial effect on L_s, the steady state content of L, particularly when F is high. (The values of the parameters used in computing these curves as listed in TABLE 2).

Increasing the flow through A while flow through B is constant provides an analogy for increases in metabolic expenditure elicited by physical activity or cold exposure. The lines in FIGURE 5 show L_s as a function of F, when total output is $1 \times$, $1.5 \times$, $2 \times$, and $2.5 \times$ the basal rate. Another impact of physical activity (not included in computing the curves of FIG. 5) is that in a situation where meals occur at fixed intervals, increased energy expenditure can be expected to cause a more extensive glycogen depletion between meals, leading to increased lipid oxidation even in the resting state.[9] (The behavior of the model for a situation in which replenishment occurs at fixed intervals is shown in FIG. 12).

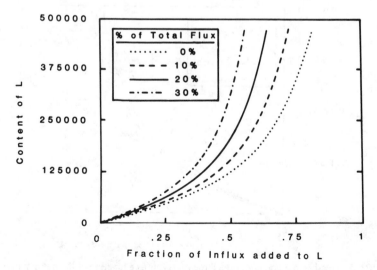

FIGURE 3. Steady state content in the large reservoir as a function of the fraction of water added to it: influence of flux through turbine B.

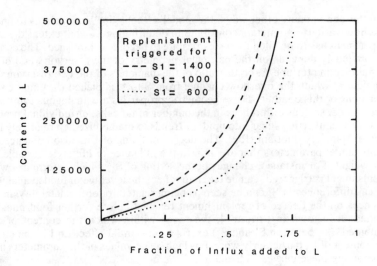

FIGURE 4. Steady state content of the large reservoir as a function of the fraction of water added to it: effect of change in the level (S_1) in the small reservoir that triggers replenishment. At the highest setting for S_1, the level in S is raised sufficiently to create some overflow from the small into the large reservoir when $F \le .2$, explaining why this curve does not approach zero when F is nil.

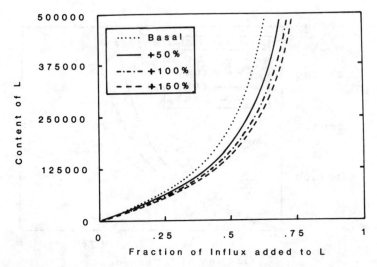

FIGURE 5. Steady state content of the large reservoir as a function of the fraction of water added to it: effect of changing the power output through turbine A while flux through turbine B is constant.

TABLE 2. Parameters Used in Computing Curves Shown in the Figures[a]

	S_1 (kcal)	F	M (kcal)	Total Flux (kcal/h)	Flux B (kcal/h)	Flux D (kcal/h)	Comments
FIGURE 3	1000	*[b]	720	60	0,6,12,18	0	‡[c]
FIGURE 4	600,1000,1400	*	1080	90	12	0	‡
FIGURE 5	1000	*	720,1080,1440,2160	60,90,120,180	12	0	‡
FIGURE 7	1400	.5	1080	90	12	0	Cycles 1–500
	1400	.25	1080	90	12	0	Cycles 501–2000
FIGURE 9	1400	.5	1080	90	12	0	Cycles 1–500
	600	.5	1080	90	12	0	Cycles 501–2000
FIGURE 10	1000	*	1080	90,99,108,117	12	0	Upper Panel, ‡
FIGURE 11	1000	*	1080	90,99,108,117	12	0,9,18,27	Lower Panel, ‡ with Regulatory feature, ‡
FIGURE 12	600,1000,1400	*	720,1080,1440,2160	60,90,120,180	12	0	with Regulatory feature and timed replenishments to restore S_2 to $1000 + 1080 \times (1 - F)$, ‡
	$S_1 = S_2 - M \times (1 - F)$						

[a] Other parameters: Cross-sectional surface of S = 40, L = 4000, S_L = 2240. Computations were based on Flux A = total Flux-Flux B-Flux D; flux from S through A = (content of S/40)/R, where R = (content of S/40 + content of L/4000)/Flux A; factor R is used to make total flux independent of changes in hydrostatic pressures.

[b] * = independent variable

[c] ‡ = cycles repeated until steady state is achieved.

It is evident from the preceding figures that the value of F appears to be of great significance in determining the steady state content of L. In the body, the contribution made by lipids to the fuel mix used for energy generation is influenced, among other factors, by changes in FFA availability.[10] FAA levels are regulated by insulin, whose concentration in the circulations is related to carbohydrate availability.[2] It is also known for the postabsorptive state that FAA levels are increased by expansion of the body's adipose tissue mass[11] and that this is accompanied by lower RQ values.[12] The model indicates that a marked decrease in the body's glycogen reserves must occur when the fat to carbohydrate ratio in the diet increases (cf. lower panels of FIG. 1), to avoid the necessity of a substantial expansion of adipose tissue, which would be needed to raise FFA levels until their average contribution to the oxidized fuel mixture becomes commensurate with the diet's fat content.

This corresponds to the situation where the average RQ is equal to the FQ^1, the FQ (food quotient) being defined as the ratio of CO_2 produced to O_2 consumed during the oxidation or a representative sample of the diet.[13] This suggests that the dietary fat content may be an important parameter in determining the degree of adiposity for which weight maintenance will tend to become established.

DISCUSSION

The curves shown in the various preceding figures indicate that the steady state content in L rises more and more steeply as F, the fraction of water falling into the large reservoir, becomes larger. This trend is enhanced by flow through turbine B (FIG. 3), but attenuated by increases in physical activity (FIG. 5). The ever more dramatic accretion of the adipose tissue mass that is suggested by these figures to be needed as fat displaces carbohydrate more and more completely in the diet is exaggerated, however, because the curves shown in these figures are generated for particular, fixed settings of S_1. In reality, glycogen levels are usually maintained in a lower range when the carbohydrate content of the diet decreases.[14] Furthermore, on diets nearly devoid of carbohydrate, the brain may obtain part of its energy from ketone bodies,[2] reducing the flow through B and hence L_s (FIG. 3).

In the model, the content of the large reservoir approaches zero as the amount of water falling into it dwindles. In animals, high carbohydrate diets containing little fat lead to higher glycogen reserves and to the induction of lipogenesis at rates sufficient to maintain, or even to accumulate reserves of body fat. This phenomenon is manifest in the model, as shown by the dashed line in the lower left corner of FIGURE 4, which does not approach zero with the highest S_1 setting for which transfer from S to L occurs. The domain of lowest F values, however, is not of great importance in discussing the regulation of body weight while mixed diets are consumed, as lipogenesis is then too limited to compensate for concomitant fat oxidation, as evident from the observations that the nonprotein RQ does not excede 1.0 even after ingesting 500 g of carbohydrate.[4,5] The curves generated by the model do, therefore, provide analogies most suitable for situations in which carbohydrate as well as fat make substantial contributions to the diet's energy content. Over the substantial range corresponding to mixed diets, the qualitative trends predicted by the model about the leverage of dietary fat on body fat content are consistent with data obtained in mice sacrificed after having been maintained *ad libitum* on synthetic diets, in which the fat to carbohydrate ratio differed while the protein content remained constant[15] (FIG. 6).

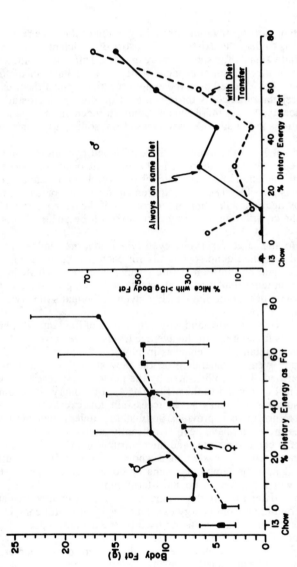

FIGURE 6. Effect of the diet's fat content on the body fat mass of *ad libitum* fed mice. Two month old males (N = 71) and female (N = 133) CD1 mice were maintained *ad libitum* for three to seven months on lab chow or on one of several synthetic diet's that contained 18% of the energy as protein, 1 to 75% as fat, and the balance as carbohydrate. The position of the points along the horizontal axis indicates the fat content of the diet consumed at the time of sacrifice. Circles and squares show the mean values for male and female mice, with vertical bars indicating one standard deviation. The incidence of obesity (>15 g of body fat) is shown for the male mice only. Closed circles are for the 71 male mice maintained constantly on the same diet, and open circles are for 100 male mice transferred for the last 2–3 months before sacrifice to high or low fat diets, after having previously been on low or high fat diets, respectively. (The effect of the diet's fat content is more readily reversible in female mice). (J. P. Flatt.[1] With permission from the *American Journal of Clinical Nutrition*.)

The usefulness of the hydraulic model is in demonstrating behaviors that are manifest in any system comprising two reservoirs of very different size that share a common outlet, as is the case for animals and humans, given their very different capacities for storing glycogen and fat.[2] The following statements illustrate this point.

1. It is evident that short-term variations in the content of the large reservoir are so minute as to defy the existence of sensors of sufficient accuracy to elicit appropriate signals for short-term responses. Difficulty in the conceptualization of mechanism(s) capable of detecting changes in the adipose tissue mass have indeed been the major objection against theories on body-weight regulation such as those centered on the "ponderostat" or set point concepts,[16-18] as these would require a mechanism capable of sensing deviations in the adipose tissue mass from some particular target value.

2. Even if based solely on the more readily envisioned responses based on sensing the relatively large short-term changes that occur in the small reservoir, achievement of a steady state where overall outflow and inflow are in balance is possible. The only requirement for such a mechanism to be able to provide for stabilization of the content of the large reservoir, as well, is that the contribution made by each reservoir be positively correlated with its content.

3. The content of the large reservoir, even when governed indirectly, is nevertheless determined quite specifically for each particular set of geometric (genetic) and circumstantial (life-style) parameters. This can account for the maintenance of a relatively stable body composition over the prolonged periods of time during which a given individual's life-style remains constant.

4. One can readily visualize how, and why, alterations of food intake habits, such as the diet's fat content, or the average levels between which glycogen stores are maintained, or changes in physical activity, can lead to changes in body weight, depending on the new steady state that must become established. This is illustrated by the model's response to a sudden decrease in F, from 0.5 to 0.25 (FIG. 7). As a corollary, it becomes evident why subjects, who may have successfully lost excess weight, are compelled to return to their previous body status, unless their life-style and/or their eating habits have been significantly altered.

5. The content of L being very large and the contribution made by S closely adjusted to its content, the system as a whole has a considerable buffer capacity (*i.e.* it absorbs temporary gains or deficits by changes in the content of L, which has almost no short-term impact). Thus, the system readily accommodates random deviations, such as those created by daily variations in food intake and energy expenditure, yet it is still compelled to reach the particular steady state imposed by the average values of the various parameters.

6. Given that replenishment occurs whenever the content of S is depleted, the steady state level maintained in the large reservoir is not dependent on total flux, but only on how changes in total flux may alter the relative contributions made by L and S (cf. FIGURES 3 and 5). Understanding the reasons for this behavior should be particularly useful because it helps to appreciate that steady states with different degrees of adiposity can be equally well-achieved among individuals with relatively low or relatively

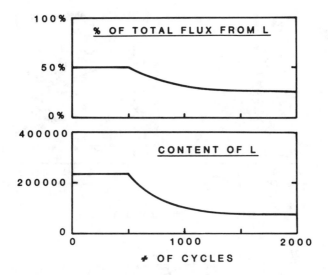

FIGURE 7. Response to a sudden change in F: the fraction of water added to the large reservoir. The time-course leading to the establishment of a new steady state is shown as a function of the number of emptying-refilling cycles that have occurred.

high rates of energy expenditure. This insight is important because of the prevailing expectation that low rates of energy expenditure are necessarily conducive to the development of obesity, whereas high rates of energy expenditure are believed to prevent excessive accumulation of body fat.

7. In view of the great discrepancies that have been observed between energy intake and energy expenditure,[19] the validity of the concept that food intake can be appropriately adjusted to energy expenditure has been questioned.[20] By combining measurements of nutrient intake and indirect calorimetric data, we have monitored the daily carbohydrate and fat balances in *ad libitum* fed mice over many consecutive 24-hour periods. Gains or losses of glycogen during a given day were statistically associated with compensatory decreases or increases in food intake during the following day (FIG. 8).[1,3] This corrective effect appeared to be sufficient to induce appropriate adjustments of the energy balance. Changes in food intake were also correlated negatively with deviations from the fat (or from the overall energy balance), but the slopes of the lines, which give a measure of the strength of possible feed-back effects, are much less steep, and days with positive or negative fat or energy balances were predictive of further gains or losses on the following day.[3] In the model, control of influx is linked to changes in the content of the small reservoir. Over brief periods, these may not be representative of alterations in the system's overall contents. If the regulation of food intake serves primarily to the preservation of the carbohydrate balance as suggested by the results described in FIGURE 8, it may also lead to adjustments of food intake that are not always consistent with expectations based on the notion that the goal of food intake regulation is the maintenance of the overall energy balance. One might speculate that metabolic feed-back effects in the control of food

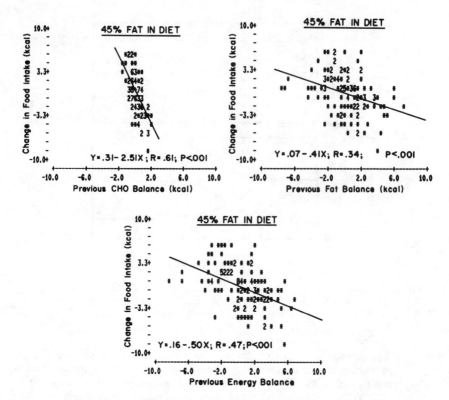

FIGURE 8. Changes in food intake in relation to the previous day's carbohydrate, fat, and energy balances in *ad libitum* fed mice. The data were obtained in five female CD1 mice whose food intake and respiratory exchange were individually determined during 28 consecutive 24-hour periods. Changes in food intake correspond to individual differences in energy intake observed on two consecutive days. (J. P. Flatt.[1] With permission from the *American Journal of Clinical Nutrition*.)

intake would be more readily apparent if one had the means to relate changes in food intake to changes in glycogen reserves, rather than to changes in the overall energy balance.

8. Weight-reducing drugs can induce weight loss initially, but their effect is usually not sustained.[21] If one considers that such drugs act by causing the energy balance to be negative, one has to conclude that they lose their effectiveness. Instead of considering that the organism becomes desensitized to their action, one can attribute this response to the fact that anorectic agents lower the body weight set point, as proposed by Stunkard.[21] In the model, this corresponds to a shift in the steady state level in L to a lower level. This could be mediated by an anorectic effect resulting in the maintenance of lower glycogen levels, (*d*-fenfluramine?) and/or to a lipolytic action (amphetamines?) capable of enhancing the oxidation of fat relative to that of glucose. FIGURE 9 shows the model's behavior when S_1 is suddenly changed to a lower setting. The figure illustrates that evolution

toward a new steady state is most rapid initially when the offset from the new steady state is greatest, and that adjustments become more gradual subsequently. This is quite similar to the observed effects of anorectic agents.[21] The limitation of their effectiveness is probably related to the fact that it is not a simple matter to appreciably alter steady state levels in a well-buffered system without causing undesirable side effects. Their action, however, may be sustained, rather than transient, and regain of the weight lost is thus to be expected when their intake is discontinued.[21]

9. There is perhaps no need to assume that obesity is due to a defect in the ability to adjust food intake to energy expenditure. Rather, one has to discover the reasons why obese subjects encounter the steady state of weight maintenance only when their adipose tissue mass has become much enlarged. Inherited differences can be mimicked in the model, for example, by changing the diameter of the large reservoir. This will greatly affect the hydrostatic pressure created by a certain volume of water in L, resulting in considerable shifts in the steady state content of the large reservoir, but without altering the nature of the basic responses involved in the control of inflow and outflow. The cause of obesity, be it inherited or induced by circumstances, would thus appear to be an insufficient rate of fatty acid oxidation relative to glucose oxidation when the adipose tissue mass is of a normal size. The notion that some alteration in the usual balance of the tone of the sympathetic, relative to the parasympathetic, nervous systems may be important in the etiology of obesity[22] could provide a concept corresponding rather well to changes in these geometric features of the model, with their powerful impact on steady state levels in the large reservoir.

10. There is considerable interest about the role that dietary-induced thermo-

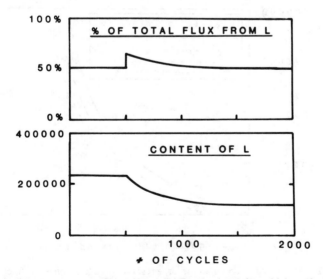

FIGURE 9. Response to a sudden change in S_1, the level for which replenishment is triggered. The time course leading to the establishment of a new steady state is shown as a function of the number of emptying-refilling cycles that have occurred.

genesis (DIT) may have in limiting the development of obesity.[23] In many animal models, ingestion of calories in excess of energy expenditure leads to an enlargement of BAT, where uncoupled oxidative phosphorylation permits the dissipation of some of the energy consumed in excess.[8,24] When this phenomenon fails to occur, animals tend more readily to become obese.[24] In humans, increases in energy expenditure by DIT appear to be much smaller than those induced by physical exertion.[23] In the model, small increments in the flux through A have only a very limited impact on the steady state level in L (FIG. 10, upper panel). Brown adipose tissue primarily oxidizes FFA,[8] rather than a mixture of glucose and

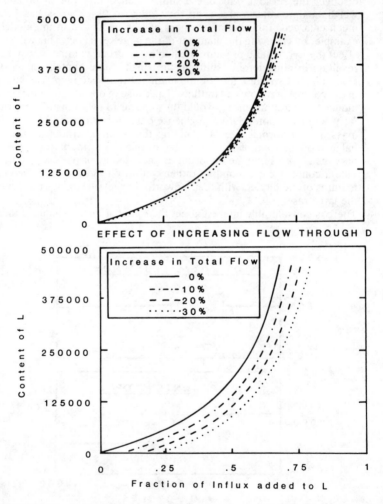

FIGURE 10. Steady state content of the large reservoir as a function of the fraction of water added to it. The upper panel shows the effect of small changes in the power output of turbine A; the lower panel describes the effect of equivalent changes in total power output caused by outflow through turbine D while flux through A is constant.

fat as does muscle. To take this into account in the model, a third turbine, D (DIT) has been included, driven exclusively by outflow from L (FIG. 2). As shown in the lower panel of FIGURE 10, equivalent increases in total flux have a much greater impact when they are brought about by initiation of flux through D, instead of merely by increased flux through A (upper panel). Thus, the role of increased oxidative activity in brown adipose tissue could be greater than one would anticipate from its minor effect on total energy expenditure. Whether BAT plays a significant role in humans remains to be established, however.[8]

11. The model suggests that the effects of minor differences in the operating conditions on the steady state levels in L become magnified when F increases, as illustrated by the widening separation of the curves calculated for different settings of S_1 (FIG. 4), or for situations in which flux through A is altered (FIG. 5). Furthermore, when F is high, deviations toward higher or lower average F values also tend to have a more considerable impact on L_s. A phenomenon of this type is apparent among *ad libitum* fed mice, as shown by increasingly wide standard deviations around the average body fat content when diets with higher fat contents are fed[15] (FIG. 6). The fact that small changes in some of the parameters should lead to increasingly large variations in L_s when F is high may help to explain why interindividual variability in the adipose tissue mass appears to be greatest among populations consuming mixed diets with a substantial fat content.[25] Greater variability can contribute to an increase in the number of individuals exceeding particular criteria for obesity, as it does in the case of mice (cf. right panel of FIG. 6).

12. Insulin resistance has been considered to be a factor favoring the development and maintenance of obesity, particularly because it may be associated with a reduction in diet-induced thermogenesis.[23,26,27] On the other hand, the induction of insulin resistance by enlargement of the adipose tissue mass[28] would be expected to reduce the oxidation of glucose relative to that of fatty acids,[12] thereby enhancing the feed-back leverage of the adipose tissue mass in promoting oxidation of fat relative to oxidation of glucose. Therefore, one should come to recognize that insulin resistance can also play a role in limiting, rather than only in promoting, further expansion of the adipose tissue mass.

The regulation of carbohydrate metabolism involves multiple control phenomena and powerful endocrine signals.[2] It seems reasonable to assume that these have biologically evolved to assure priority in metabolic regulation to the maintenance of stable glycogen levels, as required for glucose homeostasis. Changes in the relative rates of carbohydrate and fat oxidation are reflected in the RQ. In subjects consuming a western diet, the RQ generally varies between values slightly above .9 after food intake, to slightly above .8 after an overnight fast. This indicates that the ratio of fat to carbohydrate oxidation varies between 0.4 and 1.5. In the model, when F is .5, the ratio of outflow from L divided by outflow from S varies only from .8 to 1.2. This range is slightly expanded when the power demand from A is high and when replenishment occurs at fixed intervals. It is a simple matter to introduce some primitive regulatory features into the model in order to provoke greater variations in the relative contributions made by the two reservoirs during one outflow-refilling cycle, as is the case for the oxidation of fat relative to carbohydrate between meals. The impact of such a modification becomes apparent by comparing FIGURE 4 with FIGURE 11, and FIGURE 5 with

FIGURE 12. The curves in FIGURE 11 and 12 were obtained by exaggerating the effect of the hydrostatic pressure in S in computing the contributions made by the two reservoirs to the flow through A, to the extent that outflow from L varied between 0.6 and 1.6 of total flux. Under these conditions, one sees that the consequence of operating with relatively high or low levels in S becomes much greater in determining steady state level in the large reservoir (FIG. 11). Therefore, it is reasonable to expect that the availability and palatability of food, and individual responsiveness to them, through their influence on the range within which glycogen levels are maintained, should have a considerable impact in determining the size of the adipose tissue mass for which the RQ becomes equal to the FQ, as required for weight maintenance.[13] Because glycogen levels tend to be maintained at lower levels when the diet's carbohydrate content decreases,[14] one can also understand why the increase in the adipose tissue mass as a function of increasing dietary fat content (FIG. 6) is less steep than suggested by the curves that show L_s as a function of F for fixed values of S_1 (FIG. 4).

It is generally recognized that exercise effectively diminishes accumulation of body fat. In FIGURE 5 changes in the flux through turbine A, which are analogous to differences in physical activity, are seen to exert only a small effect on L_s. With the introduction of the regulatory feature discussed above, the distance between the curves obtained for different fluxes through A are expanded, particularly if one also takes into account the fact that meals are usually taken at fixed intervals (FIG. 12), with the small reservoir becoming more depleted at the end of a fixed time interval when flux through A is high. Thus the beneficial effects of exercise in the control of body weight can be attributed to the increase in fat oxidation that it induces during prolonged exertion, as well as during the resting periods following bouts of exercise.[9]

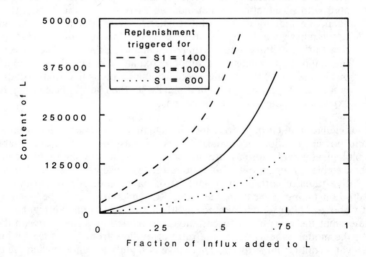

FIGURE 11. Steady state content in the large reservoir as a function of the fraction of water added to it. The effect of the hydrostatic pressure in the small reservoir on the contribution that it makes to the flux through turbine A has been amplified in order to create greater changes in the relative contributions made by the two reservoirs during one emptying-refilling cycle. The curves show the effect of changes in the setting for S_1, the level in the small reservoir for which replenishment is triggered.

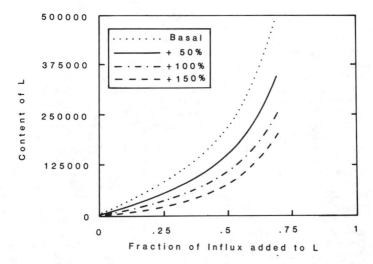

FIGURE 12. Steady state content in the large reservoir as a function of the fraction of water added to it. The effect of the hydrostatic pressure in the small reservoir on the contribution that it makes to the flux through turbine A has been amplified in order to create greater changes in the relative contributions made by the two reservoirs during one emptying-refilling cycle. Refilling occurred at fixed intervals with water additions sufficient to replenish the small reservoir to the same levels, regardless of the flow rate through A. The curves show the effect of changes in the rate of flow through turbine A on the steady state content of the large reservoir.

SUMMARY

The two-compartment model presented here suggests that weight maintenance can be achieved by a regulation of food intake geared primarily toward the maintenance of stable glycogen levels, rather than toward the preservation of the overall energy balance. This concept is reminiscent of the glucostatic theory of food intake regulation proposed by Mayer.[29] It is viewed here as being linked to changes in the body's carbohydrate stores, which represent an integration of carbohydrate and lipid fluxes, rather than to changes in blood glucose levels, whose substantial variations during the day are dependent on various circumstantial events. The model illustrates that the fat to carbohydrate ratio of the diet may have considerable potential influence on steady state body composition, even though carbohydrates and fats are both able to meet the body's energy substrate requirements. It appears that failure of appropriately reducing the range within which glycogen levels are maintained when the diet's fat content rises will require an expansion of the adipose tissue mass to raise FFA levels and fat oxidation to a rate commensurate with the proportion of fat in the diet. Maintenance of glycogen reserves below their level of saturation is made less likely by the high palatability and ubiquitous availability of foods in affluent societies. Thus, one can understand the high incidence of obesity among populations consuming mixed diets with a relatively high fat content, without having to attribute this to some defect(s) in the mechanism(s) controlling food intake.

REFERENCES

1. FLATT, J. P. 1987. Dietary fat, carbohydrate balance and weight maintenance; effects of exercise. Am. J. Clin. Nutr. **45:** 296–306.
2. CAHILL, JR., G. F. 1971. Starvation in man. Clin. Endocrinol. Metab. **5:** 397–415.
3. FLATT, J. P. 1985. Regulierung des Korpergewichtes. *In* Die Verwertung der Nahrungsenergie durch Mensch and Tier. C. Wenk, M. Kronauer, Y. Schutz & H. Bickel, Eds.: 167–181. Wissenschaftliche Verlagsgesellschaft. Stuttgart.
4. ACHESON, K. J., Y. SCHUTZ, T. BESSARD, E. RAVUSSIN, E. JEQUIER & J. P. FLATT. 1984. Nutritional influences on lipogenesis after a carbohydrate meal. Am. J. Physiol. **246:** E62–E70.
5. ACHESON, K. J., Y. SCHUTZ, T. BESSARD, J. P. FLATT & E. JEQUIER. 1987. Carbohydrate metabolism and lipogenesis in obesity. Am. J. Clin. Nutr. **45:** 78–85.
6. ELWYN, D. H., F. E. GUMP, H. N. MUNRO, M. ILES & J. M. KINNEY. 1979. Changes in nitrogen balance of depleted patients with increasing infusions of glucose. Am. J. Clin. Nutr. **32:** 1597–1611.
7. SCHUTZ, Y., K. J. ACHESON & E. JÉQUIER. 1985. Twenty-four-hour energy expenditure and thermogenesis: response to progressive carbohydrate overfeeding in man. Int. J. Obesity **9**(Suppl 2): 111–114.
8. JEAN HIMMS-HAGEN. 1985. Brown adipose tissue metabolism and thermogenesis. Annu. Rev. Nutr. **5:** 69–96.
9. BIELINSKI, R., Y. SCHUTZ & E. JÉQUIER. 1985. Energy metabolism during the post exercise recovery in man. Am. J. Clin. Nutr. **49:** 69–82.
10. RANDLE, P. J., P. B. GARLAND, E. A. NEWSHOLME & C. N. HALES. 1965. The glucose-fatty acid cycle in obesity and maturing onset diabetes mellitus. Ann. N.Y. Acad. Sci. **131:** 324–333.
11. BJORNTORP, P., H. BERGMAN, E. VARNAUSKAS & B. LINDHOLM. 1969. Lipid mobilization in relation to body composition. Metabolism **18:** 841–851.
12. GOLAY, A., J. P. FELBER, H. U. MEYER, B. CURCHOD, E. MAEDER & E. JÉQUIER. 1984. Study on lipid metabolism in obesity diabetes. Metabolism **33:** 111–116.
13. FLATT, J. P. 1978. The biochemistry of energy expenditure. *In* Recent Advances in Obesity Research. G. Bray Ed.: Vol. 2: 221–228. Newman. London.
14. HULTMAN, E. & L. H. NILSSON. 1975. Factors influencing carbohydrate metabolism in man. Nutr. Metab. **18**(Suppl 1): 45–64.
15. SALMON, D. M. W. & J. P. FLATT. 1986. Effect of dietary fat content on the incidence of obesity among *ad libitum* fed mice. Int. J. Obesity **9:** 443–449.
16. KENNEDY, G. C. 1953. The role of depot fat in the hypothalamic control of food intake in the rat. Proc. R. Soc. London **140:** 578–592.
17. CABANAC, M., R. DUCLAUX & N. H. SPECTOR. 1971. Sensory feedback in regulation of body weight: Is there a ponderstat? Nature (London) **229:** 125–127.
18. KEESEY, R. E. & S. W. CORBETT. 1984. Metabolic defense of the body weight set-point. *In* Eating and its disorders. A. J. Stunkard & E. Stellar, Eds.: 87–96. Raven Press. New York.
19. EDHOLM, O. G., J. G. FLETCHER, E. M. WIDDOWSON & R. A. MCCANE. 1955. The energy expenditure and food intake of individual man. Br. J. Nutr. **9:** 286–300.
20. GARROW, J. S. 1978. Energy Balance and Obesity in Man. 2nd ed. North Holland/Elsevier. New York.
21. STUNKARD, J. 1982. Anorectic agents lower a body weight set point. Life Sci. **30:** 2043–2055.
22. JEANRENAUD, B., S. HALIMI & G. VAN DE VERDE. 1985. Neuroendocrine disorders seen as triggers of the triad: obesity-insulin resistance abnormal glucose tolerance. 1985. *In* Diabetes Metabolism Reviews. R. A. DeFronzo, Ed. Vol. 1: 261–291. John Wiley and Sons, Inc. New York.
23. JÉQUIER, E. & Y. SCHUTZ. Does a defect in energy metabolism contribute to human obesity? 1983. *In* Recent Adv. Obesity Res. J. Hirsch & T. B. Van Itallie, Eds. **4:** 76–94. John Libbey and Company. London.
24. ROTHWELL, N. J. & M. J. STOCK. 1981. Regulation of energy balance. Annu. Rev. Nutr. **1:** 235–256.

25. BRAY, G. A. 1984. Integration of energy intake and expenditure in animals and man: The autonomic and adrenal hypothesis. Clin. Endocrinol. Metab. **13:** 521–546.
26. FELIG, P. 1984. Insulin is the mediator of feeding-related thermogenesis: insulin resistance and/or deficiency results in a thermogenic defect which contributes to the pathogenesis of obesity. Clin. Physiol. **4:** 267–273.
27. RAVUSSIN, E., K. J. ACHESON, O. VERNET, E. DANSFORTH & E. JÉQUIER. 1985. Evidence that insulin resistance is responsible for the decreased thermic effect of glucose in human obesity. J. Clin. Invest. **76:** 1268–1273.
28. FLATT, J. P. 1972. The role of the increased adipose tissue mass in the apparent insulin insensitivity of obesity. Am. J. Clin. Nutr. **25:** 1189–1192.
29. MAYER, J. 1955. Regulation of energy intake and body weight: The glucostatic theory and lipostatic hypothesis. Ann. N.Y. Acad. Sci. **63:** 15–43.

Alterations in Nutrient Intake and Utilization Caused by Disease

ROBERT A. HOERR AND VERNON R. YOUNG

*Department of Applied Biological Sciences
and the Clinical Research Center
Massachusetts Institute of Technology
Cambridge, Massachusetts 02139*

INTRODUCTION

In this conference on human obesity, a focus of discussion is the disordered control of energy intake and expenditure that results in a clinically significant gain in body fat. Here the emphasis will be briefly on the effects of major systemic illness, where the disorders of energy intake and nutrient utilization often result in profound weight loss. In fact, the consequences of serious illness, including decreased appetite, lowered food intake, and possibly increased energy expenditure are synonymous with the goals for obesity therapy.

There is extensive literature concerning the effects of disease on nutrient utilization, but the relationships between altered nutrient metabolism and the intake of food and nutrients are less well understood. For purposes of discussion, however, we will focus on two classes of disease; neoplasia, and injury together with sepsis. These conditions result in decreased food intake and major weight loss, often leading to cachexia. They are associated with qualitative and quantitative changes in energy substrate utilization (*e.g.* references 1–3). Specific examples will be used to illustrate a number of significant metabolic features that should be considered in reference to food intake regulation, because an exhaustive review of the subject is beyond our charge. Hence, a number of comprehensive reviews are provided in the references in order to give the reader an opportunity to gain relatively easy access to the more detailed literature (*e.g.* reference 4). Finally, it is hoped that by giving some attention to the consequences of systemic disease on food intake and nutrient utilization, the mechanisms of food intake regulation might be better understood and, in consequence, a more rational and effective approach to weight control in humans under various conditions might be achieved.

CANCER

There are a number of reported cases where a tumor has been found to produce weight gain or weight loss due to a direct invasion of the appetite controlling centers of the hypothalamus, but these conditions are rare.[5,6] Although weight loss is a cardinal presenting symptom of occult malignancy, many patients, both children and adults, do not necessarily exhibit weight loss at the time of diagnosis.[7,8] Nevertheless, if the tumor is not resected or does not respond to therapy, weight loss seems to be the rule. Hence, for purposes of discussion, we will attempt to focus on those possible mechanisms by which the malignancy causes weight loss.

One obvious problem resulting in a decreased food intake is when the tumor causes mechanical obstruction of the gastrointestinal tract, and this can occur at any level from the oropharynx to the terminal colon. Therapy is directed at relieving the obstruction, either surgically by resection or bypass or through irradiation and/or chemotherapy. In most patients, however, weight loss is not related to the size or location of the tumor burden, which rarely exceeds 5 percent of body weight in humans.[9] This may not be the case in rodent experimental models, where the tumor can comprise as much as half of total body weight.[10] Thus, several questions might be raised, the first of which is whether cancer patients eat less as a consequence of their disease?

The answer is usually yes, although the results of intake surveys in published studies vary widely. For example, in a study of 195 patients with various cancer diagnoses and 205 normal, age-matched controls, male patients consumed fewer calories than healthy controls, whereas female patients maintained their consumption at levels approximating their controls.[11] In a subset of male patients with lung cancer, however, those who had lost weight did not appear to eat less than those who had maintained their weight. These groups both consumed energy at about 110 percent of their calculated basal energy expenditure, as contrasted to 140 percent for the healthy controls.[11] Inasmuch as both lung cancer patient groups consumed fewer calories than control subjects, clearly the patients who did not lose weight adapted to the lower intake differently than those who experienced a loss of weight. This type of observation raises the second question: Why do some patients with cancer eat less?

The anorexia associated with malignancy can be profound, as any family member, nurse, or physician caring for these patients can attest. Appetite is a complex process that depends heavily on the sensory qualities of food. In fact, among the symptoms most frequently reported by cancer patients in one series were altered taste, altered smell, and early satiety.[12] These were reported far more often than nausea, for example. Smell aversions to food odors from meat, fowl, or chocolate[13] and also alterations in the perception and threshold of certain tastes[14] seem to be present when tested for directly. To date, however, it has not been possible to offer precise mechanisms linking these sensory changes with the metabolism of the tumor; in fact, one study suggests that the changes in taste can be entirely accounted for on the basis of age, sex, smoking history, and other related variables.[15] There have also been demonstrations that specific food aversions can be conditioned, in both animals and humans, when foods are paired with noxious therapy of irradiation or chemotherapy.[16,17] It seems, therefore, that although there may be changes in the taste and smell of food, these changes are only likely to account for a portion of the decrease in food intake.

An attractive hypothesis, relevant to the symposium discussion of obesity, is that the neoplasm produces anorexia indirectly by affecting the appetite centers in the hypothalamus, particularly the serotonergic system. Unfortunately, there are virtually no human data to support this hypothesis, other than a report of increased plasma free tryptophan levels in cancer patients.[18] We are unaware of studies in which plasma amino acid profiles have been followed in cancer patients after test meals, such as have been conducted for normal and obese patients.

A number of rat studies with the Walker 256 carcinoma, a commonly used tumor-anorexia model, suggest that the mechanism of anorexia is different from that due to centrally acting anorectic agents known to affect the appetite centers. In normal rats, the anorectic effect of d-amphetamine depends on an intact central catecholaminergic system, and that of fenfluramine depends on an intact central serotonergic system. Blockade of the noradrenergic system by way of ventral noradrenergic bundle lesions inhibits the anorexia induced by d-amphetamine, whereas the blockade of the serotonergic system by way of methergoline (a serotonin antagonist) inhibits the anorexia induced by fenfluramine. Neither of these pharmacologic treatments, however, had an effect on the anorexia of the Walker 256 tumor-transplanted rats,[19] though in other studies, the decrease in food intake after transplantation was found to correlate with increased brain tryptophan and serotonin.[20,21] These inconsistencies may reflect differences in the stage and intensity of the disease when the measurements were made.

Other agents that have increased food intake in animal models, such as oxazepam, aminoguanidine, methergoline, and amitriptyline, did not increase food intake in tumor-bearing rats,[19,21] although cyproheptadine, another serotonin antagonist, did result in a modest increase in food intake. Even if the central serotonergic system plays a role in the anorexia of cancer, there is insufficient evidence to suggest that serotonin synthesis is regulated by precursor control, under these specific pathological conditions. Nevertheless, this system is certainly subject to control by other neural and hormonal mediators.

An interesting footnote to these animal studies is that the Walker 256 tumor is sensitive to cyclophosphamide. If the animal is treated with this agent, food intake declines acutely, but returns toward normal levels if the animal's tumor responds. This leads to the discussion of another proposed mechanism for the anorexia.

In 1976, Theologides[22] predicted that the anorexia and weight loss of cancer would one day prove to be caused by factors released by the tumor itself. Since this prediction, it has been shown that tumor cells in culture release polypeptide growth factors into their conditioned medium. These same cells often have functional receptors for the secreted factors. In short, the tumor cell can produce a factor(s) that is released and subsequently promotes its own growth. For this reason, these factors have been termed "autocrine" growth factors.[23]

One such factor has been found in human lung carcinoid and in human small-cell (oat cell) carcinoma.[24] It is similar to a 27 amino acid peptide isolated in pig intestine and termed gastrin-releasing peptide (GRP), which is thought to be the mammalian analogue of bombesin. Bombesin is a tetradecapeptide, originally identified in amphibian skin, which causes the atropine-resistant release of gastrin and cholecystokinin (CCK). When used in animal experiments, it produces a dose-dependent suppression of meal size in normal weight and hypothalamically obese animals.[25] GRP also decreases meal size in rats.[26] Peripherally administered bombesin appears to have a direct central effect in contrast to CCK and glucagon, which depend on vagal afferent fibers to exert their central effects.[27] It can elicit brain site-dependent analgesia, hypothermia, and hyperglycemia through as yet undetermined mechanisms. It also constricts bronchiolar smooth muscle.

This area of investigation offers considerable promise for further unraveling the causal consequences of tumorigenesis on food intake and nutritional status. It seems likely that many tumors might express portions of the genome that are normally repressed and that the peptide fragments might be homologous with normally synthesized peptide hormones. Although the contribution by peptide mediators to appetite regulation in normal humans is not clear, it is interesting to speculate that levels of mediators produced by tumors may not be subject to normal control. They may be produced in specific locations and quantities where they may be active, so bringing about the altered food intake characteristic of patients with cancers at various organ sites.

A final question we would like to consider is, Does metabolic rate increase in cancer?

Weight loss could occur in cancer by increasing metabolic expenditure without a compensatory increase in energy intake. Abnormalities of both high and low resting energy expenditures have been reported in cancer patients.[28–30] The metabolic abnormality responsible in those cases where resting energy expenditure is truly elevated has not been elucidated. A number of alterations in energy substrate and metabolism do occur, however, including, for example, elevation of plasma glucose levels and an abnormal response to the oral glucose tolerance test, suggesting insulin resistance.[31,32] From tracer studies, it appears that there is increased gluconeogenesis and increased recycling of 3 carbon subunits to glucose.[33] This implies elevated rates of lactate production, which may become excessive as in cases of lactic acidosis in acute leukemia.[34] Glucose uptake by peripheral tissues is decreased, and muscle biopsy studies have shown reduced enzyme activities of the key enzymes regulating glycogen turnover, glycogenolysis, and oxidative metabolism.[35] In this context, insulin can be shown to stimulate protein synthesis in muscle tissue, but there is a failure to stimulate glycogen synthesis.[36] This suggests that the defect producing the insulin resistance occurs by way of a postreceptor mechanism.

The increased recycling of lactate to glucose is presumed due to tumor glycolysis. Weber[37,38] has reviewed a large body of literature and suggests that tumor cells have a decrease in the activities of the key gluconeogenic enzymes and an increase in the activities of the opposing glycolytic ones. There also seems to be an increase in the ability of tumor cells to transport glucose. Thus, tumors may have a selective advantage over normal host tissues with respect to the utilization of glucose.

The cancer-related changes in energy substrate metabolism are difficult to dissect from the contributing effects of malnutrition and therapeutic intervention. They do resemble, however, many of the metabolic changes that occur in infection and injury, as will be discussed below.

INFECTION AND INJURY

The anorexia of infection or major trauma may also be dependent on a mediator substance rather than on changes in energy substrate metabolism and status, per se. In contrast to the anorexia of cancer, the anorexia of infection may in some cases prove beneficial to the host. A degree of malnutrition may, in certain instances, actually confer some protective effect on the host by depleting certain key nutrients needed for multiplication of the infecting organism.[39]

A number of the physiological responses to acute infection, including anorexia, appear to be mediated by a specific protein produced by the reticuloendoethelial system, interleukin-1 (IL-1). IL-1 is a 17 kDa protein that is produced experimentally by injecting endotoxin or exposing monocytes to endotoxin in culture.[40] When administered directly, it produces many of the acute-phase responses to infection including fever, granulocytosis, hypoferremia and hypozincemia, skeletal muscle catabolism, and increased plasma levels of acute phase proteins like C-reactive protein, haptoglobin and fibrinogen, and of hormones like insulin and glucagon.[35] This monokine is primarily derived from phagocytic cells. It is secreted into the bloodstream and can have effects on distant organs, thus qualifying as a hormone. Blood monocytes, phagocytic lining cells of liver and spleen, macrophages of other tissues, keratinocytes, gingival and corneal epitheal cells, renal mesangial cells and brain astrocytes also produce IL-1–like molecules.[40] IL-1 produced by these localized cell types may exert its activity primarily in these tissues, and thus the levels of IL-1 in plasma might not be an adequate index of the exposure of target tissues to this protein mediator.

When IL-1, either human monocyte-drived or mouse recombinant IL-1, is administered to rats, they develop fever and short-term decrease in food intake.[41] Fever is thought to result from a direct effect of IL-1 on the anterior hypothalamus, acting by way of an abrupt increase in the synthesis of prostaglandins (prostaglandin E_2).[40] Although it has not yet been conclusively demonstrated, the anorexia of infection and other chronic inflammatory diseases in humans, as well as their associated systemic aberrations of metabolism, may well be due to the effects of this monokine.

Infection and injury are associated with a number of common metabolic responses. These include increases in the turnover and oxidation of fat and carbohydrate,[43] enhanced hepatic glucose production,[42] and augmentation in elevations in plasma insulin.[44]

In addition, a major fate of the glucose taken up appears to be due to increased glycogenesis and fat synthesis rather than direct oxidation.[45] Fat is the major oxidative fuel, and there are increases in the turnover of both glycerol and free fatty acids.[43] Among the amino acids, phenylalanine concentration in plasma almost invariably elevated, and concentrations of the branched-chain amino acids also may be elevated with reduced levels of gluconeogenic amino acids.[46] Paradoxically, these changes would actually lead one to predict an increase, rather than a decrease, in food intake.

The counter-regulatory hormones, epinephrine and glucagon, are necessary in combination to increase hepatic glucose production rates to levels seen in major infection or injury, but even these in combination sustain general change in energy substrate flux only transiently. If cortisol is added to the hormonal infusion mixture, the increased glucose production rates can be sustained.[47] The relationship, however, between the altered state of energy substrate metabolism and hormonal balance following injury and sepsis remains to be determined.

In the last year, evidence has emerged suggesting that both cancer and infection may stimulate the production of a common host-defense mediator by the reticuloendothelial system, which is different from IL-1. Cachectin is a 17 kDa protein released by macrophages when treated with endotoxin in culture.[48] When cultured adipocytes are treated with the supernatant factor, biosynthesis of acetyl-CoA carboxylase and of fatty acid synthetase is inhibited, whereas the activity of lipoprotein lipase is rapidly reduced[49] due possibly to an inhibition of the synthesis or intracellular processing of the enzyme.[49] Thus, after exposure to the factor, the adipocyte could no longer synthesize fatty acids by the *de novo* pathway or obtain them from the extracellular millieu.

In addition to cachectin, a tumor necrosis factor (TNF) is released by macrophages in response not only to endotoxin but also to tumor cells. It exhibits tumoricidal activity that can be blocked by specific antisera.[50] This protein mediator also has a molecular mass of 17 kDa. Recently, marked homology between cachectin and human tumor necrosis factor was reported,[51] suggesting that TNF and cachectin may be the same protein or under the same transcriptional control. Furthermore, a recent *Lancet* editorial[48] speculated that in cancer patients, the reticuloendothelial cell system might synthesize the factor(s) in response to tumor invasion, even if the tumor was resistant to its action. Chronic, inappropriate synthesis of cachectin/tumor necrosis factor would then lead to cachexia, but the metabolic basis for the weight loss remains to be determined in humans.

CONCLUSION

Both cancer and infection produce weight loss in humans, the effects of which produce major morbidity and mortality. Two processes appear responsible for the weight loss: anorexia with decreased food intake, and altered energy substrate metabolism that uses fat and amino acids preferentially over glucose. New developments suggest that both of these processes could be mediated by peptide or protein factors long hypothesized but not previously known. Tumors produce peptide molecules similar to gut hormones that modulate satiety. Infecting organisms and tumors both trigger the immune system to produce protein molecules that have multisystem effects throughout the body, including anorexia and some of the metabolic alterations that are characteristic of weight-losing patients with either cancer or infection. A better understanding of how these mediators lead to anorexia and weight loss in human disease may ultimately lead to improved understanding of how energy intake and utilization are regulated in normal and obese individuals, and also to new therapeutic alternatives.

REFERENCES

1. GIL, K. M., R. A. FORSE, J. ASKANAZI, C. WEISSMAN & J. M. KINNEY. 1985. Energy metabolism in stress. *In* Substrate and Energy Metabolism. J. S. Garrow & D. Halliday, Eds.: 203–211. J. Libbey. London.
2. LITTLE, R. A. 1985. Heat production after injury. Br. Med. Bull. **41:** 226–231.
3. FRAYR, K. N. 1985. Substrate turnover after injury. Br. Med. Bull. **41:** 232–239.
4. VAN EYS, J. 1985. Nutrition and cancer: physiological relationships. Ann. Rev. Nutr. **5:** 435–61.
5. BRAY, G. A. & T. F. GALLAGHER JR. 1975. Manifestations of hypothalamic obesity in man. Medicine (Baltimore) **54:** 301–330.
6. KAZAN, H. 1958. Anorexia and severe inanition associated with a tumor involving the hypothalamus. Arch. Dis. Child. **33:** 257–260.
7. VAN EYS, J. 1979. Malnutrition in children with cancer: incidence and consequence. Cancer (Philadelphia) **43:** 2030–2035.
8. DEWYS, W. D. *et al.* (Eastern Cooperative Oncology Group). 1980. Prognostic effect of weight loss prior to chemotherapy in cancer patient. Am. J. Med. **69:** 491–497.
9. COSTA, G. 1977. Cachexia, the metabolic component of neoplastic disease. Cancer Res. **37:** 2327–2335.
10. WATERHOUSE, C. 1963. Nutritional disorders in neoplastic disease. J. Chronic Dis. **16:** 637–644.
11. COSTA, G., P. BEWLEY, M. ARAGON & J. SIEBOLD. 1981. Anorexia and weight loss in cancer patients. Cancer Treat. Rep. **65** (suppl. 5): 3–7.
12. DEWYS, W. D., G. COSTA & R. HENKIN. 1981. Clinical parameters related to anorexia. Cancer Treat. Rep. **65** (suppl. 5): 49–52.
13. VICKERS, Z. M., S. S. NIELSEN & A. THEOLOGIDES. 1981. Odor aversions in cancer patients. Minn. Med. **64:** 227–279.
14. DEWYS, W. D. & K. WALTERS. 1975. Abnormalities of taste sensation in patients with cancer. Cancer (Philadelphia) **36:** 1888–1896.
15. HEBER, D., L. O. BYERLY & R. T. CHLEBOWSKI. 1985. Metabolic abnormalities in the cancer patient. Cancer (Philadelphia) **55:** 225–229.
16. BERNSTEIN, I. L. 1985. Learned food aversions in the progression of cancer and its treatment. Ann. N.Y. Acad. Sci. **443:** 365–380.
17. SMITH, J. D. & J. T. BLUMSACK. 1981. Learned taste aversion as a factor in cancer therapy. Cancer Treat. Rep. **65** (suppl. 5): 37–47.
18. KRAUSE, R., C. HUMPHREY, M. VON MEYENFELDT, H. JAMES & J. E. FISCHER. 1981. A central mechanism for anorexia in cancer: a hypothesis. Cancer Treat. Rep. **65:**(suppl. 5): 15–21.

19. GARATTINI, S. & A. GUAITANI. 1981. Animal models for the study of cancer-induced anorexia. Cancer Treat. Rep. **65** (suppl. 5): 23–25.
20. NICHOLS, M., R. P. MAICKEL & G. K. YIM. 1983. Increased central serotonergic activity associated with nocturnal anorexia induced by Walker 256 carcinoma. Life Sci. **32:** 1819–1825.
21. VON MEYENFELDT, M., W. T. CHANCE & J. E. FISCHER. 1982. Correlation of changes in brain indoleamine metabolism with onset of anorexia in rats. Am. J. Surgery. **143:** 133–138.
22. THEOLOGIDES, A. 1976. Anorexia-producing intermediary metabolites. Am. J. Clin. Nutr. **29:** 552–558.
23. SPORN, M. B. & A. B. ROBERT. 1985. Autocrine growth factors and cancer. Nature (London) **313:** 745–747.
24. BOSTWICK, D. G., K. A. ROTH, C. J. EVANS, J. D. BARCHAS & K. G. BENSCH. 1984. Gastrin-releasing peptide, a mammalian analog of bombesin, is present in human neoroendrocrine lung tumors. Am. J. Patho. **117:** 195–200.
25. SMITH, G. P., C. JAMES & J. GIBBS. 1981. Abdominal vagotomy does not block the satiety effect of bombesin in the rat. Peptides (Fatetteville) **2:** 409–411.
26. STEIN, L. J. & S. C. WOODS. 1982. Gastrin releasing peptide reduces meal size in rats. Peptides (Fatetteville) **3:** 833–835.
27. MORLEY, J. E., A. S. LEVINE, B. A. GOSNELL & C. J. BILLINGTON. 1984. Neuropeptides and appetite: contribution of neuropharmacological modeling. Fed. Proc. Fed. Am. Soc. Exp. Biol. **43:** 2903–2907.
28. KNOX, L. S., L. O. CROSBY, I. D. FEURER, G. P. BUZBY, C. L. MILLER et al. 1983. Ann. Surg. **197:** 152–162.
29. WARNOLD, I., K. LUNDHOLM & T. SCHERSTEN. 1978. Energy balance and body composition in cancer patients. Cancer Res. **38:** 1801–1807.
30. YOUNG, V. R. 1977. Energy metabolism and requirements in the cancer patient. Cancer Res. **38:** 2336–2347.
31. MARKS, P. A. & J. BISHOP. 1957. The glucose metabolism of patients with malignant disease and of normal subjects as studied by means of an intravenous glucose tolerance test. J. Clin. Invest. **36:** 254–264.
32. LUNDHOLM, K., A.-C. BYLUND & T. SCHERSTEN. 1977. Glucose tolerance in relation to skeletal muscle enzyme activities in cancer patients. Scand. J. Clin. Lab. Invest. **37:** 267–272.
33. WATERHOUSE, C., N. JEANPRETRE & J. KEILSON. 1979. Gluconeogenesis from alanine in patients with progressive malignant disease. Cancer Res. **39:** 1968–1972.
34. WATERHOUSE, C. 1974. Lactate metabolism in patients with cancer. Cancer (Brussels) **33:** 66–71.
35. LUNDHOLM, K., S. EDSTROM, L. EKMAN et al. 1978. A comparative study of the influence of malignant tumor on host metabolism in mice and man. Cancer (Brussels) **42:** 453–461.
36. LUNDHOLM, K., S. EDSTROM, L. EKMAN, I. KARLBERG & T. SCHERSTEN. 1981. Metabolism in peripheral tissues in cancer patients. Cancer Treat. Rep. **65** (suppl. 5): 79–83.
37. WEBER, G. 1977. Enzymology of cancer cells (first of two parts). N. Eng. J. Med. **296:** 486–493.
38. WEBER, G. 1977. Enzymology of cancer cells (second of two parts). N. Eng. J. Med. **296:** 541–551.
39. MURRAY, M. J. & A. B. MURRAY. 1979. Anorexia of infection as a mechanism of host defense. Am. J. Clin. Nutr. **32:** 593–596.
40. DINARELLO, C. A. 1984. Interleukin-1 and the pathogenesis of the acute-phase response. N. Engl. J. Med. **311:** 1413–1418.
41. MCCARTHY, D. O., M. J. KLUGER & A. J. VANDER. 1985. Suppression of food intake during infection: is interluekin-1 involved? Am. J. Clin. Nutr. **42:** 1179–1182.
42. WOLFE, R. R. 1985. Glucose metabolism in burn injury. J. Burn Care Rehabil. **6:** 408–418.
43. SHAW, J. H. F., S. KLEIN & R. R. WOLFE. Assessment of alanine, urea and glucose

interrelationships in normal subjects and in patients with sepsis with stable isotope tracers. Surgery 97: 557–567.

44. WOLFE, R. R., M. J. DURKOT, J. R. ALLSOP et al. 1979. Glucose metabolism in severely burned patients. Metab. Clin. Exp. 28: 1031–1039.

45. WOLFE, R. R., T. F. O'DONNELL, M. D. STONE, D. A. RICHMOND & J. F. BURKE. 1980. Investigation of factors determining the optimal glucose infusion rate in total parenteral nutrition. Metab. Clin. Exp. 29: 892–900.

46. LUND P. & D. H. WILLIAMSON. 1985. Inter-tissue nitrogen fluxes. Br. Med. Bull. 41: 251–256.

47. GELFAND, R. A., R. A. DEFRONZO & R. GUSBERG. 1983. Metabolic alterations associated with major injury and infection. In New Aspects of Clinical Nutrition. G. Kleinberger & E. Dentach, Eds.: 211–239. Karger. Basel.

48. Editorial. 1985. Cachectin. Lancet 2: 312–313.

49. PEKALA, P. H., S. R. PRICE, C. A. HORN, B. E. HOM, J. MOSS & A. CERAMI. 1984. Model for cachexia in chronic disease: secretory products of endotoxin-stimulated macrophages induce a catabolic state in 3T3-L1 adipocytes. Trans. Assoc. Am. Physicians 97: 251–259.

50. MATTHEWS, N. 1983. Effect on human monocyte killing of tumour cells of antibody raised against an extracellular monocyte cytotoxin. Immunology 48: 321–327.

51. BEUTLER, B., D. GREENWALD, J. D. HOLMES, M. CHANG, U.-C. E. PAN, J. MATHISON, R. ULEVITCH & A. CERAMI. 1985. Identity of tumor necrosis factor and the macrophage-secreted factor cachectin. Nature (London) 316: 552.

The Effect of Gut Peptides on Hunger, Satiety, and Food Intake in Humans[a]

GERARD P. SMITH AND JAMES GIBBS

Department of Psychiatry
Cornell University Medical College
and
the Eating Disorders Institute
New York Hospital-Cornell Medical Center
Westchester Division
White Plains, New York 10605

A number of peptides synthesized and secreted by gastrointestinal cells have been shown to possess significant effects on food intake and on perceptions of hunger and satiety in humans. In this paper, we review the available literature on these effects and emphasize the current obstacles for the therapeutic application of peptides to the problem of obesity.

STIMULATION OF FOOD INTAKE

Insulin is the only gut peptide known to stimulate hunger and to increase food intake. Barbour[1] was the first to report this effect of insulin in his study of malnourished children. Barbour observed large effects. For example, one child who was given small doses of insulin 20 minutes prior to a meal, three times a day, complained of hunger until the child was eating 3000 calories a day. This child was described as having a ravenous appetite. This observation stimulated a number of studies in the subsequent decade.

Appel et al.[2] observed increased appetite and food intake in undernourished psychotic adults treated with insulin. In a study of seven malnourished adult patients, Short[3] noticed increased appetite in all and an increase in body weight in five. Short also noted the important fact that there is a delay of about 30 minutes between the administration of insulin and the report of increased appetite.

The best evidence that insulin increases hunger was obtained by Silverstone and Besser in 1971.[4] They administered insulin intravenously to 15 men and 15 women after an overnight fast. Using a visual analog scale for hunger, subjects reported increased hunger about 30 minutes after insulin administration. This increase in hunger remained elevated for about 90 minutes. Thus, they confirmed with modern techniques the delay between the onset of hunger and the decrease in blood sugar produced by insulin.

The mechanism appears to be glucoprivation, that is, decreased glucose utilization. The evidence for this is that the administration of the glucose analogue, 2-deoxyglucose (2-DG), which produces glucoprivation without hypoglycemia, also stimulated hunger and increased food intake.[5] The effect the glucoprivation pro-

[a] This research was supported by Research Scientist Award MH-00149 and Research Grant Awards MH-40010 and MH-15455 (G. P. Smith) and Research Scientist Development Award MH-70874 and Research Grant Award AM-33248 (J. Gibbs).

132

duced by insulin and 2-DG appears to be independent of the autonomic nervous system because vagotomy does not block the effect of insulin on hunger in humans,[6] and vagotomy or high cervical cord section that disconnects the peripheral sympathetic nervous system from the brain does not block the stimulation of hunger and food intake by 2-DG.[5]

Thus, insulin increases hunger and increases food intake in humans within a short time after injection. These reliable effects appear to be obtained with doses of insulin that are pharmacological because they produce the metabolic emergency of hypoglycemia. There is no evidence at this time to implicate insulin in the psychobiological process that underlies the awareness of hunger and the initiation of eating under normal circumstances.

TABLE 1. Inhibition of Food Intake by Gut Peptides in Humans[a]

Experiment	Number	Treatment	Intake
Schulman et al.[9]	10	glucagon 1 mg, i.m.[b]	decreased
Penick and Hinkle[7]	10	glucagon 1 mg, i.m.	decreased
Penick and Hinkle[8]	4	glucagon 1 mg, i.m.	decreased
Clayton and Librik[10]	1	glucagon 2 mg, i.m.	decreased
Sturdevant and Goetz[16]	10	CCK (20% pure), i.v.[c]	
		23 ng kg^{-1}	decreased (12%)
		2.3 ng kg^{-1} min^{-1}	increased (22%)
Greenway and Bray[17]	14	CCK-8, i.v. and s.c.[d]	
		20–80 ng kg^{-1}	no change
Kissileff et al.[12]	12	CCK-8, i.v.	
		4 ng kg^{-1} min^{-1}	decreased (18%)
Pi-Sunyer et al.[18]	8	CCK-8, i.v.	
		4 ng kg^{-1} min^{-1}	decreased (13%)
Stacher et al.[11]	16	CCK-8, i.v.	
		4.6 ng kg^{-1} min^{-1}	decreased (17%)
		9.2 ng kg^{-1} min^{-1}	decreased (50%)
Shaw et al.[13]	11	CCK-8	
		2 mcg bolus	decreased (12%)
		+5 mcg infusion	
Murrahainen et al.[15]	8	Bombesin, i.v.	
		4 ng kg^{-1} min^{-1}	decreased (16%)

[a] The dose of 20% CCK used by Sturdevant and Goetz has been converted to the equivalent weight of CCK-8 to facilitate comparison. All decreases were statistically significant.
[b] i.m. = intramuscular
[c] i.v. = intravenous
[d] s.c. = subcutaneous

INHIBITION OF FOOD INTAKE

Glucagon was the first gut peptide to be shown to inhibit food intake (TABLE 1). This was demonstrated after acute injection[7] as well as after repeated injections prior to each meal.[7-10]

Although the injection of glucagon was accompanied by slight nausea in some instances (TABLE 2) and by glycosuria in 1 of 2 subjects that received repeated injections, the occurrence of nausea was not a sufficient explanation for the decrease in food intake. It is not clear from the published studies whether the

TABLE 2. Side Effects of Gut Peptides That Inhibit Food Intake

Experiment	Treatment	Side Effects[a]
Schulman et al.[9]	glucagon 1 mg, i.m.	none 0/10
Penick and Hinkle[7]	glucagon 1 mg, i.m. (acute)	slight nausea[b]
	glucagon 1 mg, i.m. (chronic)	glycosuria 1/2
Penick and Hinkle[8]	glucagon 1 mg, i.m.	none 0/4
Clayton and Librik[10]	glucagon 2 mg, i.m.	slight nausea 1/1
Thompson and Amberg[19]	CCK-8 1 ng kg^{-1} min^{-1} (30 min)	very mild nausea 1/12
	CCK-8 4 ng kg^{-1} min^{-1} (30 min)	very mild nausea 1/12
	CCK-8 4 ng kg^{-1} min^{-1} (30 min)	mild nausea and cramps 1/50
Kissileff et al.[12]	CCK-8 4 ng kg^{-1} min^{-1} (16–27 min)	slightly stomach sick 5/12[c]
Pi-Sunyer et al.[18]	CCK-8 4 ng kg^{-1} min^{-1} (19–27 min)	slightly stomach sick 3/8[c]
Stacher et al.[11]	CCK-8 4.6 ng kg^{-1} min^{-1} (15 min)	none 0/8
	9.2 ng kg^{-1} min^{-1} (15 min)	none 0/8
Shaw et al.[13]	CCK-8 2 mcg bolus +	mild nausea during bolus 11/11
	5 mcg (45 min)	none during infusion 0/11
Murrahainen et al.[15]	bombesin	slightly stomach sick 5/8[c]

[a] The fractions in the column of Side Effects refer to the ratio of subjects that had the side effect to the total number of subjects.

[b] Penick and Hinkle did not report the number of the 8 subjects that had nausea; they reported slight nausea in 15 of 29 experiments.

[c] Indicates that there was no significant correlation between the side effect and the inhibition of food intake.

inhibition of food intake by glucagon was accompanied by normal feelings of postprandial satiety.

The most intensively studied peptide for the inhibition of food intake is cholecystokinin. In five of six studies, cholecystokinin octapeptide (CCK-8) or an impure preparation of cholecystokinin produced a significant decrease in food intake in lean subjects (TABLE 1). This effect was also observed in obese subjects[18] and was dose-related in the only study that varied doses.[11] This inhibition of food intake was sometimes accompanied by mild nausea or abdominal distress, but these symptoms were not correlated with the decrease in food intake (TABLE 2). Kisseleff et al.[12] reported that after meals that were decreased in size by CCK-8, subjects did not advance the time of their afternoon snack nor did they report increased hunger prior to their evening meal.

The satiety effect of CCK-8 was not observed in five vagotomized men.[13] This suggests that vagal afferent fibers mediate the satiating effect of CCK-8 in humans just as they have been proposed to do in rats.[14]

The most recent peptide to be investigated is bombesin. Murrahainen et al.[15] reported that an infusion of bombesin decreased food intake in the identical paradigm in which CCK-8 had decreased food intake. There were slight side effects, but these could not be correlated with the decreased food intake.

PHYSIOLOGICAL SIGNIFICANCE AND THERAPEUTIC POTENTIAL

Despite the consistent inhibitory effects observed with glucagon, CCK-8, and bombesin, the role of the gut peptides in the control of food intake remains uncertain. There is no evidence at the present time to consider the effects of these peptides on food intake to be physiological functions of the endogenous peptides. On the other hand, until the appropriate experiments are carried out, the gut hormone hypothesis[20] that suggested that gut peptides were short-term satiety signals remains heuristic.

Given their consistent efficacy for decreasing food intake, the possibility that the peptides could be used for therapeutic purposes is worth considering. Although the peptides have usually been administered in exogenous form, it is quite possible that when selective releasing agents for individual peptides are identified, these agents, if calorically trivial, could be used to release the endogenous peptides and presumably produce the same inhibitory effect on meal size. Until such releasing agents are discovered, exogenous peptides will have to be administered. At the present time, however, there are several obstacles for the application of these peptides in the control of food intake in humans. These include the lack of an orally active form, the question of the safety of chronic treatment, the question of efficacy against preferred foods, and the lack of compelling evidence for efficacy for weight loss. All of these obstacles could be overcome by further work. Given the current compelling evidence for the efficacy of these peptides in reducing food intake at a single meal without producing clinically significant side effects, further investigation seems worthwhile and is likely to produce knowledge concerning the therapeutic usefulness of these peptides as well as their putative role in the normal process of satiation.

ACKNOWLEDGEMENT

We thank Mrs. Marion Jacobson for typing this manuscript.

REFERENCES

1. BARBOUR, O. 1924. Use of insulin in undernourished non-diabetic children. Arch. Pediatr. **41:** 707–711.
2. APPEL, K. E., C. B. FARR & H. K. MARSHALL. 1928. Insulin therapy in undernourished psychotic patients: Preliminary report. J. Am. Med. Assoc. **22:** 1788–1789.
3. SHORT, J. J. 1929. Increasing weight with insulin. J. Lab. Clin. Med. **14:** 330–335.
4. SILVERSTONE, T. & M. BESSER. 1971. Insulin, blood sugar and hunger. Postgrad. Med. J. **47:** 427–429.
5. THOMPSON, D. A. & R. G. CAMPBELL. 1978. Experimental hunger in man: Behavioral and metabolic correlates of intracellular glucopenia. *In* Central Mechanisms of Anorectic Drugs. S. Garritini & R. Samanin, Eds.: 437–450. Raven Press. New York.

6. GROSSMAN, M. I. & I. F. STEIN JR. 1948. Vagotomy and the hunger producing action of insulin in man. J. Appl. Physiol. **1:** 263–269.
7. PENICK, S. B. & L. E. HINKLE JR. 1961. Depression of food intake in healthy subjects by glucagon. N. Engl. J. Med. **264:** 893–897.
8. PENICK, S. B. & L. E. HINKLE JR. 1963. The effect of glucagon, phenmetrazine and epinephrine on hunger, food intake and plasma nonesterified fatty acids. Am. J. Clin. Nutr. **13:** 110–114.
9. SCHULMAN, J. L., J. L. CARLETON, G. WHITNEY & J. C. WHITEHORN. 1957. Effect of glucagon on food intake and body weight in man. J. Appl. Physiol. **11:** 419–421.
10. CLAYTON, G. W. & L. LIBRIK. 1963. Therapy of exogenous obesity in childhood and adolescence. Pediatr. Clin. North Am. **10:** 99–107.
11. STACHER, G. H., G. STEINRINGER, G. SCHMIERER, C. SCHNEIDER & S. WINKLEHNER. 1982. Cholecystokinin octapeptide decreases intake of solid food in man. Peptides **3:** 133–136.
12. KISSILEFF, H. R., F. X. PI-SUNYER, J. THORNTON & G. P. SMITH. 1981. Cholecystokinin-octapeptide (CCK-8) decreases food intake in man. Am. J. Clin. Nutr. **34:** 154–160.
13. SHAW, M. J., J. J. HUGHES, J. E. MORLEY, A. S. LEVINE, S. E. SILVERS & R. B. SCHAFFER. 1985. Cholecystokinin octapeptide action on gastric emptying and food intake in normal and vagotomized man. *In* Neuronal Cholecystokinin. J. J. Vanderhaeghen & J. N. Crawley, Eds.: **448:** 640–641. Ann. N.Y. Acad. Sci.
14. SMITH, G. P., C. JEROME & R. NORGREN. 1985. Afferent axons in abdominal vagus mediate satiety effect of cholecystokinin in rats. Am. J. Physiol. **249:** R638–R641.
15. MURRAHAINEN, N. E., H. R. KISSILEFF, J. THORNTON & F. X. PI-SUNYER. 1983. Bombesin: another peptide that inhibits feeding in man. Soc. Neurosci. (Abstr.) **9:** 183.
16. STURDEVANT, R. A. L. & H. GOETZ. 1976. Cholecystokinin both stimulates and inhibits human food intake. Nature (London) **261:** 713–715.
17. GREENWAY, F. L. & G. A. BRAY. 1977. Cholecystokinin and satiety. Life Sci. **21:** 769–771.
18. PI-SUNYER, F. X., H. R. KISSILEFF, J. THORNTON & G. P. SMITH. 1982. C-terminal octapeptide of cholecystokinin decreases food intake in obese men. Physiol. Behav. **29:** 627–630.
19. THOMPSON, W. M. & J. R. AMBERG. 1978. Use of the C-terminal octapeptide of cholecystokinin in clinical radiology I. The gallbladder. Gastrointest. Radiol. **3:** 191–194.
20. GIBBS, J., R. C. YOUNG & G. P. SMITH. 1973. Cholecystokinin decreases food intake in rats. J. Comp. Physiol. Psychol. **84:** 488–495.

Hypothalamic Neurotransmitters in Relation to Normal and Disturbed Eating Patterns[a]

SARAH F. LEIBOWITZ

The Rockefeller University
New York, New York 10021

An integrated hypothesis for explaining eating behavior must consider the organism as a whole, the multiple brain neurotransmitters and structures involved, and the diverse variables that have impact on the expression of the behavior. In this review, we will examine a variety of brain monoamines and neuropeptides, in terms of their impact on eating, and also relate these neurochemical systems to peripheral autonomic and endocrine functions. We will propose how these central and peripheral systems may interact under normal and generally stable conditions, as well as how they may help to maintain energy or nutritional homeostasis under stressful conditions, in particular, food deprivation.

ROLE OF THE HYPOTHALAMUS

The hypothalamus is particularly rich with biologically active substances, such as putative neurotransmitters and neurohormones. Although this structure does not operate autonomously in the control of eating behavior, it is known to have a major responsibility in producing appropriate quantitative and qualitative adjustments in food intake and appetite for specific nutrients, in response to the complex sensory and metabolic information that it receives regarding the nutritional status of the organism. Thus, it is not surprising that neurochemical substances, applied directly into the hypothalamus of conscious and freely moving animals, are found in this structure, as opposed to other forebrain sites, to be particularly effective in altering food intake. Fully satiated animals can be made to eat and even binge on a particular diet, and food-deprived animals can be made to stop eating and even rest in the presence of food.

Important biochemical studies have yielded encouraging evidence that these behavioral changes induced by exogenously administered neurotransmitters or drugs reflect similar patterns of behavior that occur naturally through the action of endogenous neurotransmitters. The relevance of these findings to our understanding of human eating disorders becomes particularly apparent in numerous pharmacological studies (*e.g.*, with antidepressants, antipsychotics, stimulants, and certain peptides), which reveal similar drug-related responses in animals and in humans.[1-5] Possible similarities between animal and human neurotransmitter systems are further suggested by analyses of human cerebrospinal fluid, which reveal

[a] This study was supported in part by USPHS Grant MH-22879 from the National Institute of Mental Health and by funds from the Whitehall Foundation.

specific disturbances in brain or hypothalamic neurochemical function in association with abnormal eating patterns.[6,7]

INTRACEREBRAL INJECTION STUDIES

When administered directly into the brain, four classes of neurotransmitters have been found to influence eating in a stimulatory manner, whereas a considerably larger number of substances are shown to inhibit eating. The evidence for a physiological role of the stimulatory neurotransmitters in control of natural feeding is stronger than that for the inhibitory substances. This is, in part, due to the fact that more critical studies have, to date, been performed on these stimulatory substances, but also due to some additional evidence that the feeding-inhibitory responses, at least in some cases, may not be behaviorally and/or anatomically specific. Concerns of specificity must be carefully and systematically addressed before hypotheses of physiological function become tenable.

EATING-STIMULATORY NEUROTRANSMITTERS

The feeding-stimulatory neurotransmitters include catecholamine (CA) and norepinephrine (NE), acting by way of α_2-noradrenergic receptors, and three classes of neuropeptides, namely, the opioids (β-endorphin, enkephalin, and dynorphin), the pancreatic polypeptides (neuropeptide Y [NPY] and peptide YY), and galanin. Injections of these substances directly into the rat hypothalamus potentiate eating in satiated subjects.[3,4,8-13] These responses are dose-related and, on a molar basis, their order of potency appears to be pancreatic polypeptides $\geq$ NE > galanin = opioid peptides. Chronic hypothalamic injections of NPY or NE are effective in potentiating daily food intake and, particularly in the case of NPY, producing a profound increase in body weight and body fat composition.[14,15]

Tests in different nuclei of the hypothalamus reveal strong sensitivity in the medial paraventricular nucleus (PVN) to all four classes of these endogenous substances. Whereas other hypothalamic sites besides the PVN are relatively insensitive to NE, the neuropeptides, in contrast, with the possible exception of galanin, appear to be less anatomically specific in their action, exerting reliable effects at multiple hypothalamic sites. With a few exceptions, extra hypothalamic structures are generally unresponsive to each of these neurotransmitters that potentiate eating.

EATING-INHIBITORY NEUROTRANSMITTERS

The feeding-inhibitory neurotransmitters in the brain include the monoamines,[3,16,17] in particular, dopamine (DA), serotonin (5-HT), and under certain conditions, NE and epinephrine (EPI) (acting by way of β-adrenergic receptors), and a long list of gut-brain peptides, most notably cholecystokinin (CCK), neurotensin (NT), calcitonin (CT), and glucagon.[11,18,19] Extensive mapping and lesion studies with the three CAs, tested in hungry rats, indicate that they act within the hypothalamus, in particular the lateral (perifornical) area, to inhibit eating. Serotonin, by contrast, appears to be effective in the medial hypothalamus as opposed to laterally, although further studies will need to be conducted to establish extra-hypothalamic sensitivity. Few such mapping studies have been conducted with the peptides, and limited evidence available to date demonstrates that exogenously administered peptides are apparently effective in multiple brain sites, including medial as well as lateral hypothalamic nuclei and both forebrain and hindbrain sites (Stanley & Leibowitz, unpublished data).

MACRONUTRIENT SELECTION

What is most striking about these neurotransmitter effects on eating is that they are characterized by a specific change in macronutrient selection, rather than simply an increase or decrease in total food intake. This specificity argues for a physiological function in regulation of diet composition. In particular, PVN injection of NE in the rat causes a selective increase in carbohydrate ingestion, in association with little or no change in fat and in some cases a suppression of protein.[4,20] A constant carbohydrate craving can be seen in animals receiving chronic stimulation with NE. A similar pattern of diet preference is produced by NPY and peptide YY, which can induce satiated rats to eat in 2 to 4 hours of the light cycle what they normally eat in 24 hours.[21,22] This raises the possibility that NE and NPY, which are known to coexist in medullary projections that innervate the PVN,[23] may be acting through a similar medial hypothalamic system that specifically controls carbohydrate intake. Interestingly, this contrasts with the peptide, galanin, which stimulates fat intake to a greater extent than carbohydrate intake,[24] and also the opioid peptides which, by way of μ, δ, and k receptors, enhance ingestion of fat and, to some extent, protein, while actually suppressing the relative proportion of carbohydrate ingested.[4] Based on this evidence, it seems that these hypothalamic noradrenergic and neuropeptide systems may participate and interact in coordinating the pattern of carbohydrate, protein, and fat meals consumed by the animal. Physiological studies have shown that, in addition to total calorie intake, macronutrient selection and their pattern and ratio are regulated aspects of eating behavior.[25]

The brain monoamines, which act to suppress eating, may also participate in this process of controlling diet composition. This is indicated by the evidence that peripheral and hypothalamic injection of the CA-releasing drug amphetamine, and lateral hypothalamic administration of the CA, cause a preferential decrease in protein consumption, whereas dopamine-receptor blockade preferentially stimulates protein ingestion.[25,26] This pattern of effects, suggesting a role of lateral hypothalamic CA in producing satiety for protein, contrasts with that observed for 5-HT, indicating that this monoamine in the medial hypothalamus may selectively suppress carbohydrate intake while sparing protein intake.[16,27,28] The feeding inhibitory effects of central peptides have yet to be systematically explored in a dietary self-selection paradigm.

ENDOCRINE PARAMETERS

Two hormones, in particular, are believed to be important for the expression of these hypothalamic neurotransmitter effects on nutrient intake. These hormones are the adrenal glucocorticoid, corticosterone, and the pancreatic hormone, insulin, both of which appear to function synergistically with the central

neurotransmitters. The strongest evidence has been obtained for PVN NE-elic-
ited eating, which is abolished by adrenalectomy and attenuated by dissection of
vagal fibers to the pancreas.[29-31] Although the opioids and pancreatic polypeptides
have not yet been tested in vagotomized animals, the eating-stimulatory effects of
NPY and the μ agonist morphine in the PVN[32,33] are found to be significantly
reduced in adrenalectomized rats and restored after corticosterone replacement.
Both corticosterone and insulin have long been known to be involved in the
control of food intake, and it now appears that these hormones may work in close
association with specific neurotransmitters in the hypothalamus. In fact, a strong
positive correlation has been detected between circulating levels of corticosterone
(2 to 15 μg%) and the amount of food consumed in response to NE in the rat.[4]
Recent studies indicate that PVN administration of NE, as well as NPY, dramatically enhances the release of corticosterone into the circulation of awake and
freely moving rats,[34] and systemic corticosterone injection is itself effective in
stimulating eating, particularly of carbohydrate.[35]

MONOAMINE-PEPTIDE INTERACTIONS

Evidence has been obtained for both an association and a dissociation between
NE and the peptides in these hypothalamic systems. The possibility of a close
interaction in control of food intake is consistent with the apparent anatomical
overlap of these systems, as well as their dependence upon corticosterone. In
addition, eating induced by opiate stimulation is antagonized by α-adrenergic as
well as opiate receptor antagonists[36,37] and has a similar circadian rhythm to that
observed with NE.[38] Also, a strong selective preference for carbohydrate, like
that shown for NE, can be seen with both NPY and peptide YY.[21]
    Whereas this evidence argues for some degree of association, there are other
results suggesting that these neurotransmitters may in part function independently. For example, galanin and opiate agonists, in contrast to NE, preferentially
stimulate fat or protein intake (see above), and this effect of the opiates is unaffected by local neurotoxin lesions of noradrenergic innervation to the medial
hypothalamus.[39] Similarly, even though NPY acts like NE in the stimulation of
carbohydrate ingestion, its feeding response remains intact after α-receptor blockade,[11,22] as well as after knife-cut damage to descending periventricular fiber
projections that are critical to NE's action (Stanley & Leibowitz, unpublished
data). Based on this evidence and the fact that the opioids and pancreatic polypeptides work in other hypothalamic areas (besides the PVN) that are unresponsive to NE, it may be concluded that the peptides may function both in association
with and independently of endogenous NE, depending upon brain area and possibly the circumstances through which they become activated.
    The brain peptides that inhibit eating have similarly been investigated in terms
of their potential interaction with endogenous CA in the control of appetite. For
example, these peptides have been shown to have a potent suppressive effect on
food ingestion induced by PVN NE injection.[11,40,41] The peptides NT and CCK
also affect the release of endogenous NE, exerting opposite effects in the medial
versus lateral hypothalamus that depend upon the nutritional state of the animal.[42]
Additional evidence indicates that these peptides may similarly interact with dopaminergic and β-adrenergic systems,[43,44] possibly within the lateral hypothalamus where they evoke satiety,[4] and also with hypothalamic opioid systems, which
potentiate food consumption.[45]

PHYSIOLOGICAL FUNCTION

Regarding NE function within the hypothalamus, the available evidence has generated the hypothesis that this neurotransmitter system, as part of its overall effort to rapidly replenish body energy stores, becomes physiologically activated under conditions involving energy expenditure, for example, during food deprivation, stress, and at the start of the active period of the diurnal cycle. Circadian patterns of eating place particular demands on body energy stores, such that at the end of the inactive cycle during which little food is ingested, hepatic glycogen stores are low and blood glucose levels may actually decline.[46] Several studies suggest the PVN NE is called upon, at this particular time, to initiate the eating process and thereby restore carbohydrate reserves. Specifically, in the nocturnal rat, the burst of eating that normally occurs at the beginning of the dark period is found to be associated with 1) a sharp unimodal peak of circulating corticosterone, α_2-receptor density exclusively in the PVN, and α_2-receptor responsiveness to PVN NE and clonidine infusion;[38,47,48] 2) a release of medial hypothalamic NE in association with eating;[49,50] and 3) a natural increase in meal size, rate of eating, and preference for carbohydrate.[46,51,52] A similar circadian rhythm of opiate-induced feeding[32] suggests that this system may also become activated at the start of the dark cycle.

In addition to the circadian rhythm of feeding, it is likely that NE, and possibly the neuropeptides as well, may be essential in the mediation of compensatory eating behavior induced by episodes of food deprivation. In addition to increased food intake, food deprivation is found to enhance the release of hypothalamic or PVN NE and to cause a rapid, dramatic, and site-specific down regulation of α_2-receptors in the PVN.[53-55] This latter effect, which occurs in close association with a decline in blood glucose,[46,53] can be seen with a very brief period of food deprivation (less than 3 hours), particularly at the beginning of the dark cycle, and can be reversed by refeeding. The opiates are well-known for their analgesic properties, and it is also known that food deprivation, like stress, decreases nociception and potentiates hypothalamic opiate activity.[10,56,57] Work from this laboratory[4,35,58] has recently demonstrated that animals with PVN lesions, or after adrenalectomy, exhibit particular disturbances in carbohydrate ingestion, in their ability to produce adequate compensatory eating in response to food deprivation, in their adrenal release of corticosterone, and also in their responsiveness to NE and opiate stimulation (see above). This evidence confirms the importance of these hypothalamic, adrenal-dependent neurotransmitter systems in monitoring and replenishing energy stores after acute food deprivation.

REFERENCES

1. GIBBS, J. & G. P. SMITH. 1984. The neuroendocrinology of postprandial satiety. *In* Frontiers in Neuroendocrinology. L. Martini & W. F. Ganong, Eds.: **8:** 223–246. Raven Press. New York.
2. JOHNSON, C., M. STUCKEY & J. MITCHELL. 1983. J. Nerv. Ment. Dis. **171:** 524–534.
3. LEIBOWITZ, S. F. 1980. Neurochemical systems of the hypothalamus in control of feeding and drinking behavior and water-electrolyte excretion. *In* Handbook of the Hypothalamus. P. J. Morgane & J. Panksepp, Eds.: **3A:** 299–437. Marcel Dekker. New York.
4. LEIBOWITZ, S. F. 1986. Fed. Proc. Fed. Am. Soc. Exp. Biol. **45:** 1396–1403.
5. SILVERSTONE, T., ED. 1982. Drugs and Appetite. Academic Press. New York.

6. KAYE, W. H., M. H. EBERT, H. E. GWIRTSMAN & S. R. WEISS. 1984. Am. J. Psychiatry **141:** 1598–1601.
7. KAYE, W. H., D. C. JIMERSON, C. R. LAKE & M. H. EBERT. 1984. Psychiatry Res. **14:** 333–342.
8. KYRKOULI, S. E., B. G. STANLEY & S. F. LEIBOWITZ. 1986. Eur. J. Pharmacol. **122:** 159–160.
9. LEIBOWITZ, S. F. 1978. Pharmacol. Biochem. Behav. **8:** 163–175.
10. MORLEY, J. E., A. S. LEVINE, G. K. YIM & M. T. LOWY. 1983. Neurosci. Biobehav. Rev. **7:** 281–305.
11. MORLEY, J. E., A. S. LEVINE, B. A. GOSNELL & D. D. KRAHN. 1985. Brain Res. Bull. **14:** 511–520.
12. STANLEY, B. G. & S. F. LEIBOWITZ. 1984. Life Sci. **35:** 2635–2642.
13. STANLEY, B. G., A. S. CHIN & S. F. LEIBOWITZ. 1985. Brain Res. Bull. **14:** 521–524.
14. LICHTENSTEIN, S. S., C. MARNESCU & S. F. LEIBOWITZ. 1984. Brain Res. Bull. **13:** 591–595.
15. STANLEY, B. G., S. E. KYRKOULI, S. LAMPERT & S. F. LEIBOWITZ. 1985. Neurosci. Abstr. **11:** 36.
16. BLUNDELL, J. E. 1984. Neuropharmacology **23:** 1537–1552.
17. LEIBOWITZ, S. F. & G. SHOR-POSNER. 1986. Appetite 7(Suppl.): 1–14.
18. INOKUCHI, A., Y. OOMURA & H. NISHIMURA. 1984. Physiol. Behav. **33:** 397–400.
19. STANLEY, B. G., B. G. HOEBEL & S. F. LEIBOWITZ. 1983. Peptides **4:** 493–500.
20. LEIBOWITZ, S. F., G. F. WEISS, F. YEE & J. B. TRETTER. 1985. Brain Res. Bull. **14:** 561–568.
21. STANLEY, B. G., D. R. DANIEL, A. S. CHIN & S. F. LEIBOWITZ. 1985. Peptides **6:** 1205–1211.
22. STANLEY, B. G. & S. F. LEIBOWITZ. 1985. Proc. Natl. Acad. Sci. USA **82:** 3940–3943.
23. EVERITT, B. J., T. HÖKFELT, L. TERENIUS, K. TATEMOTO, V. MUTT & M. GOLDSTEIN. 1984. Neurosci. **11:** 443–462.
24. TEMPEL, D. L., K. J. LEIBOWITZ, D. SMITH & S. F. LEIBOWITZ. 1986. Neurosci. Abstr. **12:** 594.
25. BLUNDELL, J. E. 1983. Problems and processes underlying the control of food selection and nutrient intake. *In* Nutrition and the Brain. R. J. Wurtman & J. J. Wurtman, Eds.: **6:** 163–222. Raven Press. New York.
26. LEIBOWITZ, S. F., G. SHOR-POSNER, C. MACLOW & J. A. GRINKER. 1986. Brain Res. Bull. **17:** 681–689.
27. SHOR-POSNER, G., J. A. GRINKER, C. MARINESCU & S. F. LEIBOWITZ. 1986. Brain Res. Bull. **17:** 663–671.
28. WURTMAN, R. J. & J. J. WURTMAN. 1984. Nutrients, neurotransmitter synthesis, and the control of food intake. *In* Eating and Its Disorders (Series: Association for Research in Nervous and Mental Disease). **62:** 77–96. Raven Press. New York.
29. LEIBOWITZ, S. F., C. R. ROLAND, L. HOR & V. SQUILLARI. 1984. Physiol. Behav. **32:** 857–864.
30. ROLAND, C. R., P. BHAKTHAVATSALAM & S. F. LEIBOWITZ. 1986. Neuroendocrinology **42:** 296–305.
31. SAWCHENKO, P. E., R. M. GOLD & S. F. LEIBOWITZ. 1981. Brain Res. **225:** 249–269.
32. BHAKTHAVATSALAM P. & S. F. LEIBOWITZ. 1986. Pharmacol. Biochem. Behav. **24:** 911–917.
33. STANLEY, B. G., D. LANTHIER, A. S. CHIN & S. F. LEIBOWITZ. 1986. Neurosci. Abstr. **12:** 592.
34. LEIBOWITZ, S. F., S. DIAZ & L. SPENCER. 1986. Neurosci. Abstr.: 782.
35. BHAKTHAVATSALAM, P. & S. F. LEIBOWITZ. 1986. Am. J. Physiol. In press.
36. LEIBOWITZ, S. F. & L. HOR. 1982. Peptides **3:** 421–428.
37. TEPPERMAN, F. S., M. HIRSCH & C. W. GOWDEY. 1981. Pharmacol. Biochem. Behav. **15:** 555–558.
38. BHAKTHAVATSALAM, P. & S. F. LEIBOWITZ. 1986. Am. J. Physiol. **250:** R83–R88.
39. SHOR-POSNER, G., A. AZAR, R. FILART, D. TEMPEL & S. F. LEIBOWITZ. 1986. Pharmacol. Biochem. Behav. **24:** 931–939.

40. MYERS, R. D. & M. L. MCCALEB. 1981. Neurosci. 6: 645–655.
41. STANLEY, B. G., S. F. LEIBOWITZ, N. EPPEL et al. 1985. Brain Res. 343: 297–304.
42. MYERS, R. D. 1985. Psychopharmacol. Bull. 21: 406–411.
43. HÖKFELT, T., B. J. EVERETT, E. THEODORSSON-NORHEIM & M. GOLDSTEIN. 1984. J. Comp. Neurol. 222: 543–559.
44. KOCHMAN, R. L., T. R. GREY & J. D. HIRSCH. 1984. Peptides 5: 499–502.
45. MORLEY, J. E., A. S. LEVINE, J. KNEIP et al. 1983. Pharmacol. Biochem. Behav. 19: 577–582.
46. LEMAGNEN, J. 1981. Behav. Brain Sci. 4: 561–607.
47. KRIEGER, D. & H. HAUSER. 1978. Proc. Natl. Acad. Sci. USA 75: 1577–1581.
48. JHANWAR-UNIYAL, M., C. R. ROLAND & S. F. LEIBOWITZ. 1986. Life Sci. 38: 473–482.
49. MARTIN, G. E. & R. D. MYERS. 1975. Am. J. Physiol. 229: 1547–1555.
50. VAN DER GUGTEN, J. & J. L. SLANGEN. 1977. Pharmacol. Biochem. Behav. 7: 211–219.
51. JOHNSON, D. J., E. T. S. LI, D. V. COSCINA & G. H. ANDERSON. 1979. Physiol. Behav. 22: 777–780.
52. TEMPEL, D., P. BHAKTHAVATSALAM, G. SHOR-POSNER et al. 1985. Proc. 56th EPA Meeting. Boston, MA.
53. CHAFETZ, M. D., K. PARKO, S. DIAZ & S. F. LEIBOWITZ. 1986. Brain Res. 384: 404–408.
54. JHANWAR-UNIYAL, M. & S. F. LEIBOWITZ. 1986. Brain Res. Bull. 17: 889–896.
55. JHANWAR-UNIYAL, M., F. FLEISCHER, B. E. LEVIN & S. F. LEIBOWITZ. 1982. Soc. Neurosci. Abstr. 8: 711.
56. GAMBERT, S. R., T. L. GARTHWAITE, C. H. PONTZER & T. C. HAGEN. 1980. Science 210: 1271–1272.
57. MCGIVERN, R. F. & G. G. BERNTSON. 1980. Science 210: 210–211.
58. SHOR-POSNER, G., A. P. AZAR, M. JHANWAR-UNIYAL, R. FILART & S. F. LEIBOWITZ. 1986. Pharmacol. Biochem. Behav. 25: 381–392.

Nutritional Manipulations for Altering Food Intake

Towards a Causal Model of Experimental Obesity

J. E. BLUNDELL

Biopsychology Group
Psychology Department
University of Leeds
Leeds, LS2 9JT, United Kingdom

ANIMAL MODELS FOR THE STUDY OF OBESITY AND APPETITE

For more than 40 years, researchers have carried out experimental investigations on the food consumption and body weight regulation of laboratory animals in order to throw light upon mechanisms that may contribute to our understanding of the genesis of human obesity, the maintenance of excessive body weight, the apparent resistance of obesity to treatment, and to the development of new therapies. Different types of experimental strategies may be required for these separate objectives. A smaller number of studies has been concerned with the experimental models of underweight and with the treatment of abnormalities involving weight loss. Considering obesity, Mayer[1] has distinguished between the traumatic, hereditary, and environmental factors in the etiology of obesity. Each of these factors has been associated with the use of particular models. More recently Sclafani[2] has reviewed experimental models for body weight changes and has drawn up a classification system.[3] This system distinguishes between treatments that give rise to obesity relatively independently of the available diet and those manipulations that are diet-dependent. The first category includes genetic obesities, whereas the second category clearly includes all nutritional treatments. Some treatments such as ovariectomy or medial hypothalamic lesions fall on the spectrum midway between the diet-dependent and diet-independent extremes. This review will be concerned only with the diet-dependent alterations.

DIETARY MANIPULATIONS

The phenomena of dietary obesity and dietary-induced overeating have been the subject of fairly recent and extensive reviews.[4,5] The objective of this contribution is to draw attention to newer findings, to consider dietary manipulations not normally associated with obesity, and to highlight important implications of these studies.

High Fat Diets

Rats,[6] mice,[7] and dogs[8] become obese when offered high fat diets (up to 65% fat) *ad libitum*. Although the actual weight of food consumed may be reduced, the greater caloric density of fatty foods is sufficient to lead to increased body weight and fat deposition.[9,10] It is also known that large increases in fat cell number occur when rats are fed a high fat diet.[11] This can be contrasted with the adjustments seen in hypothalamically lesioned rats fed a chow diet where the obesity is due almost entirely to adipocyte hypertrophy.[12] Moreover, after nine weeks of high-fat feeding, adipocyte hyperplasia is not reversed by a further 20 weeks on laboratory chow,[11] which usually contains less than 5% fat. This amount of time on chow does, however, allow fat cell size to return to normal.[13] Rats fed a high fat diet for six months displayed a degree of hyperplasia that produced a permanent 20% increase in body weight.[14] Consequently for the rat, the total amount of fat in the diet exerts a marked effect not only on body weight and total body fat, but also upon adipocyte dynamics. By combining dietary fat manipulations with other physiological treatments it becomes possible to produce an adult animal displaying either hypertrophy or hyperplasia of fat cells. In turn, these preparations can serve as test models to examine the effects of putative treatments for obesity.

Carbohydrate Supplements

One way to increase carbohydrate intake is to mix the material with the standard diet. Some years ago the rationale for doing this was that the sweet taste of the carbohydrate (normally sucrose, fructose, or glucose) would enhance the palatability of the standard diet and therefore promote consumption. This technique, however, is not successful in augmenting caloric intake or increasing body weight; moreover, with additions of sucrose in the diet, rats may actually consume less food but increase the percentage of body fat (e.g., reference 15). A different technique, which does lead to increases in caloric intake and weight gain, is to provide the palatable carbohydrate as a solution separate from the standard laboratory chow. With sucrose given in a 32% solution, it has been demonstrated that daily caloric intake rises by approximately 20%, and rats increase body weight by 43% over three and a half months. In addition, it appears that rats with access to sucrose solutions have a higher percentage of body fat.[16] Increases in body weight of adult rats can be brought about by giving animals access to solutions of glucose, fructose, or maltose. The belief, however, that animals consume these solutions because of the high palatability afforded by the sweet taste is questioned by observation that 62% sucrose solutions are not ingested in greater amounts than the much less sweet glucose.[5] In addition, rats will consume as much bland-tasting saccharide powder (dextrin) as a sweet-tasting sucrose solution.[17] More recently it has been demonstrated that rats will consume equal amounts of 32% solutions of sweet-tasting sucrose or bland-tasting polycose, which is minimally sweet but equicaloric with sucrose and glucose.[18] The polycose-induced hyperphagia induced a weight gain equal to that of sucrose supplemented rats. Polycose administered as a powder or as a powder mixed with laboratory chow, however, did not lead to overconsumption.[19] The importance of the particular form of the dietary manipulation illustrates the potency of contextual factors determining intake.[20,21] The capacity of both polycose and sucrose to increase weight gain, however, under the appropriate circumstances, suggests the existence of the different carbohydrate tastes that aid in the identification of starch-rich and sugar-rich foods.[22] Also, rats avidly respond to polycose in short-term taste tests.[22]

Cafeteria Diets

A procedure in which various aspects of the diet, energy density, variety, and palatability, are manipulated can produce dramatic increases in energy intake and body weight and has led to the establishment of an interesting model of obesity.[4,23,24] Rats can be offered a number of snack foods such as biscuits, cheese, salami, and sweets or more mundane foods like bread and lard. These items may be presented together or serially. The effects generated by this type of dietary manipulation are illustrated in FIGURE 1. It is noticeable that the cafeteria procedure brings about changes not only in body weight and daily food intake but also

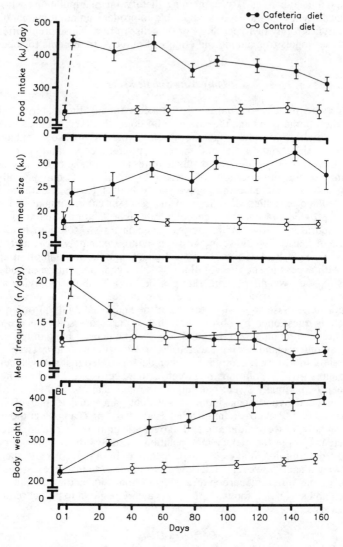

FIGURE 1. Changes in body weight, daily energy intake, meal size, and meal frequency during the development of dietary-induced obesity using a cafeteria diet of three foods plus laboratory chow.

in eating parameters such as meal size and meal frequency.[25] As with other forms of experimental obesity, developmental aspects are prominent with the trajectory of body weight reflecting a dynamic and plateau phase. Further analysis of the structure of feeding has revealed that the features of variety and palatability play separate but overlapping roles in the enhancement of calorie intake and in the profile of meal taking.[26,27] One prominent feature of the eating pattern is the maintained increase in average meal size during the dynamic and plateau phases of obesity. Although some studies have regarded the cafeteria model as generating a form of reversible obesity,[28] under certain conditions a persistent elevation of body weight occurs.[25,17,29] The persistence of the obesity appears to be related to the duration of exposure to the cafeteria diet, the amount of fat in the diet and, ultimately, probably to the degree of hyperplasia engendered. This form of obesity has already been used as a model for the examination of putative treatments such as pharmacotherapy, and it is clear that drugs vary in their capacity to suppress intake of a cafeteria diet[30] and in their capacity to suppress weight gain during the dynamic and plateau phases.[31]

Diet Selection and Nutrient Choice

The essence of dietary selection in experimental studies is to present animals with the opportunity of making choices among dietary items offered simultaneously (not sequentially). This procedure may appear similar to the cafeteria model, but whereas cafeteria feeding (as designated previously) allows animals to choose from assorted snack food items varying widely in energy density, nutrient composition, and sensory aspects, the diet selection paradigm usually offers alternatives containing systematically varied proportions of macro- and micronutrients (e.g. reference 32). In recent years, the technique has usually involved choices between pure sources of fat, protein, and carbohydrate (plus vitamins) or between diets containing precise amounts of these macronutrients. The purpose of this type of experimental design is to determine the quantities and proportions of particular nutrients that are voluntarily self-selected by an animal. Why should this procedure be useful in the study of obesity? One reason is that it is often claimed that obese human beings display strong preference for certain macronutrients such as carbohydrates[33] or fat.[34] Therefore an experimental preparation in which nutrient (or dietary) preferences can be examined during obesity is useful. Indeed it has been demonstrated that dietary selection is invariably altered during the development of obesity brought about by surgical treatments of the hypothalamus. The particular form of the selection pattern, however, appears to depend upon a number of contextual variables. Some researchers have found that hyperphagic rats with lesions of the medial hypothalamus prefer high fat rather than high carbohydrate diets[35] or, if choosing between pure macronutrient sources, increase fat intake and decrease protein intake.[36] A further study that compared the overeating induced by medial hypothalamic lesions, paraventricular nucleus lesions, and parasagittal medial hypothalamic knife cuts found that all preparations overate by increasing carbohydrate intake.[37] In contrast to the other treatments, however, paraventricular lesioned animals failed to increase protein intake proportionately and therefore displayed a diminution in protein energy percent. The difference observed between this study[37] and the previous one[36] was attributed to the decreased water intake following medial hypothalamic lesions,[36] which would tend to favor the selection of fat.[38] In one further study,[39] which used equicaloric composite diets in which fat proportions were held constant, medial hypothalamic lesions brought about overeating and weight gain through an increase in consumption of the high carbohydrate (low protein) diet while a normal level of protein intake was preserved. In a different obesity preparation (the ob/ob mouse), replacement of dietary carbohydrate by fat lowered the percentage of energy self-selected as protein.[40] Consequently, it appears that during overeating and weight gain, dietary selection is usually modulated. Of course this does not necessarily mean that there has been a change in the mechanisms regulating nutrient intake; since sensory factors (taste, texture) are altered vicariously when nutrient values change, a new pattern of selection may arise from disturbed sensory preferences rather than through an obligatory demand to alter the supply of nutrients. Moreover, a similar qualification can be made of apparent nutrient preferences in humans; selection of particular dietary commodities may be on the basis of sensory aspects rather than nutrient composition.

Two major inferences may be drawn from the description of the above studies. First, nutrient intakes are markedly influenced by the contextual qualities of the diet. For example, fat intake may be enhanced when fat is mixed with a chow diet, decreased if offered as a pure source, or increased if water consumption is simultaneously reduced. Does this mean that dietary preferences (and selection) are so capricious as to be of little value in understanding their significance for obesity? My view is that this is not the case, but it is clear that the particular dietary selection paradigm must be chosen carefully and according to the specific objectives of the experiment. Second, the modulation of dietary preferences according to the degree of obesity suggests that treatments for obesity are likely to bring about alterations in nutrient consumption. In certain cases this could lead to nutrient imbalance. Accordingly, the dietary selection procedure can be usefully employed to evaluate the effect of obesity treatments upon nutrient intake.

INDIVIDUALITY OF APPETITES AND PRONENESS TO OBESITY

In all studies of experimentally induced obesity by means of nutritional manipulations, it is noticeable that there is considerable variability in individual responsiveness. Some animals are very susceptible to the development of obesity, whereas others appear resistant. What factors could account for the variability in the responses of animals to dietary manipulations?

Cephalic Phase Responsiveness

The concept of cephalic phase response refers to physiological changes that are brought into play rapidly by way of central nervous system mechanisms when eating is imminent. Cephalic responses can be regarded as a preparatory phase during which time physiological events take place that anticipate the handling of incoming nutrients.[41] The elements of the cephalic phase include salivation, gastric responses, pancreatic secretions, and intestinal events. The cephalic-phase insulin response has been widely studied in animals and humans. Interestingly the strength of this response may be a useful diagnostic indicator of susceptibility to obesity. In apparently identical rats of the same breed, age and sex cephalic-phase insulin secretion was stimulated by placing the artificial sweetener saccharine in the mouth. The rats could be divided into two groups on the basis of the degree of the rise in blood insulin. Moreover, when subsequently placed on a cafeteria diet, the good responders gained weight at a significantly higher rate than the poor responders.[42] It is worth noting that obese subjects can display an elevation of cephalic phase plasma insulin four times greater than lean subjects.[43] Consequently the sensitivity of the cephalic-phase insulin response could be related to the amplitude of appetite induction by food and to the susceptibility to gain weight.

Natural Eating Profile

The way in which animals (or humans) normally eat may be related to alterations in energy intake observed when the variety and palatability of food are enhanced. This possibility can be readily tested in rats in which the pattern of meal taking is monitored before they are placed on an alternative diet. When this investigation was carried out the rats were classified as gorgers or nibblers according to the measured average meal size.[44] While eating standard laboratory chow, the rats did not display differences in body weight gain, but when they were offered a high fat sugar mix in addition to chow, the gorgers showed a more rapid rate of weight gain than the nibblers. Moreover, there was a significant positive correlation (+.54) between meal size and fat cell number.[44] Consequently, the natural feeding profile predicted the susceptibility to accumulate weight following nutritional manipulation. This observation is interesting because meal size is markedly increased during the dynamic and plateau phases of cafeteria-induced obesity,[25] and it has also been reported that some obese humans display a pattern of eating characterized by the daily consumption of a small number of large meals.[45] If the tendency to consume large meals represents a meaningful indicator of appetite, then individual differences in this parameter will be a significant vulnerability factor in the development of obesity.

Patterns of Diet Selection

In those experimental designs in which animals are offered choices and where the selection of dietary commodities can be accurately measured, it is noticeable that there is a marked variability in individual response patterns. For example, it has been reported that for rats allowed to self-select from purified components "even though all of the essentials may be present, not all of the rats eat them. Even two series of animals similar in their genetic and physiological background, and tested under the same conditions do not exhibit the same pattern of selection."[46] Considerable interanimal variation has been shown in a number of experiments,[47,48] even to the extent that some rats, when offered a pure protein source of casein, refused to eat and eventually died.[49] In addition, Lat[50] has reported distinct subgroups. It was believed that underlying biochemical factors were responsible for determining two basic patterns designated as glucogenic or gluconeogenic, depending on the relative proportions of fat, carbohydrate, and protein regularly consumed. It also appeared that the different patterns of selection were associated with differing general drive levels assumed to reflect different excitability levels of the central nervous system. In other words, there exist different types of rats showing different personalities that are associated with different patterns of nutrient selection.

Data from the studies of diet selection show clearly that animals, just as much as humans, show great individuality in the expression of appetite. It has been noted earlier that the induction of obesity leads to alterations in diet selection. It therefore seems very likely that the direction of individual appetites, that is, the type of nutrient selection pattern, would either facilitate or retard the development of obesity. The natural style of diet selection may constitute either a vulnerability factor or a protection factor for obesity.

IMPLICATIONS

A number of conclusions may be drawn from the preceding brief description of nutritional manipulations in experimental animal models.

(a) Obesity can be readily induced in normal animals that have not undergone any neurological or physiological treatments. Moreover, even allowing for possible compensatory responses in energy output and the opposing action of such phenomena as diet-induced thermogenesis, the alteration of dietary factors alone can lead to dramatic weight gains and increases in body fat.

(b) Although an increase in total caloric intake may, under some circumstances, be sufficient for weight gain, the nutrient composition of the diet is important. High fat or high sugar diets or combinations of these components represent potent obesity-inducing manipulations. Two factors are implicated. First, nutrients that raise the palatability of the diet will promote consumption, and nutrients that promote hyperplasia of fat cells will lead to irreversible or refractory obesity.

(c) Dietary induction of obesity appears to display a dynamic phase of rapid weight accumulation and a plateau phase of weight maintenance (at an upper limit of body weight) or a much slower rate of weight gain. These phases represent the stages of getting fat and staying fat. The characteristics and properties of these two stages may be quite different.

(d) In the face of dietary manipulations, there is considerable variability in the strength of response of individual animals. Not all animals respond by gaining weight. Some subjects are more vulnerable than others to the obesity-promoting effects of diets. This vulnerability or proneness may be diagnosed and is reflected in a potent cephalic-phase response or a natural meal pattern dominated by large meals. Other diagnostic indices may be revealed later. Individual differences are a significant component of both experimental dietary-induced obesity and natural human obesity.

(e) Dietary models provide a means of studying the natural history of obesity from its inception through to its ultimate stage. In addition, these models permit the examination of circumstances and variables that may facilitate or amplify weight gain or that may protect animals from the insidious accumulation of weight. Facilitatory factors may include the presence of drugs such as tranquilizers,[52] whereas a protective agent could be physical exercise.[53]

(f) Dietary models form an important testing ground for potential treatments of obesity. In the absence of definitive evidence about the causal agents responsible for human obesity, it may be assumed that dietary factors play a significant role. Therefore, experimental models in which dietary factors are paramount have high external validity.[54] Such models may be particularly useful in evaluating the effects of drugs acting by way of peripheral[55] or central mechanisms.[30,31]

(g) The study of experimental dietary obesity has forced a consideration of the status and role of different causal factors contributing to the development and/or maintenance of obesity. These factors may have the status of vulnerability factors, provoking agents, facilitating agents or protective factors (see next section).

TOWARDS A CAUSAL MODEL OF OBESITY

It is frequently asserted and generally agreed that obesity is a condition under multifactorial influences. Today, few people argue that there is a single dominant cause for the increase in body fat or for its maintenance. It is often assumed, however, that the contributing factors have the same etiological status and that they exercise an equal influence within the matrix of variables affecting body weight. One valuable feature of animal models is that variables can be experimentally controlled and their effects monitored over long periods of time, especially during the development of obesity. It is important to note that the full course of the development of obesity in humans cannot be studied, although brief investigations of the simulated onset may be carried out (*e.g.* reference 51).

One prominent feature of the studies described here is that they allow the separation of factors with different functions in the genesis of obesity. Mention has already been made (see above) of the distinctions that may be drawn between vulnerability, protection, provoking, and amplification factors. These terms reflect the differing assumptions that underly the operation of a disposition to develop obesity (vulnerability factor) and an agency that actually induces the condition (provoking factor). Similarly, other variables may operate so as to intensify the action of a provoking agent (amplification factor) or to impede the effect of such an agent (protection factor). Consequently a system can be constructed to illustrate how these various categories of factors might interact (FIGURE 2). This matrix of interacting variables represents an attempt to develop a causal model of obesity that recognizes the multiple etiology of the condition by assigning roles to particular causal agencies. The idea of causality embodied here is similar to that inherent in certain models of psychopathology (see reference 56). A causal model such as this proposes that obesity arises from combinations of factors rather than from unique causes. Indeed the causal idea is embodied in interactions between variables. The model suggests that there are few, if any, sufficient conditions for the development of obesity, but that there may be numerous necessary conditions.

Using this causal model (FIG. 2), it is possible to define the combination of factors that should lead to the most severe obesity. For example, an Osborne-Mendel rat (susceptible background factor) displaying a profile of large meals (vulnerability factor) offered a high fat/high sugar diet (provoking agent) with a long exposure to the diet (amplification factor) and prevented from taking exercise (low protection factor) should lead to rapid and massive obesity. Similarly, a set of circumstances could be defined that would either prevent the onset of obesity or militate against further weight increase once the process of fat accumulation had begun.

In addition to assigning functional roles to particular categories of causal factors, the model also possesses a number of other features. First it permits a clear perception of those factors that lead to the development of obesity and those that maintain the condition once achieved. For example, a vulnerability factor may be important in establishing obesity but have little further effect once a level of body fat has been deposited. This idea emphasizes the significance of the temporal arrangement of the factors. It can be inferred that some factors may have separate roles according to the order in which they occur. For example, a stressor may function as a vulnerability factor if present before the onset of a provoking agent or as an amplification factor if it occurs afterwards. Similarly, a protection factor such as physical exercise may function as an antivulnerability factor if it takes place before the onset of provoking agents or as an antiamplification factor if it arises later.

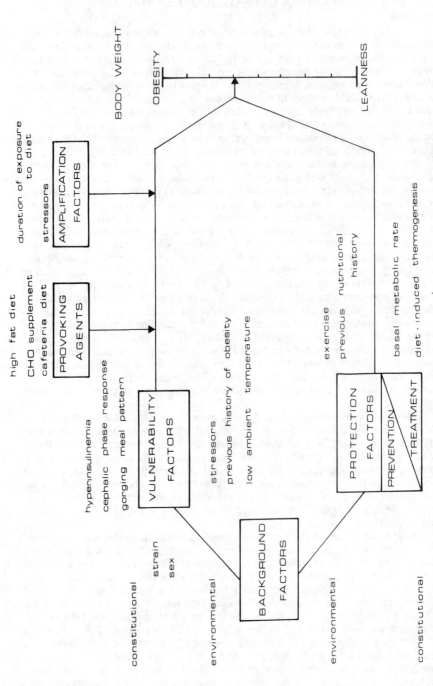

FIGURE 2. Conceptualization of a causal model for experimentally induced obesity. The model assigns separate roles to particular factors contributing to the development or maintenance of obesity.

Second, the intended conceptual clarification offered by this causal model suggests certain testable hypotheses. Many of these hypotheses relate to the manner of the interaction between various types of factors. For example, does a protection factor (such as physical exercise) impede equally the development of obesity with different types of provoking agents? Does an amplification factor (such as stress) exert a similar enhancing effect in combination with different types of vulnerability factors or different provoking agents?

Third, the model raises questions about the nature of strategies underlying the treatment of obesity and the use of animal models to evaluate new forms of therapy. In broad terms, should treatment attempt to diminish the potency of vulnerability factors, to lessen the action of provoking agents, to decrease the effect of amplification factors, or to increase the strength of protection factors? Would the most effective form of therapy involve treatments dealing simultaneously with different types of factors? What combination of treatments would work best? For example, how effective would be increasing a protection factor (such as exercise) in combination with a drug treatment to lessen the impact of a provoking agent? In pharmacotherapy, would the presence of a drug-based protection factor be sufficient to offset the effect of strong provoking agents? Alternatively, would drugs intended to blunt the action of provoking agents be equally effective against the inductive effect of high fat, high carbohydrate, cafeteria or other types of provocative diets?

This attempt to conceptualize the arrangement of causal factors contributing to obesity has been provoked by a consideration of the effects of nutritional manipulations. It is clear, however, that other experimental treatments can be inserted into the arrangement of factors embraced by the model. For example, lesions of the ventromedial nucleus, parasagittal knife cuts, paraventricular nucleus lesions, or other interventions could all be regarded as vulnerability factors whose effect is only fully realized in the presence of certain provoking agents or amplification factors, or in the absence of protection factors. In this way the model builds upon the diet-dependency dimension proposed by Sclafani[3] and embraces the hereditary, traumatic, and environmental factors set out by Mayer.[1] It is intended that this scheme will provide a basis for the rational use of animal models in understanding obesity. A similar conceptualization for human obesity could help in the development of therapeutic strategies.

REFERENCES

1. MAYER, J. 1953. Genetic, traumatic and environmental factors in the etiology of obesity. Physiol. Rev. 33: 472–508.
2. SCLAFANI, A. 1981. Extremes in body weight in experimental animal preparations. In The Body Weight Regulatory System: Normal and Disturbed Mechanisms. L. A. Cioffi, W. P. T. James & T. B. Van Itallie, Eds.: 153–160. Raven Press. New York.
3. SCLAFANI, A. 1984. Animal models of obesity: classification and characterisation. Int. J. Obesity. 8: 491–508.
4. SCLAFANI, A. 1978. Dietary obesity. In Recent Advances in Obesity Research II. G. Bray, Ed.: 123–132. Newman. London.
5. KANAREK, R. B. & E. HIRSCH. 1977. Dietary-induced overeating in experimental animals. Fed. Proc. Fed. Am. Soc. Exp. Biol. 36: 154–158.
6. INGLE, D. J. 1949. A simple means of producing obesity in the rat. Proc. Soc. Exp. Biol. Med. 72: 604–605.
7. LEMONNIER, D. 1972. Effect of age, sex and site on the cellularity of the adipose tissue in mice and rats rendered obese by a high fat diet. J. Clin. Invest. 51: 2907–2915.
8. ROMSOS, D. R., M. J. HORNSHUTT & G. A. LEVEILLE. 1978. Influence of dietary fat

and carbohydrate on food intake, body weight and body fat of adult dogs. Proc. Soc. Exp. Med. **157:** 278–281.

9. JEN, K. L. C. 1980. The effect of high fat diet on the behavioural patterns of male rats. Physiol. Behav. **25:** 373–381.

10. WOOD, J. D. & J. T. REID. 1975. The influence of dietary fat on fat metabolism and body fat deposition in meal-feeding and nibbling rats. Br. J. Nutr. **34:** 15–24.

11. FAUST, I. M., P. R. JOHNSON, J. S. STERN & J. HIRSCH. 1978. Diet-induced adipocyte number increase in adult rats: a new model of obesity. Am. J. Physiol. **235:** E279–E286.

12. FAUST, I. M., J. TRISCARI, A. SCLAFANI, W. H. MILLER & A. C. SULLIVAN. 1980. Moderate adipocyte hyperplasia in the chow-fed VMH rat. Fed. Proc. Fed. Am. Soc. Exp. Biol. **39:** 887.

13. FAUST, I. M. 1981. Factors which affect adipocyte formation in the rat. *In* Recent Advances in Obesity Research: III. P. Bjorntorp, M. Cairella & A. N. Howard, Eds.: 52–57. Libby. London.

14. FAUST, I. M. 1980. Nutrition and the fat cell. Int. J. Obesity **4:** 314–321.

15. ALLEN, R. J. L. & J. S. LEAHY. 1966. Some effects of dietary dextrose, fructose, liquid glucose and sucrose in the adult male rat. Br. J. Nutr. **20:** 339–347.

16. KANAREK, R. B. & R. MARKS-KAUFMANN. 1979. Developmental aspects of sucrose-induced obesity in rats. Physiol. Behav. **23:** 881–885.

17. HILL, W., T. W. CASTONGUAY & G. H. COLLIER. 1980. Taste or Diet Balancing? Physiol. Behav. **24:** 765–767.

18. SCLAFANI, A. & S. XENAKIS. 1984. Sucrose and polysaccharide induced obesity in the rat. Physiol. Behav. **32:** 169–174.

19. SCLAFANI, A. & S. XENAKIS. 1984. Influence of diet form on the hyperphagia-promoting effect of polysaccharide in rats. Life Sci. **34:** 1253–1259.

20. HILL, A., P. ROGERS & J. BLUNDELL. 1983. Effect of an anorexic drug (d-Fenfluramine) on body weight and food intake during the dynamic and plateau phases of dietary-induced obesity in rats: more potent drug action in obese animals. Proceeding of IV Int. Cong. on Obesity. 11A. New York, Oct. 5–8.

21. MCARTHUR, R. A. & J. E. BLUNDELL. 1986. Dietary self-selection of protein and energy is altered by the texture of the diets. Physiol. Behav. **38:** 315–319.

22. SCLAFANI, A. 1987. Carbohydrate taste, appetite and obesity: an overview. Neurosci. Biobehav. Rev. **11.** In press.

23. SCLAFANI, A. & D. SPRINGER. 1976. Dietary obesity in adult rats: similarities to hypothalamic and human obesity syndromes. Physiol. Behav. **17:** 461–471.

24. SCLAFANI, A. & A. N. GORMAN. 1977. Effects of age, sex and prior body weight on the development of dietary obesity in adult rats. Physiol. Behav. **18:** 1021–1026.

25. ROGERS, P. J. & J. E. BLUNDELL. 1984. Meal patterns and food selection during the development of obesity in rats fed a cafeteria diet. Neurosci. Biobehav. Rev. **8:** 441–453.

26. ROGERS, P. J. & J. E. BLUNDELL. 1980. Investigation of food selection and meal parameters during the development of dietary induced obesity. Appetite. **1:** 85.

27. ROGERS, P. J. 1985. Returning 'cafeteria-fed' rats to a chow diet: negative contrast and effects of obesity on feeding behaviour. Physiol. Behav. **35:** 493–499.

28. ROTHWELL, N. J. & M. J. STOCK. 1979. A role for brown adipose tissue in diet-induced thermogenesis. Nature (London) **281:** 31–35.

29. ROLLS, B. J., E. A. ROWE & R. C. TURNER. 1980. Persistent obesity in rats following a period of consumption of a mixed energy diet. J. Physiol. (London) **298:** 415–427.

30. BOWDEN, C. R., K. D. WHITE & G. F. TUTWILER. 1985. Energy intake of cafeteria-diet and chow-fed rats in response to amphetamine, fenfluramine, (-)-hydroxycitrate, and naloxone. J. Obesity Wt. Reg. **1:** 5–13.

31. BLUNDELL, J. E. & A. J. HILL. 1985. Effect of dextrofenfluramine on feeding and body weight: relationship with food composition and palatability. *In* Metabolic Complications of Human Obesities. J. Vague, B. Guy-Grand & P. Bjorntorp, Eds.: 199–206. Elsevier. Nordholland.

32. BLUNDELL, J. E. 1983. Process and problems underlying the control of food selection and nutrient intake. *In* Nutrition and the Brain. R. J. Wurtman & J. J. Wurtman, Eds.: **6:** 164–221. Raven Press. New York.

33. WURTMAN, J. J. 1985. Neurotransmitter control of carbohydrate consumption. Ann. N. Y. Acad. Sci. **443:** 145–151.
34. DREWNOWSKI, A. & M. R. C. GREENWOOD. 1983. Cream and sugar: human preferences for high-fat foods. Physiol. Behav. **30:** 629–633.
35. ANDIK, I., J. BANK & S. DONHOFER. 1957. The effect of hypothalamic lesions on intake and selection of foods by rats. Arch. Exp. Pathol. Pharmakol. **231:** 55–62.
36. KANAREK, R. B., P. G. FELDMAN & C. HANES. 1981. Pattern of dietary self-selection in VMH-lesioned rats. Physiol. Behav. **27:** 337–343.
37. SCLAFANI, A. & P. F. ARAVICH. 1983. Macronutrient self-selection in three forms of hypothalamic obesity. Am. J. Physiol. **244:** R686–R694.
38. OVERMANN, S. R. & M. G. YANG. 1973. Adaptation to water restriction through dietary selection in weanling rats. Physiol. Behav. **11:** 781–786.
39. ANDERSON, G. H., C. LEPROHON, J. W. CHAMBERS & D. V. COSCINA. 1979. Intact regulation of protein intake during the development of hypothalamic or genetic obesity in rats. Physiol. Behav. **23:** 751–755.
40. CHEE, K. M., D. R. ROMSOS & W. G. BERGEN. 1981. Effects of dietary fat on protein intake regulation in young obese and lean mice. J. Nutr. **111:** 668–677.
41. POWLEY, J. 1977. The ventromedial hypothalamic syndrome, satiety and a cephalic phase hypothesis. Psychol. Rev. **84:** 89–126.
42. JEANRENAUD, B., P. ASSIMACOPOULOS-JEANNET, M. CRETTAZ, H. R. BERTHOUD, D. A. BEREITER & F. ROHNER-JEANRENAUD. 1981. Experimental obesities: a progressive pathology with reference to the potential importance of the CNS in hyperinsulinaemia. *In* Recent Advances in Obesity Research. P. Bjorntorp, M. Cairella & A. N. Howard, Eds.: 159–171. Libby. London.
43. SJOSTROM, L., G. GARELLICK, M. KROTKIEVSKY & A. LUYCKX. 1980. Peripheral insulin in response to the sight and smell of food. Metab. Clin. Exp. **29:** 901–909.
44. DREWNOWSKI, A., A. E. COHEN, I. M. FAUST & J. A. GRINKER. 1984. Meal-taking behaviour is related to predisposition to dietary obesity in the rat. Physiol. Behav. **32:** 61–67.
45. KULESZA, W. 1982. Dietary intake in obese women. Appetite **3:** 61–68.
46. PILGRIM, F. & R. PATTON. 1947. Patterns of self-selection of purified dietary components by the rat. J. Comp. Physiol. Psychol. **40:** 343–348.
47. LEATHWOOD, P. D. & D. V. M. ASHLEY. 1983. Strategies of protein selection by weanling and adult rats. Appetite **4:** 97–112.
48. MCARTHUR, R. A. & J. E. BLUNDELL. 1983. Protein and carbohydrate self-selection: modification of the effects of fenfluramine and amphetamine by age and feeding regimen. Appetite **4:** 113–124.
49. KON, S. 1931. The self-selection of food constituents by the rat. Biochemical J. **25:** 473–481.
50. LAT, J. 1967. Self-selection of dietary components. *In* Handbook of Physiology. F. Code, Ed. Vol. 1: Alimentary Canal. American Physiology Society. Washington, D.C.
51. SIMS, E. A. H., R. F. GOLDMAN, C. M. GLUCK, E. S. HORTON, P. C. KELLEHER & D. W. ROWE. 1968. Experimental obesity in man. Trans. Assoc. Am. Physicians **81:** 153–170.
52. BLUNDELL, J. E. & P. J. ROGERS. 1978. Pharmacological approaches to the understanding of obesity. Psychiatr. Clin. N. Am. **1:** 629–650.
53. APPLEGATE, E. A., D. E. UPTON & J. S. STERN. 1982. Food intake, body composition and blood lipids following treadmill exercise in male and female rats. Physiol. Behav. **28:** 917–920.
54. BLUNDELL, J. E. & A. J. HILL. 1980. Behavioural pharmacology of feeding: relevance of animal experiments for studies in man. *In* Pharmacology of Eating Disorders: Theoretical and Clinical Advances. M. O. Carruba & J. E. Blundell, Eds. 51–70. Raven Press. New York.
55. SULLIVAN, A. 1987. New developments in pharmacological treatments. *In* Human Obesity. R. J. Wurtman & J. J. Wurtman, Eds. Ann. N. Y. Acad. Sci. This volume.
56. BROWN, G. W. & T. HARRIS. 1978. Social origins of depression. A study of psychiatric disorder in women. Tavistock. London.

From Fenfluramine Racemate to d-Fenfluramine

Specificity and Potency of the Effects on the Serotoninergic System and Food Intake

SILVIO GARATTINI, TIZIANA MENNINI,
AND ROSARIO SAMANIN

Istituto di Ricerche Farmacologiche "Mario Negri"
20157 Milan, Italy

INTRODUCTION

Considerable evidence suggests that serotonin (5-HT) in the brain acts to suppress feeding in laboratory animals. The suggestion is based mainly on the fact that 5-HT injections in certain brain areas and various indirect and direct agonists at central serotoninergic synapses cause marked reduction of food intake in various animal species.[1-4] Recently, reduction of central 5-HT function by a selective neurotoxin for 5-HT neurons or 8-OH-DPAT, a 5-HT$_{1A}$ agonist, was found to increase eating in sated rats,[5] confirming that 5-HT–containing neurons act by tonically inhibiting feeding in this animal species.

There is as yet no direct evidence of this in humans, although the fact that fenfluramine, a releaser and uptake inhibitor of 5-HT[2,6,7] causes anorexia in humans makes this likely. The fact, however, that fenfluramine also affects catecholamines in the brain (although at doses higher than those affecting 5-HT) and that catecholamines are involved in the anorectic activity of other phenylethylamines such as amphetamine and diethylpropion[2,3,6,7] makes it uncertain which endogenous compound mediates the anorectic effect of fenfluramine in humans. A good opportunity for clarifying this issue is offered by the finding that the d and l isomers of fenfluramine and its active metabolite, norfenfluramine, have different biochemical and functional effects, with the d isomer showing more potency and specificity in its effects on the serotoninergic system and food intake.[4,7]

The present study is aimed at providing, through *in vitro* and *in vivo* studies, further evidence that the d isomer of fenfluramine specifically and potently affects 5-HT mechanisms and food intake in the rat. It also shows that 5-HT$_1$ receptors are preferentially involved in the anorectic effect of d-fenfluramine. The ability of d-fenfluramine (d-F) to cause a marked inhibition of various types of hyperphagia, including those resistant to amphetamine, is also discussed. Finally, the characteristics, brain regional distribution, and pharmacological characterization of [^{3}H]d-F binding in the rat are shown. We hope that these sites may help in developing novel and more potent strategies in the pharmacological treatment of clinical obesity.

156

IN VITRO STUDIES ON MONOAMINE MECHANISMS

The effects of d and l isomers of fenfluramine and norfenfluramine on various monoamine mechanisms are shown in TABLE 1. The l forms were found slightly more potent than the d forms in displacing 5-HT_1 binding sites, whereas d-norfenfluramine (d-NF) was more active at 5-HT_2 binding sites. However, IC_{50} for fenfluramine isomers and metabolites were considerably higher than for known 5-HT receptor agonists and antagonists (IC_{50} in μM for 5-HT on 5-HT_1 and metergoline on 5-HT_2 binding was 0.002). d-F was the least active compound at both

TABLE 1. Effects of the Stereoisomers of Fenfluramine and Norfenfluramine on Monoamine Mechanisms[a]

Amine Mechanisms	d-F	d-NF	l-F	l-NF
Binding (IC_{50} μM)				
5-HT_1	7.0	4.2	2.7	2.2
5-HT_2	>30.0	2.2	4.5	3.0
D_2	>30.0	>30.0	>30.0	>30.0
βNA	>30.0	10.0	>30.0	6.0
α_1NA	>30.0	>30.0	5.4	15.0
α_2NA	25.0	17.0	>30.0	20.0
Uptake (IC_{50} μM)				
NA	10.0	1.8	13.0	—
DA	20.0	17.0	38.0	—
5-HT	0.5	1.4	8.9	14.0
Release SC_{25}				
5-HT (normal)	5.0	1.0	3.0	2.0
5-HT (reserpine)[b]	>100.0	0.2	1.0	2.0

[a] [³H]5-HT uptake, release, and binding were studied according to the method described by Mennini et al.[8,9,10] Data are means of four replications varying less than 10%. IC_{50} are the drug concentrations producing 50% inhibition of uptake or binding, and are calculated from the log dose-effect plot of the data, using three to four drug concentrations. SC_{25} are the drug concentrations stimulating [³H]5-HT release by 25%, calculated from the log dose-effect plot of the data using three drugs concentrations. % release stimulation = (% release with drugs/ % release of controls × 100) − 100. Data for CA binding are IC_{50} μM, obtained from three to four replications varying less than 5%. 5-HT₂ and CA receptor binding was determined as described by Mennini et al.[11] using the following ligands: [³H]Spiperone (5-HT₂ and D₂), [³H]dihydroalprenolol (βNA), [³H]WB4101 (α_1NA), and [³H]Clonidine (α_2NA).
[b] The animals received 10 mg/kg reserpine intraperitoneally 18 h before death.

binding sites. Fenfluramine isomers and metabolites did not significantly affect D_2-receptor binding to rat brain membranes, whereas some weak effects were found with certain compounds on β, alpha$_1$, and alpha$_2$ noradrenaline (NA) binding. In particular, fenfluramine metabolites appeared to be more active than fenfluramine in displacing β NA binding and l isomers of fenfluramine, and norfenfluramine, unlike the d isomers, showed some activity on alpha$_1$ NA binding. With the exception of l-fenfluramine (l-F), the various compounds inhibited the alpha$_2$ binding with IC_{50} of about 20 μM.

d-Fenfluramine was a powerful inhibitor of 5-HT uptake into nerve endings, as shown by the fact that at 0.5 μM it caused 50% inhibition of the accumulation of [^{3}H]5-HT into the synaptosomes of rat brain. d-NF, l-F, and l-norfenfluramine (l-NF) were less potent than d-F as 5-HT uptake inhibitors, showing IC$_{50}$ values of 1.4, 8.9, and 14.0 μM respectively. Fenfluramine isomers and metabolites were much less potent in inhibiting the uptake of noradrenaline (NA) and dopamine (DA) into nerve endings, with the exception of d-NF's effect on NA uptake (IC$_{50}$ = 1.8 μM). Fenfluramine isomers and metabolites significantly increased the release of [^{3}H]5-HT in the rat brain synaptosomes with SC$_{25}$ ranging from 1 to 5 μM. The effects of d-F and d-NF on [^{3}H]5-HT release markedly differed in brain synaptosomes of rats given an intraperitoneal injection of 10 mg/kg reserpine 18 h before the experiments, whereas the effect of l isomers was not appreciably affected. In these conditions d-F practically lost its ability to release [^{3}H]5-HT (SC$_{25}$ higher than 100 μM), whereas the effect of d-NF was actually potentiated (SC$_{25}$ 0.2 μM). These data can be interpreted as showing that d-F uses a granular pool sensitive to reserpine to release 5-HT from nerve terminals, whereas d-NF may preferentially use a reserpine-insensitive compartment.

The data show that d-F is particularly potent in inhibiting 5-HT uptake and that d-NF is potent in releasing 5-HT from a reserpine-insensitive pool. Because substantial amounts of d-NF, which persist for a long time even after a single dose of fenfluramine, are found in the brain after d-F's administration,[7] the findings suggest that a long-lasting increase of 5-HT availability at central synapses occurs in animals treated with d-F. As regards the effects of the various compounds on catecholamine receptor binding and uptake, no major differences were found, with the possible exception of l isomers of fenfluramine and norfenfluramine, which unlike d isomers, showed some activity in displacing alpha$_1$ NA binding. As we will see in the next paragraph, the l isomer of fenfluramine preferentially affects catecholamine metabolism in the rat brain by a mechanism that is not yet clarified, but that seems to involve a blockade of catecholamine-dependent behavior in this species.[12]

EFFECTS ON MONOAMINE METABOLISM AND 5-HT SYNTHESIS

As shown in TABLE 2, an oral administration of 2.5 and 5.0 mg/kg d-F significantly reduced the brain levels of 5-hydroxyindole acetic acid (5-HIAA), the major metabolite of 5-HT, with no effect on the metabolism of NA and DA measured as 3-methoxy-4-hydroxyphenylethylene glycol sulphate (MHPG-SO$_4$) and dihydroxyphenylacetic acid (DOPAC), respectively. By contrast, 2.5 and 5 mg/kg p.o. l-F significantly increased MHPG-SO$_4$ and DOPAC with no effect on 5-HIAA. The peak of d-F's effect on 5-HIAA was observed at 4 h after injection, whereas 1 h was the peak time for the effect of l-F on catecholamine metabolites.[13]

In order to get further information on the potency of the two isomers in affecting central 5-HT mechanisms, we measured the accumulation of 5-hydro-tryptophan after decarboxylase inhibition in rats 1 h after treatment with various doses of d-F and l-F. As shown in TABLE 3, an oral dose of 2.5 mg/kg d-F significantly reduced 5-HT synthesis in the hypothalamus and brainstem, whereas the same effects were observed with 10 mg/kg p.o. l-F. Because 2.5 mg/kg d-F and 10 mg/kg l-F correspond to equiactive anorectic doses (about 80% reduction of food intake), the results indicate that nearly maximal anorexia with d- and l-F is associated with decreased 5-HT synthesis in the rat brain. It should be noted, however, that the anorectic effect of 2.5 mg/kg i.p. d-F, but not that of 10 mg/kg

TABLE 2. Effects of d and l isomers of Fenfluramine on Monoamine Metabolism in the Rat Brain[a]

Dose (mg/kg p.o.)	5-HIAA	Percent of controls MHPG-SO$_4$	DOPAC
d-F 2.5	74 ± 4[c]	96 ± 4	85 ± 4
d-F 5.0	70 ± 7[c]	95 ± 5	89 ± 4
l-F 2.5	93 ± 14	137 ± 14[b]	126 ± 9[c]
l-F 5.0	86 ± 7	140 ± 5[c]	136 ± 10[c]

[a] 5-HIAA was measured 4 h after injection by the method of Wightman et al.[14] MHPG-SO$_4$ and DOPAC were measured 1 h after injection according to Kohno et al.[15] and Achilli et al.[16] respectively.
[b] p < 0.05
[c] p < 0.01 vs control (Dunnett's test).

TABLE 3. Effects of d- and l-Fenfluramine on 5-Hydroxytryptophan (5-HTP) Accumulation in the Hypothalamus and Brain Stem of Rats[a]

Drug	mg/kg	5-HTP ng/g Hypothalamus	Brain Stem
Control	—	178 ± 8	176 ± 7
d-F	1.25	164 ± 11	180 ± 6
d-F	2.50	142 ± 9[b]	136 ± 6[c]
d-F	5.00	107 ± 7[c]	120 ± 4[c]
Control	—	208 ± 12	163 ± 14
l-F	5.00	170 ± 11	157 ± 5
l-F	10.00	134 ± 9[c]	103 ± 5[c]

[a] The animals were killed 30 minutes after intraperitoneal injection of 100 mg/kg NSD 1015. Fenfluramine was administered orally 30 minutes before NSD 1015. 5-HTP levels were measured according to the method of Di Paolo et al.[17] with slight modifications. Each value is the mean ± SEM of six determinations.
[b] p < 0.05
[c] p < 0.01 compared with controls (Dunnett's test).

TABLE 4. Effect of Blockade of 5-HT Receptors on Anorexia by d-F and l-F in Rats[a]

Treatment	mg/kg p.o.	1 h food intake ± SEM Vehicle	Metergoline
Saline	—	8.6 ± 1.1	6.7 ± 0.5
d-F	2.5	2.4 ± 0.6[c]	6.2 ± 0.7[d]
l-F	10.0	2.2 ± 0.5[c]	3.4 ± 0.8[b]

[a] Female rats weighing 200 g were trained over two weeks to eat their food during a daily 4 h period (11:00–15:00 h). Metergoline 1 mg/kg i.p. was injected 2 h before d-fenfluramine or l-fenfluramine. d-Fenfluramine and l-fenfluramine were administered 1 h before the feeding test. Each value represents the mean of 7 rats. F interaction (ANOVA 2 × 2) was significant for the d-fenfluramine group (p < 0.02) but not for l-fenfluramine.
[b] p < 0.05 versus respective saline group.
[c] p < 0.01 versus respective saline group.
[d] p < 0.01 versus vehicle group.

l-F, was prevented by metergoline, a 5-HT antagonist (TABLE 4), suggesting that mechanisms other than 5-HT are involved in decrease of food intake caused by the *l* isomer of fenfluramine. Because *d*-F anorexia depends on its ability to increase the availability of 5-HT at central receptors, the reduction of 5-HT synthesis is probably secondary to stimulation of auto- and/or postsynaptic 5-HT receptors through inhibition of uptake and increased release.

EVIDENCE AGAINST A ROLE OF 5-HT₂ RECEPTORS IN MEDIATING THE ANORECTIC ACTIVITY OF *d*-FENFLURAMINE

In order to evaluate the possible role of 5-HT_2 receptors in the reduction of food intake caused by *d*-F in rats, we compared two serotonin antagonists: metergoline, a competitive antagonist of 5-HT_1 receptors[18] with similar *in vitro* affinity for both 5-HT_1 and 5-HT_2 receptors,[19] and ritanserin, a potent and selective 5-HT_2 receptor antagonist.[20] We measured the *in vivo* occupancy of cortical 5-HT_2 receptors[21] in rats at the same treatment schedule used to measure the inhibition of food intake exerted by *d*-F.[22] The data reported in FIGURE 1 show that doses of the two antagonists that result in the same *in vivo* occupancy of 5-HT_2 receptors (about 50%) produced respectively maximal inhibition (metergoline, 1 mg/kg) or no significant inhibition (ritanserin, 0.5 mg/kg) of the anorectic effect of *d*-F. These results clearly argue against a role of 5-HT_2 receptors in mediating the anorectic effect of *d*-F.

EFFECTS OF *d*-FENFLURAMINE AND *d*-AMPHETAMINE ON VARIOUS FORMS OF HYPERPHAGIA IN RATS

Although *d*-amphetamine is equally or even more potent than *d*-fenfluramine in inhibiting food intake of starved rats or the intake of palatable food by sated

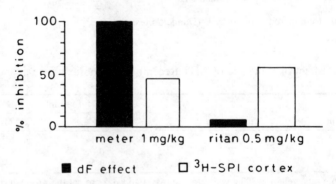

FIGURE 1. Metergoline (meter)(1 mg/kg) was given i.p. 150 min before the experiments; ritanserin (ritan)(0.5 mg/kg i.p.) 30 min before. For food intake experiments, rats were treated i.p. with 2.5 mg/kg of *d*-fenfluramine, as described in detail elsewhere.[10] For *in vivo* occupancy of 5-HT_2 receptors, rats were injected i.v. with 50 μCi of [³H]spiperone[21] ([³H]SPI). Data are calculated as percent inhibition of *d*-F effect on food intake and percent inhibition of specific [³H]spiperone binding in cortex, and are means of four animals per group.

TABLE 5. Effect of *d*-Fenfluramine and *d*-Amphetamine on Various Hyperphagias in Rats

Type of Hyperphagia	*d*-Fenfluramine	*d*-Amphetamine
Food intake of starved rats	$++^b$	$++^b$
Intake of palatable food by sated rats	$++^b$	$+++^a$
Eating induced by neuropeptide Y in the paraventricular nucleus of the hypothalamus	$++^b$	$+^c$
Eating induced by tail pinch	$++^b$	$-^d$
Eating induced by insulin glucoprivation	$++^b$	$-^d$
Eating induced by muscimol	$+++^a$	$-^d$

^{a} $+++$ = very active
^{b} $++$ = active
^{c} $+$ = moderately active
^{d} $-$ = inactive (up to 2.5 mg/kg i.p.)

rats,[23,24] it is unable to modify the eating associated with stressful stimuli or caused by muscimol injection in the nucleus raphe dorsalis.[3,24,25] By contrast, in this latter form of eating, *d*-F is more effective on food intake of starved rats.[24] Of particular interest is the finding that 5-HT injection in the nucleus accumbens blocks hyperphagia caused by muscimol injection in the raphe dorsalis but has no effect on eating by food-deprived rats.[26] The fact that the injection of *d*-NF in the nucleus accumbens also inhibits eating induced by muscimol injection in the raphe dorsalis but not that of starved rats[26] suggests that this area plays a role in the inhibitory effects of 5-HT and serotoninergic drugs on particular types of overeating not associated with nutritional deficits. Recently, we have studied the effect of *d*-F and *d*-amphetamine on eating caused by the injection of neuropeptide Y in the paraventricular nucleus of the hypothalamus in rats and found that both drugs inhibited this type of eating, with *d*-F being slightly more effective. TABLE 5 summarizes the effects of *d*-F and *d*-amphetamine on the various types of hyperphagia. The main conclusion of these studies is that the effectiveness of anorectic drugs may depend on the mechanism primarily involved in a particular eating disorder. The difficulty of recognizing the intrinsic factors affecting the action of different anorectics may be one reason for the limited success of available drugs. The effectiveness of *d*-F in various models of hyperphagia, however, should encourage the use of this drug for the long-term control of clinical hyperphagia and obesity.

[³H]*d*-FENFLURAMINE BINDING

Binding Characterization

High affinity[³H]*d*-fenfluramine binding (specific activity 16 Ci/nmol, Commissariat à l'Energie Atomique) has been characterized in rat brain membranes, incubated at 37°C for 90 minutes in 50 mM Tris HCl buffer, pH 7.4, containing 0.1% ascorbic acid. As shown in FIGURE 2, the specific binding, determined with

Kinetics of ^{3}H-dFenfluramine binding

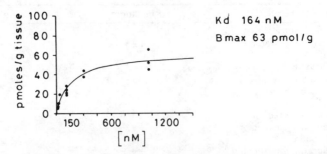

Kd 164 nM

Bmax 63 pmol/g

FIGURE 2. Saturation curve of [^{3}H]d-fenfluramine binding was obtained by incubating [^{3}H]d-F (8–1000 nM) at 37°C for 90 minutes, in presence or absence of 10 μM d-F to determine nonspecific binding. Crude membrane preparations of rat brain (15 mg original wet weight) were used in final incubation volume of 1 ml. Kinetic parameters (K$_d$ and B max) were determined by nonlinear fitting of the experimental points.

10 μM cold d-fenfluramine, is saturable, with K$_d$ 163.7 ± 27.4 nM and B max of 63.0 ± 3.7 pmoles/g tissue. It is inhibited dose-dependently (5–120 mM) by NaCl added *in vitro*, with IC$_{50}$ of about 5 mM. TABLE 6 reports the pharmacological characterization of [^{3}H]d-fenfluramine binding in rat whole brain, excluding cerebellum. It appears to be highly stereospecific, since the l-isomer has affinity one order of magnitude lower than the d form. It is shared with the same affinity by the normetabolite. The most active compounds in inhibiting [^{3}H]d-fenfluramine binding are imipramine and fluoxetine, followed by other tricyclic and nontricyclic 5-HT uptake inhibitors. Among the other compounds examined, belonging to different pharmacological classes, only desipramine and clonidine inhibit [^{3}H]d-fenfluramine binding, although at micromolar concentrations.

Regional Distribution

TABLE 7 reports the regional distribution of [^{3}H]d-fenfluramine binding, 2 minutes after i.v. injection of 53.7 μCi/rat. Nonspecific binding was calculated in parallel samples after *in vitro* dissociation (90 minutes at 37°C) of total [^{3}H]d-fenfluramine bound in presence of 10 μM cold d-fenfluramine. It can be seen that the regional distribution of [^{3}H]d-fenfluramine binding does not parallel the endogenous concentrations of serotonin, being high in cerebellum and low in striatum.

Comparison with [^{3}H]Imipramine Binding

Several differences can be found between [^{3}H]d-fenfluramine and [^{3}H]imipramine binding. First the effect of sodium: [^{3}H]imipramine binding is enhanced by sodium,[27] whereas [^{3}H]d-fenfluramine binding is inhibited by NaCl, resembling in this respect [^{3}H]d-amphetamine binding, which is also inhibited by sodium.[28] This similarity is casual, however, because d-amphetamine does not inhibit [^{3}H]d-fenfluramine binding at the highest concentration tested (100 μM). Another important difference between [³H]d-fenfluramine and [³H]imipramine binding is the relation to presynaptic serotonin nerve endings: although the regional distribution of [³H]imipramine binding closely parallels that of endogenous serotonin,[29] the regional distribution of [³H]d-fenfluramine binding does not. Moreover, some discrepancies exist between the drug's inhibition of the two ligands. In fact, LM5008, a potent inhibitor of serotonin uptake devoid of anorectic activity,[30] is

TABLE 6. Drugs Inhibition of [³H]d-Fenfluramine Binding[a]

			$-\log IC_{50}$	SEM
Fenfluramine Analogues		d-Fenfluramine	6.79	0.41
		d-Norfenfluramine	6.68	0.43
		l-Fenfluramine	5.78	0.30
		l-Norfenfluramine	5.83	0.16
5-HT Uptake Inhibitors		Imipramine	7.25	0.42
		Fluoxetine	6.91	0.29
		Amitriptyline	6.18	0.22
		Citalopram	6.13	0.22
		Chlorimipramine	6.04	0.52
		LM 5008	6.01	0.32
Drugs Active at 5-HT Receptors	5HT-1	Serotonin	3.52	0.23
	5HT-1 A	8-OH DPAT	5.86	0.16
	5HT-1 B	RU 24969	3.92	0.23
	5HT-2	Spiperone	5.06	0.35
	5HT-2	Ketanserin	5.37	0.28
		Trazodone	5.95	0.16
		Metergoline	5.54	0.28
		Quipazine	4.45	0.24
		mCPP	3.82	0.27
		d-LSD	3.76	0.25
NA Agents		Desipramine	6.04	0.52
		Clonidine	6.03	0.52
		(−) Propanolol	5.80	0.24
		Phentolamine	3.71	0.26
		Isoproterenol	<4.00	
		Prazosin	<4.00	
		(−) Noradrenaline	<4.00	
DA Agents		Apomorphine	<4.00	
		d-Amphetamine	<4.00	
		Nomifensine	<4.00	
		(+) Butaclamol	<4.00	
		Dopamine	<4.00	
GABAergic Agents		GABA	<4.00	
		Muscimol	<4.00	
		Diazepam	<4.00	
Others		Reserpine	5.94	0.77
		Verapamil	5.26	0.33
		Mepyramine	5.15	0.24
		Pargyline	4.60	0.29
		Atropine	4.02	0.22

[a] IC_{50} (drug concentration producing half maximal inhibition of total [³H]d-fenfluramine binding) were determined by incubating 10 nM [³H]d-fenfluramine in the presence of four to six drug concentrations for 90 min at 37°C with a crude rat membrane preparation (15 mg original wet weight). Samples were filtered through Whatman GF/B glass fiber filters and counted for radioactivity content.

TABLE 7. Regional Distribution of [³H]d-Fenfluramine Binding and 5-HT Levels in the Rat Brain[a]

	[³H]d-Fenfluramine Binding (fmoles/mg protein)	5-HT Concentrations (ng/g tissue)
Cortex	36.5 ± 9.5	254 ± 12
Cerebellum	31.6 ± 5.7	66 ± 10
Brainstem	32.9 ± 9.7	333 ± 27
Hippocampus	18.9 ± 6.4	186 ± 13
Striatum	13.1 ± 1.7	324 ± 26
Hypothalamus	25.8 ± 11.4	716 ± 20

[a] [³H]fenfluramine binding in vivo was determined 2 min after i.v. injection of 50 μCi/rat. Brain regions were homogenized, and aliquots of the homogenate were filtered on Whatman GF/B glass fiber filters. Others were incubated for 90 min at 37°C to determine nonspecific binding and then filtered as described. 5-HT concentrations were determined by high performance liquid chromatography with electrochemical detection (HPLCED).[13] Data are means ± SD of three to four animals per group.

one of the most potent inhibitors of [³H]imipramine binding,[31] but is poorly active on [³H]d-fenfluramine binding. Taken together, these points suggest that the binding sites for [³H]d-fenfluramine, different from those of [³H]imipramine, are not related to the serotonin uptake carrier. The possibility that these sites represent the target of action of drugs that exert anorectic activity acting on serotonin is under investigation.

CONCLUSION

Fenfluramine, used as an anorexigenic drug in obese people, has contributed considerably to the hypothesis of a role of 5-HT in feeding. The fact that the d isomer of fenfluramine releases 5-HT from nerve terminals and inhibits its reuptake more potently and specifically than the racemate and is more potent in causing anorexia in rats and reducing body weight in obese patients confirms that brain 5-HT has an inhibitory role on feeding in several animal species, including humans. The demonstration of high-affinity [³H]d-fenfluramine binding to rat brain membranes, which is displaced by some drugs using 5-HT to cause anorexia, together with the fact that 5-HT$_1$ are preferentially involved in d-fenfluramine's anorexia, may help in developing novel and potent strategies for the treatment of clinical hyperphagia. Besides its use as an appetite suppressant in obese people, d-fenfluramine may constitute a very valuable tool for improving our knowledge of the functional role of 5-HT in the central nervous system and in the periphery.

SUMMARY

Experiments using the binding of various ligands for monoamines to rat brain membranes and synaptosomal preparations for studying monoamine uptake and release have shown that d-fenfluramine is more potent than the l isomer in inhibiting 5-HT uptake, whereas d-norfenfluramine preferentially releases 5-HT from a reserpine-insensitive compartment. Studies on brain monoamine metabolism in intact animals have shown that the d and l isomers of fenfluramine at relatively low doses have a specific action on brain 5-HT and catecholamines, respectively. Based on the different ability of metergoline and ritanserin to displace 5-HT$_2$ binding to rat brain membranes and to antagonize d-fenfluramine's anorexia, evidence has been provided that d-fenfluramine preferentially uses 5-HT$_1$ sites in the rat brain to cause anorexia in this animal species. Finally, characteristics, regional distribution, and pharmacological characterization of a high-affinity [^{3}H]d-fenfluramine binding to rat brain membranes have been described. This binding appears to be different from 5-HT uptake sites ([^{3}H]imipramine binding) and 5-HT receptors and is not regionally related to the endogenous levels of 5-HT in the rat brain. It is, however, preferentially displaced by some agents using 5-HT to cause anorexia in rats, raising the possibility that it is somewhat related to 5-HT mechanisms involved in feeding control.

REFERENCES

1. BLUNDELL, J. E. 1977. Int. J. Obesity 1: 15–42.
2. GARATTINI, S. & R. SAMANIN. 1976. In Dahlem Workshop on Appetite and Food Intake. T. Silverstone, Ed.: 83–108.
3. SAMANIN, R. & S. GARATTINI. 1982. In Drugs and Appetite. T. Silverstone, Ed.: 23–39. Academic Press. London.
4. SAMANIN, R. 1983. In Biochemical Pharmacology of Obesity. P. B. Curtis-Prior, Ed.: 339–356. Elsevier. Amsterdam.
5. BENDOTTI, C. & R. SAMANIN. 1986. Eur. J. Pharmacol. 121: 147–150.
6. GARATTINI, S., W. BUCZKO, A. JORI & R. SAMANIN. 1975. Postgrad. Med. J. 51 suppl. 1: 27–35.
7. GARATTINI, S., S. CACCIA, T. MENNINI, R. SAMANIN, S. CONSOLO & H. LADINSKY. 1979. Curr. Med. Res. Opin. 6 suppl. 1: 15–27.
8. MENNINI, T., E. BORRONI, R. SAMANIN & S. GARATTINI. 1981. Neurochem. Int. 3: 289–294.
9. MENNINI, T., R. PATACCINI & R. SAMANIN. 1978. Br. J. Pharmacol. 64: 75–82.
10. MENNINI, T., S. GARATTINI & S. CACCIA. 1985. Psychopharmacology 85: 111–114.
11. CECI, A., S. GARATTINI, M. GOBBI & T. MENNINI. 1986. Br. J. Pharmacol. 88: 269–275.
12. BENDOTTI, C., F. BORSINI, M. G. ZANINI, R. SAMANIN & S. GARATTINI. 1980. Pharmacol. Res. Commun. 12: 567–574.
13. INVERNIZZI, R., C. BERETTERA, S. GARATTINI & R. SAMANIN. 1986. Eur. J. Pharmacol. 120: 9–15.
14. WIGHTMAN, R. M., P. M. PLOTSKY, E. STROPE, R. DELCORE JR. & R. N. ADAMS. 1977. Brain. Res. 131: 345–349.
15. KOHNO, Y., K. MATSUO, M. TANAKA, T. FURUKAWA & N. NAGASAKI. 1979. Anal. Biochem. 97: 352–358.
16. ACHILLI, G., C. PEREGO, F. PONZIO & S. ALGERI. 1983. Res. Commun. Chem. Pathol. Pharmacol. 40: 67–72.
17. DI PAOLO, T., A. DUPONT, P. SAVARD & M. DAIGLE. 1983. Can. J. Physiol. Pharmacol. 61: 530–534.
18. DE BLASI, A. & T. MENNINI. 1983. Life Sci. 32: 2585–2588.
19. PEROUTKA, S. J., R. M. LEBOVITZ & S. H. SNYDER. 1981. Science 212: 827–829.
20. LEYSEN, J. E., W. GOMMEREN, P. VAN GOMPEL, J. WYNANTS, P. F. M. JANSSEN & P. M. LADURON. 1985. Mol. Pharmacol. 27: 600–611.
21. BARONE, D., F. LUZZANI, A. ASSANDRI, G. GALLIANI, T. MENNINI & S. GARATTINI. 1985. Eur. J. Pharmacol. 116: 63–74.
22. SAMANIN, R., T. MENNINI, A. FERRARIS, C. BENDOTTI, F. BORSINI & S. GARATTINI. 1979. Naunyn-Schmiedeberg's Arch. Pharmakol. 308: 159–163.

23. Borsini, F., C. Bendotti & R. Samanin. 1985. Int. J. Obesity 9: 277–283.
24. Borsini, F., C. Bendotti, B. Przewlocka & R. Samanin. 1983. Eur. J. Pharmacol. 94: 109–115.
25. Carruba, M. O., S. Ricciardi, P. Spano & P. Mantegazza. 1985. Life Sci. 36: 1739–1749.
26. Bendotti, C., S. Garattini & R. Samanin. J. Pharm. Pharmacol. In press.
27. Severson, J. A. 1986. Neurobiol. Aging 7: 83–87.
28. Hauger, R. L., B. Hulihan-Giblin, P. Skolnick & S. M. Paul. 1984. Life Sci. 34: 771–782.
29. Palkovits, M., R. Raisman, M. Briley & S. Z. Langer. 1981. Brain Res. 210: 493–498.
30. Samanin, R., S. Caccia, C. Bendotti, F. Borsini, E. Borroni, R. Invernizzi, R. Pataccini & T. Mennini. 1980. Psychopharmacology 68: 99–104.
31. Gobbi, M., C. Taddei & T. Mennini. Submitted for publication to Life Sci.

The Place of Animal Models and Animal Experimentation in the Study of Food Intake Regulation and Obesity in Humans

RAY W. FULLER AND TERENCE T. YEN

Lilly Research Laboratories
Eli Lilly and Company
Lilly Corporate Center
Indianapolis, Indiana 46285

INTRODUCTION

Progress in understanding and treating human disease has depended heavily on animal research. In some cases, pathologic conditions in animals are used in a true sense as models of the human disease, even though the similarities between the conditions may be only superficial.

Animal studies related to obesity can have multiple purposes and may require an obese animal as a model of an obese human or may be done in nonobese animals. Animal studies may be aimed at elucidating etiologic factors in obesity or metabolic abnormalities associated with obesity; animals may be used to study the neurotransmitters involved in the regulation of food intake or pharmacokinetic properties of drugs that are clinical candidates for treating obesity, as examples. The investigative purpose must be defined when nonhuman experimental subjects are chosen. This paper considers some similarities and differences between animal models of obesity and obese humans with respect to genetics, control of food intake, intermediary metabolism, and therapeutic approaches to obesity.

Obese Animals as Models of Human Obesity

Obese animals may represent models of obesity in humans in certain respects but not others. For example, a genetically obese mouse might not be an appropriate model for studying the inheritance of obesity in humans in a general sense, for hereditary is not as important a factor in human obesity generally as it is in these mice. On the other hand, metabolic abnormalities and drug responses in genetically obese mice may be the same as in obese humans.

Obesity can have different origins and etiologies in animals just as it can in humans. In animals, obesity can be genetic, or it can be induced by chemical, surgical, or dietary means.[1,2] Several commonly used animal models of obesity are listed in TABLE 1. In addition to genetically obese mice and rats, a smaller amount of study has been done in other species. Obesity can be induced by increasing caloric intake forcibly, by enhancing the palatability of food available, or by manipulations such as tail-pressure stress[3] to increase feeding. When the palatability of food is enhanced by use of the so-called cafeteria diet, the lack of homogeneity of the diet introduces difficulty in estimating the types of nutrients and amount of calories that are ingested. Mechanical or drug-induced lesions in

TABLE 1. Commonly Used Animal Models of Obesity

Cause of Obesity	Type of Model
Genetic	Single gene mutations: Dominant: Yellow mouse (A^y, A^{vy}) Recessive: Obese mouse (ob) Diabetic mouse (db,db^{2J}) Fatty rat (fa) Polygenic mutations: New Zealand obese mouse (NZO) KK mouse
Diet-induced	Forced feeding Palatability-induced feeding ("cafeteria" diet) Stress-induced overeating (tail pressure)
Lesion-induced	Mechanical lesion Knife cut Electrolytic Radio frequency Chemical lesion Gold thioglucose Monosodium glutamate 6-Hydroxydopamine 5,7-Dihydroxytryptamine
Drug-induced	Insulin p-Chlorophenylalanine Antidepressant drugs Anxiolytic drugs

hypothalamic areas that regulate feeding reliably result in hyperphagia and obesity.

Obese animals can be used for screening antiobesity drugs without regard to the mechanism of action of those drugs. Compounds can be screened initially for their ability to reduce body weight in obese animals; compounds with various mechanisms could be found in this way, as distinct from specific screens for appetite suppression, enhanced thermogenesis, or other defined actions.

Animals as Experimental Subjects

Besides the various animal models of obesity that are used, normal nonobese animals are used in obesity research in a variety of ways, including the study of neurotransmitters and brain regions involved in regulating total caloric intake and nutrient selection; the study of metabolism as influenced by dietary alterations, as a function of biological rhythms; and the study of drug effects on food intake and on metabolism, as well as the study of other pharmacologic actions, pharmacokinetics, and metabolism of drugs that are candidates for treating obesity.

The effect of a drug that reduces food intake may be the same in a nonobese animal as in an obese animal. But a drug that acts to correct an impaired response of the sympathetic nervous system to overfeeding, for example, may necessarily have to be studied in obese animals.

GENETICS

Genetically transmitted obesity in animals can be caused by single gene mutations or polygenic mutations. Obesity due to single gene mutations is inherited recessively, such as the obese gene (ob) and the diabetes gene (db) in mice and the fatty gene (fa) in rats, or dominantly such as some of the yellow alleles at the agouti locus in mice.[4] Examples of obesity that are polygenic in origin include NZO mice and KK mice.[4]

Genetics of obesity has been studied most extensively in mice, where numerous spontaneous mutations predispose to obesity and where breeding experiments can be done with ease and relatively quickly. Some mutations, functioning either as structural genes or regulatory genes and distinctively located on different chromosomes, may control the same biochemical site that leads to the development of obesity. Other mutations probably control different sites. The primary biochemical mechanism controlled by any of the mutations that cause obesity in animals is not known, but in some of the genetically obese animals, hypothalamic lesions in the regions of the satiety center may be responsible for the obesity syndrome.[5]

The genetics of obesity in humans is less clear,[6] probably due to the heterogeneous nature of the obese population, where various etiologic factors are involved. Human obesity has been considered in two categories: childhood obesity and maturity-onset obesity (middle-age obesity).[7] In mice, models for both types of obesity are available.[8]

CONTROL OF FOOD INTAKE

The control of food intake is complex and involves numerous brain neurotransmitters.[9-12] Overeating may cause obesity, and reduction of food intake is a means of treating obesity, so an understanding of mechanisms involved in the control of food intake in laboratory animals and in humans is a major goal. Both the amount of food consumed (frequency and duration of meals) and the selection of nutrients appear to be regulated.

Central and Peripheral Mechanisms

The central nervous system undoubtedly plays a dominant role in the control of food intake, but many peripheral mechanisms may be components of this control or adjunctive controls. Peripheral organs such as the gut, liver, and brown adipose tissue (BAT) have been suggested to have important roles in the overall control of food intake.

Signals to the Brain from the Periphery

The hypothalamus, as an integrating center that regulates energy balance (intake, deposition, utilization), responds to various signals including blood-borne dietary constituents and hormonal and neural messages.[10] Bombesin and cholecystokinin are examples of peptides present in the gastrointestinal tract of rats and primates that may act as satiety signals to the brain.[13,14] Decreases in blood glucose concentration have long been thought to be a signal to the brain for initiating food intake.[15] A possible role of glucoreceptors that are present in the liver and that relay neural messages to the brain in the control of feeding behavior has also been suggested.[16] Bellinger *et al.*[17] have found no effect of liver denervation on feeding behavior in rats, but liver glucoreceptors may influence feeding behavior in rabbits.[18] This is an example of possible species differences in mechanisms that control overall energy balance, including food ingestion, and in most instances, data from humans are more sparse than data from laboratory animals.

Heat production by BAT thermogenesis has been suggested as a possible feedback signal for satiety,[19] and heat production from amphetamine-stimulated thermogenesis[20] might be a cue that mediates amphetamine-induced anorexia. Chemical sympathectomy of BAT, expected to prevent or attenuate the stimulation of BAT thermogenesis, was found not to attenuate amphetamine-induced anorexia, however.[21] Substantial evidence indicates that a direct action in the hypothalamus mediates amphetamine-induced anorexia.[22]

Brain Regions and Brain Neurotransmitters Involved in Control of Food Intake

Earlier anatomical and chemical studies provided evidence for the dual-center hypothesis of the control of feeding in animals, that is, the lateral hypothalamus being the feeding center and the ventromedial hypothalamus the satiety center.[23] This hypothesis, still controversial, led to the study of physiological compounds as regulators of food intake. Neurotransmitters such as dopamine, norepinephrine, serotonin and gamma-aminobutyric acid; peptides such as cholecystokinin, pancreatic polypeptide, and endorphins; and metabolites such as glucose and fatty acids are among the mediators proposed to play a role in hunger and satiety.[9,11,12,24,25] The overall integration of various pathways involved in regulating feeding is still poorly understood.

The increase of β-endorphin levels in the pituitary of obese rodents[26] and of concentrations of norepinephrine and serotonin, but not dopamine, in the brains of genetically obese rodents[27-29] are possibly related to the hyperphagia in these animals. Recently, the number of dopamine receptors in the brains of obese animals were reported to be increased.[30] Because little is known about brain neurotransmitter concentrations and receptors in humans, it is difficult to interpret the relevance to human obesity of these findings in animals.

Control of Food Intake as One Component of Body-Weight Management

The hypothalamus matches energy intake to energy expenditure despite variation in energy utilization. The lipostatic theory of energy balance regulation by the hypothalamus has suggested that long-term food intake is controlled to prevent the accumulation of excess body fat.[25] Such a theory is analogous to a glucostatic theory that food intake and metabolism are regulated to maintain stable blood glucose levels. The lipostatic theory relates to the concept of a set point, a predetermined body weight that the animal maintains by regulating caloric intake and utilization. The brain may sense numerous signals that reflect the nutritional state and the metabolic state of the animal in order to integrate the choice of nutrients, initiation and cessation of feeding, storage and utilization of calories, and mobilization of energy storage forms. Difficult as it is to measure and correlate all of these events in laboratory animals, it may be impossible to do so in humans, given the inaccessibility of tissue sites like fat, liver, and brain. Even in laboratory animals, only a few parameters usually are measured within a given experimental paradigm. We often try to draw an enormously complex picture from sketches of only a few parts.

Patterns of feeding and choices of nutrient intake in addition to amount of food consumed may give important clues about how food intake is regulated and about alterations associated with obesity. For instance, the diurnal variations of food intake reported in normal mice may be absent in obese mice.[31] When a choice of diet is given, obese mice and rats prefer a high-fat diet to a high-carbohydrate or a high-protein diet,[32,33] unlike the carbohydrate-craving syndrome reported in humans, sometimes associated with obesity or with depression.[34,35] Interest in food choice in experimental animals has been enhanced by recent evidence that brain serotonin may play an important role in regulating the choice as well as the amount of foods consumed.[36,37] Some success in extrapolating animal data on food selection to humans has been met. For instance, fenfluramine, a drug that enhances serotonin function by release of serotonin, is reported to suppress selectively the intake of carbohydrates in rats[36] and in humans.[38]

Identifying specific neuronal systems and receptors that regulate feeding choice and frequency may have to be done first in laboratory animals. A new approach to identifying receptors involved in feeding regulation is the use of tritiated amphetamine to label binding sites in brain where receptors are located that are involved in the control of food intake.[39] Various studies indicate that these sites probably are not associated with amine uptake carriers.[40] The relative affinities of phenylethylamines for the sites were highly correlated with the appetite-suppressant potencies of the drugs.[41] The number of sites increased in hypothalamus during the onset of obesity in ob/ob mice and remained high.[42] Food deprivation reduced the number of these amphetamine-binding sites in hypothalamus and brain stem but not in other brain regions,[43] and the decrease was rapidly reversed by refeeding. A precise role of these binding sites in physiological regulation of food intake or in pharmacologic intervention has yet to be established. But if such binding sites are shown to occur in human brain, further studies in animals will deserve high priority with possible relevance to human obesity and/or eating disorders.

METABOLISM

Obesity is a problem of excess energy storage. Obesity could be caused by hyperphagia in some people, but in most, overeating produces only limited obesity.[44] An increased efficiency of energy storage, of unknown etiology, is usually required to produce obesity. Differences in metabolic or other events have often been identified in obese animals compared to their lean counterparts. Altered lipogenesis, hyperglycemia, endocrine abnormalities, adipocyte hyperplasia, increased lipoprotein lipase activities, to name a few, have been found in some obese animals. Understanding the relationships among these various abnormalities and defining which are the causes and which are the effects of obesity has been difficult. One reason for the current high level of interest in thermogenesis is that faulty thermogenic responses have been identified in genetic strains of animals even before obesity has developed.[45,46]

Thermogenesis as a Means of Energy Utilization

Thermogenesis in BAT has been known for some time, but only in the past few years has there been an explosion of interest in this phenomenon as a regulator of energy homeostasis.[47] The idea that BAT thermogenesis has an important role in energy utilization in laboratory animals is now widely accepted. According to Foster,[48] BAT thermogenesis may account for as much as one-third of the overall metabolic rate in some animal species. There are fewer data in humans, and debate continues about the importance of BAT thermogenesis in humans.[49-52]

Influence of Food Intake on Metabolic Events: Diet-Induced Thermogenesis

Just as there has been general debate about the physiologic importance of BAT thermogenesis in humans as compared to laboratory animals, there is specific controversy about whether abnormalities in diet-induced thermogenesis exist in humans and whether they play an important role in human obesity as they appear to do in some obese animals. Rothwell and Stock[53] have discussed the role of diet-induced thermogenesis in obese rats and mice and have argued persuasively for a potential importance of diet-induced thermogenesis in human obesity, but there is not yet sufficient evidence to convince all investigators.[54]

Sympathetic Nerve Input as a Regulator of Thermogenesis

Sympathetic nerve input to the BAT regulates thermogenesis and energy utilization in laboratory animals,[55] but most evidence comes from studies that are difficult or impossible to do in humans. Fasting or caloric restriction is associated with reduced norepinephrine turnover in interscapular BAT in the rat, whereas overfeeding is associated with increased norepinephrine turnover.[56] The composition of the diet as well as total caloric intake affects norepinephrine turnover in BAT and other sympathetically innervated organs in rats.[57] Drugs that decrease sympathetic nerve function by depleting norepinephrine from nerve terminals caused an increase in body fat content along with reduced metabolic rate and increased efficiency of energy utilization in mice.[58] Drugs that increase sympathetic nerve input to the BAT increased metabolic rate and reduced body weight in obese animals.[59]

There is still inadequate evidence that the sympathetic nervous system is the predominant controller of diet-induced thermogenesis in humans.[51,60,61] Even in animals, the importance of the sympathetic nervous system in regulating BAT thermogenesis does not imply a lack of other control mechanisms. Hormones that appear to modulate thermogenesis or the noradrenergic regulation of thermogenesis include thyroid hormone, glucocorticoids, and insulin.[47]

Impaired Thermogenesis in Obesity

Impaired thermogenesis, especially diet-induced thermogenesis, has been proposed to play a major role in the development of genetic[62,63] and lesion-induced[63,64] obesity in laboratory animals. Defective thermogenesis in obese animals may result from insufficient sympathetic input to BAT. Altered norepinephrine turnover in BAT in ob/ob mice, fa/fa rats, and in obese rats with hypothalamic lesions points to defective sympathetic function as a cause of impaired thermogenesis.[65] Some workers[66] but not others[60] have reported evidence for impaired thermogenesis in obese humans. Finer et al.[67] found the thermogenic response to norepinephrine infusion to be reduced after weight loss in obese humans and suggested that previous contradictory data about norepinephrine-induced thermogenesis in human obesity might have resulted because subjects were studied under different dietary conditions. In some cases the reduction in noradrenergic function associated with obesity seems to be specific for BAT,[68] which would decrease the likelihood of finding such an abnormality in humans by measuring blood or urinary catecholamines or their metabolites.

DRUG INTERVENTION

All of the currently marketed antiobesity drugs are appetite suppressants, but other classes of drugs are being developed for trials and potential use in treating human obesity, based on studies in laboratory animals.

Sites of Drug Action

In addition to suppression of food intake, other sites of drug intervention have been proposed and tested in animal models of obesity. Compounds that stimulate thermogenesis,[69–72] that inhibit lipogenesis,[73] absorption,[74] or digestive enzymes,[75,76] or that prevent gastric emptying[77] are under development.

Mechanisms of Appetite Suppression

The effects of amphetamine-type anorectics are probably mediated by dopamine or perhaps norepinephrine,[22,78] whereas the effects of some other anorectic drugs, for example, fenfluramine,[79] fluoxetine,[80,81] zimelidine[82] and femoxetine[83] are mediated by serotonin. Because both types of drugs reduce food intake in animals and in humans, animal models are useful in studying the activities of anorectic drugs in these classes. Generally the amphetamine-related drugs that release catecholamines cause increased locomotor activity in laboratory animals and are associated with CNS side effects and sometimes abuse potential in humans; furthermore, tolerance may develop rapidly to their appetite-suppressant effect. Drugs acting through a serotonergic mechanism do not change locomotor activity in animals and have no apparent abuse potential in humans. Fluoxetine is a serotonin uptake inhibitor that reduces food intake and body weight in animals.[80,81] In clinical trials in depressed and nondepressed obese subjects, fluoxetine caused statistically significant weight loss.

Some of the appetite suppressant drugs have recently been demonstrated to be thermogenic.[59] One example is ephedrine, which showed antiobesity efficacy both in animals[84–86] and in humans,[87,88] again illustrating the predictive value of animal data.

Compounds that increase gamma-aminobutyric acid concentrations in the brain[89] and opiate antagonists[90–92] are appetite suppressants in animals. No clinical trials of GABA antagonists in obesity have been reported, and naltrexone, an opiate antagonist, failed to show long-term efficacy in humans.[93,94] Differences across species lines in the effects of some agents on food intake[12] illustrate that the neuronal circuitry controlling feeding is not likely to be identical in all species; thus all types of anorexic drugs that are effective in rats and mice may not produce anorexia in humans.

Mechanisms of Thermogenesis Stimulation

Animal studies on diet-induced thermogenesis in BAT and especially on defects in obese animals suggested that a potential site of drug action in the treatment of human obesity is enhancement of thermogenesis. Even while the investigation continues into whether obese humans have a defect in diet-induced thermogenesis as obese animals do, the identification and development of drugs that stimulate thermogenesis has progressed.

Theoretically, drugs could promote thermogenesis either by mimicking the effect of the sympathetic neurotransmitter, norepinephrine, on fat cells or by enhancing the effectiveness of the sympathetic nervous system, such as by releasing norepinephrine, by increasing the amount of norepinephrine available for release, or by blocking norepinephrine inactivation. All types of these drugs have been tried in laboratory animals.

The sympathetic stimulation of BAT thermogenesis is mediated by β receptors on brown fat cells. Recently there has been debate about the nature of these β receptors in rats. Arch et al.[95] suggested that a novel type of β receptor is involved, but Levin and Sullivan[96] presented evidence that a $\beta 1$ receptor is primarily responsible for thermogenesis in BAT of rats. Since β receptors that mediate BAT thermogenesis represent a potential target site for antiobesity drugs, it will be important to have information on the nature of these β receptors in human BAT.

OVERVIEW: CORRELATIONS BETWEEN ANIMALS AND HUMANS

Experimentation in obese and nonobese laboratory animals should continue to make important contributions to the understanding of human obesity. In this research, investigators must be aware that some findings in obese animals are likely to have more relevance to human obesity than others. Not all types of obese animals can be expected to be alike, anymore than all obesity in humans has the same origin. Findings in animal studies are important guides to research into human obesity nonetheless. If causes of obesity are identified in animals, these will open avenues of research to identify causes in humans. Drugs to treat obesity ordinarily have to be tested first for this purpose in animals, and such testing should be done with consideration of how the results will predict what would happen in humans. The benefits may be better appetite suppressant drugs that do not have severe adverse effects and that do not lose efficacy before the therapeutic goal is reached, drugs that promote energy expenditure through enhanced thermogenesis or perhaps other means, or drugs that act at other stages of the energy intake and utilization cycle.

REFERENCES

1. BRAY, G. A. & D. A. YORK. 1979. Hypothalamic and genetic obesity in experimental animals: an autonomic and endocrine hypothesis. Physiol. Rev. **59:** 719–809.
2. ROBBINS, T. W., B. J. EVERITT & B. J. SAHAKIAN. 1981. Stress-induced eating in animals. In The Body Weight Regulatory System: Normal and Disturbed Mecha-

nisms. L. A. Cioffi, W. P. T. James & T. B. Van Itallie, Eds.: 289–297. Raven Press. New York.

3. ROWLAND, N. E. & S. M. ANTELMAN. 1976. Stress-induced hyperphagia and obesity in rats: A possible model for understanding human obesity. Science 191: 310–312.

4. COLEMAN, D. L. 1978. Obesity and diabetes: two mutant genes causing diabetes-obesity syndromes in mice. Diabetologia 14: 141–148.

5. COLEMAN, D. L. 1973. Effects of parabiosis of obese with diabetes and normal mice. Diabetologia 9: 294–298.

6. BRAY, G. A. 1981. The inheritance of corpulence. In The Body Weight Regulatory System: Normal and Disturbed Mechanisms. L. A. Cioffi, W. P. T. James & T. B. Van Itallie, Eds.: 185–195. Raven Press. New York.

7. SJÖSTRÖM, L. & P. BJÖRNTORP. 1974. Body composition and adipose tissue cellularity in human obesity. Acta Med. Scand. 195: 201–211.

8. YEN, T. T., J. A. ALLAN, P-L. YU, M. A. ACTON & D. V. PEARSON. 1976. Triacyl-glycerol contents and in vivo lipogenesis of ob/ob, db/db and A^{vy}/a mice. Biochim. Biophys. Acta 441: 213–220.

9. BLUNDELL, J. E. 1984. Serotonin and appetite. Neuropharmacology 23: 1537–1551.

10. ANDERSON, G. H.. E. T. S. LI & N. T. GLANVILLE. 1984. Brain mechanisms and the quantitative and qualitative aspects of food intake. Brain Res. Bull. 12: 167–173.

11. LEIBOWITZ, S. F. 1986. Brain monoamines and peptides: role in the control of eating behavior. Fed. Proc. Fed. Am. Soc. Exp. Biol. 45: 1396–1403.

12. MORLEY, J. E., A. S. LEVINE, B. A. GOSNELL & C. J. BILLINGTON. 1984. Neuropeptides and appetite: contribution of neuropharmacological modeling. Fed. Proc. Fed. Am. Soc. Exp. Biol. 43: 2903–2907.

13. GIBBS, J. & G. P. SMITH. 1986. Satiety: the roles of peptides from the stomach and the intestine. Fed. Proc. Fed. Am. Soc. Exp. Biol. 45: 1391–1395.

14. McHUGH, R. P. & T. H. MORAN. 1986. The stomach, cholecystokinin, and satiety. Fed. Proc. Fed. Am. Soc. Exp. Biol. 45: 1384–1390.

15. CAMPFIELD, L. A., P. BRANDON & F. J. SMITH. 1985. On-line continuous measurement of blood glucose and meal pattern in free-feeding rats: the role of glucose in meal initiation. Brain Res. Bull. 14: 605–616.

16. RUSSEK, M. 1981. Current status of the hepatostatic theory of food intake control. Appetite 2: 137–143.

17. BELLINGER, L. L., V. E. MENDEL, F. E. WILLIAMS & T. W. CASTONGUAY. 1984. The effect of liver denervation on meal patterns, body weight and body composition of rats. Physiol. Behav. 33: 661–667.

18. NOVIN D., D. A. VANDERWEELE & M. REZEK. 1973. Infusion of 2-deoxy-D-glucose into the hepatic-portal system causes eating: evidence for peripheral glucoreceptors. Science 181: 858–860.

19. GLICK, Z. V. 1982. Inverse relationship between brown fat thermogenesis and meal size: The thermostatic control of food intake revisited. Physiol. Behav. 29: 1137–1140.

20. WELLMAN, P. J. 1983. Influence of amphetamine on brown adipose tissue thermogenesis. Res. Commun. Chem. Pathol. Pharmacol. 41: 173–176.

21. FREEMAN, P. H., P. J. WELLMAN & D. E. CLARK. 1985. Effects of guanethidine sympathectomy on feeding, drinking, weight gain and amphetamine anorexia in the rat. Physiol. Behav. 35: 473–477.

22. McCABE, J. T. & S. F. LEIBOWITZ. 1984. Determination of the course of brainstem catecholamine fibers mediating amphetamine anorexia. Brain Res. 311: 211–224.

23. CAWTHORNE, M. A. 1982. Control of food intake. Mol. Aspects Med. 5: 293–400.

24. KELLY, J. & S. P. GROSSMAN. 1980. GABA and hypothalamic feeding systems. Brain Res. Bull. 5: 237–244.

25. HARRIS, R. B. S. & R. J. MARTIN. 1984. Lipostatic theory of energy balance: Concepts and signals. Nutr. Behav. 1: 253–275.

26. MARGULES, D. L., B. MOISSET & M. J. LEWIS. 1978. β-Endorphin is associated with overeating in genetically obese mice (ob/ob) and rats (fa/fa). Science 202: 988–991.

27. CRUCE, J. A. F., N. B. THOA & D. M. JACOBOWITZ. 1976. Catecholamines in the brains of genetically obese rats. Brain Res. 101: 165–170.

28. LORDEN, J. F. & G. A. OLTMANS. 1977. Hypothalamic and pituitary catecholamine levels in genetically obese mice (ob/ob). Brain Res. 131: 162–166.
29. FELDMAN, J. M., J. A. BLALOCK & R. T. ZERN. 1979. Elevated hypothalamic norepinephrine content in mice with the hereditary obese-hyperglycemic syndrome. Horm. Res. 11: 170–178.
30. EL-REFAI, M. F. & T. M. CHAN. 1986. Possible involvement of a hypothalamic dopaminergic receptor in development of genetic obesity in mice. Biochim. Biophys. Acta 880: 16–25.
31. BAILEY, C. J., T. W. ATKINS, M. J. CONNER, C. G. MANLEY & A. J. MATTY. 1975. Diurnal variations of food consumption, plasma glucose and plasma insulin concentrations in lean and obese hyperglycemic mice. Horm. Res. 6: 380–386.
32. ROMSOS, D. R. & D. FERGUSON. 1982. Self-selected intake of carbohydrate, fat, and protein by obese (ob/ob) and lean mice. Physiol. Behav. 28: 301–305.
33. CASTONGUAY, T. W., N. E. ROWLAND & J. S. STERN. 1985. Nutritional influences on dietary selection patterns of obese and lean Zucker rats. Brain Res. Bull. 14: 625–631.
34. HOPKINSON, G. 1981. A neurochemical theory of appetite and weight changes in depressive states. Acta Psychiat. Scand. 64: 217–225.
35. WURTMAN, J. J., R. J. WURTMAN, J. H. GROWDON, P. HENRY, A. LIPSCOMB & S. H. ZEISEL. 1981. Carbohydrate craving in obese people: suppression by treatments affecting serotoninergic transmission. Int. J. Eating Disorders 1: 2–15.
36. WURTMAN, J. J. & R. J. WURTMAN. 1979. Fenfluramine and other serotoninergic drugs depress food intake and carbohydrate consumption while sparing protein consumption. Curr. Med. Res. Opin. 6, Suppl. 1: 28–33.
37. LI, E. T. S. & G. H. ANDERSON. 1984. 5-Hydroxytryptamine: A modulator of food composition but not quantity? Life Sci. 34: 2453–2460.
38. WURTMAN, J. J. & R. J. WURTMAN. 1985. d-Fenfluramine selectively decreases carbohydrate but not protein intake in obese subjects. Int. J. Obesity 8: 79–84.
39. HAUGER, R. L., B. HULIHAN-GIBLIN, P. SKOLNICK & S. M. PAUL. 1984. Characteristics of [³H-](+)-amphetamine binding sites in the rat central nervous system. Life Sci. 34: 771–782.
40. HULIHAN-GIBLIN, B., R. L. HAUGER, A. JANOWSKY & S. M. PAUL. 1985. Dopaminergic denervation increases [³H-](+)-amphetamine binding in the rat striatum. Eur. J. Pharmacol. 113: 141–142.
41. PAUL, S. M., B. HULIHAN-GIBLIN & P. SKOLNICK. 1982. (+)-Amphetamine binding to rat hypothalamus: Relation to anorexic potency of phenylethylamines. Science 218: 487–490.
42. HAUGER, R., B. HULIHAN-GIBLIN & S. M. PAUL. 1986. Increased number of hypothalamic [³H-](+)-amphetamine binding sites in genetically obese (ob/ob) mice. Neuropharmacology 25: 327–330.
43. HAUGER, R., B. HULIHAN-GIBLIN, I. ANGEL, M. D. LUU, A. JANOWSKY, P. SKOLNICK & S. M. PAUL. 1986. Glucose regulates [³H](+)-amphetamine binding and Na+K+ ATPase activity in the hypothalamus: A proposed mechanism for the glucostatic control of feeding and satiety. Brain Res. Bull. 16: 281–288.
44. SIMS, E. A. H., E. DANFORTH JR., E. S. HORTON, G. A. BRAY, J. A. GLENNON & L. B. SALANS. 1973. Endocrine and metabolic effects of experimental obesity in man. Recent Prog. Horm. Res. 29: 457–496.
45. TRAYHURN, P., P. L. THURLBY & W. P. T. JAMES. 1977. Thermogenic defect in pre-obese ob/ob mice. Nature (London) 266: 60–63.
46. GODBOLE, V., D. A. YORK & D. P. BLOXHAM. 1978. Developmental changes in the fatty (fa/fa) rat: evidence for defective thermogenesis preceding the hyperlipogenesis and hyperinsulinemia. Diabetologia 15: 41–44.
47. HIMMS-HAGEN, J. 1985. Brown adipose tissue metabolism and thermogenesis. Annu. Rev. Nutr. 5: 69–94.
48. FOSTER, D. O. 1984. Quantitative contribution of brown adipose tissue thermogenesis to overall metabolism. Can. J. Biochem. Cell Biol. 62: 618–622.
49. HIMMS-HAGEN, J. 1984. Brown adipose tissue thermogenesis as an energy buffer. Implications for obesity. N. Engl. J. Med. 311: 1549–1558.

50. JÉQUIER, E. & Y. SCHUTZ. 1985. New evidence for a thermogenic defect in human obesity. Int. J. Obesity 9, Suppl. 2: 2–17.
51. SJÖSTRÖM, L. 1985. Catecholamine sensitivity with respect to metabolic rate in man. Int. J. Obesity 9, Suppl. 2: 123–129.
52. KATZEFF, H. L., M. O'CONNELL, E. S. HORTON, E. DANFORTH JR., J. B. YOUNG & L. LANDSBERG. 1986. Metabolic studies in human obesity during overnutrition and undernutrition: thermogenic and hormonal responses to norepinephrine. Metab. Clin. Exp. 35: 166–175.
53. ROTHWELL, N. J. & M. J. STOCK. 1983. Luxuskonsumption, diet-induced thermogenesis and brown fat: the case in favour. Clin. Sci. 64: 19–23.
54. HERVEY, G. R. & G. TOBIN. 1983. Luxuskonsumption, diet-induced thermogenesis and brown fat: a critical review. Clin. Sci. 64: 7–18.
55. LANDSBERG, L. & J. B. YOUNG. 1984. The role of the sympathoadrenal system in modulating energy expenditure. Clin. Endocrinol. Metabol. 13: 475–498.
56. LANDSBERG, L., M. E. SAVILLE & J. B. YOUNG. 1984. Sympathoadrenal system and regulation of thermogenesis. Am. J. Physiol. 247: E181–E189.
57. VANDER TUIG, J. G. & D. R. ROMSOS. 1984. Effects of dietary carbohydrate, fat, and protein on norepinephrine turnover in rats. Metab. Clin. Exp. 33: 26–33.
58. DULLOO, A. G. & D. S. MILLER. 1985. Increased body fat due to elevated energetic efficiency following chronic administration of inhibitors of sympathetic nervous system activity. Metab. Clin. Exp. 34: 1061–1065.
59. DULLOO, A. G. & D. S. MILLER. 1984. Thermogenic drugs for the treatment of obesity: sympathetic stimulants in animal models. Br. J. Nutr. 52: 179–196.
60. KATZEFF, H. L. & R. DANIELS. 1985. The sympathetic nervous system in human obesity. Int. J. Obesity 9, Suppl. 2: 131–137.
61. WELLE, S. 1985. Evidence that the sympathetic nervous system does not regulate dietary thermogenesis in humans. Int. J. Obesity 9, Suppl. 2: 115–121.
62. TRIANDAFILLOU, J. & J. HIMMS-HAGEN. 1983. Brown adipose tissue in genetically obese (fa/fa) rats: response to cold and diet. Am. J. Physiol. 244: E145–E150.
63. HIMMS-HAGEN, J. 1985. Defective brown adipose tissue thermogenesis in obese mice. Int. J. Obesity 9, Suppl. 2: 17–24.
64. SAITO, M., Y. MINOKOSHI & T. SHIMAZU. 1985. Brown adipose tissue after ventromedial hypothalamic lesions in rats. Am. J. Physiol. 248: 20–25.
65. ROMSOS, D. R. 1985. Norepinephrine turnover in obese mice and rats. Int. J. Obesity 9, Suppl. 2: 55–62.
66. JUNG, R. T., P. S. SHETTY, W. P. T. JAMES, M. H. BARRAND & B. A. CALLINGHAM. 1979. Reduced thermogenesis in obesity. Nature (London) 279: 322–323.
67. FINER, N., P. C. SWAN & F. T. MITCHELL. 1985. Suppression of norepinephrine-induced thermogenesis in human obesity by diet and weight loss. Int. J. Obesity 9: 121–126.
68. YORK, D. A., D. MARCHINGTON, S. J. HOLT & J. ALLARS. 1985. Regulation of sympathetic activity in lean and obese Zucker (fa/fa) rats. Am. J. Physiol. 249: E299–E305.
69. MEIER, M. K., L. ALIG, M. E. BÜRGI-SAVILLE & M. MÜLLER. 1984. Phenethanolamine derivatives with calorigenic and antidiabetic qualities. Int. J. Obesity 8, Suppl. 1: 215–225.
70. ARCH, J. R. S., A. T. AINSWORTH, R. D. M. ELLIS, V. PIERCY, V. E. THODY, P. L. THURLBY, C. WILSON, S. WILSON & P. YOUNG. 1984. Treatment of obesity with thermogenic β-adrenoceptor agonists: studies on BRL 26830A in rodents. Int. J. Obesity 8, Suppl. 1: 1–11.
71. YEN, T. T. 1984. The antiobesity and metabolic activities of LY79771 in obese and normal mice. Int. J. Obesity 8: 69–78.
72. YEN, T. T., M. M. MCKEE & N. B. STAMM. 1984. Thermogenesis and weight control. Int. J. Obesity 8, Suppl. 1: 65–78.
73. TRISCARI, J. & A. C. SULLIVAN. 1984. Antiobesity effects of a novel lipid synthesis inhibitor (Ro 22-0654). Life Sci. 34: 2433–2442.
74. DREWNOWSKI, A., J. A. GRINKER, R. GRUEN & A. C. SULLIVAN. 1985. Effects of inhibitors of carbohydrate absorption or lipid metabolism on meal patterns of Zucker rats. Pharmacol. Biochem. Behav. 23: 811–821.

75. JANDACEK, R. J. 1984. Studies with sucrose polyester. Int. J. Obesity 8, Suppl. 1: 13–21.
76. PULS, W., H. P. KRAUSE, L. MÜLLER, H. SCHUTT, R. SITT & G. THOMAS. 1984. Inhibitors of the rate of carbohydrate and lipid absorption by the intestine. Int. J. Obesity 8, Suppl. 1: 181–190.
77. TRISCARI, J. & A. C. SULLIVAN. 1981. Studies on the mechanism of action of a novel anorectic agent, (−)-threo-chlorocitric acid. Pharmacol. Biochem. Behav. 15: 311–318.
78. SULLIVAN, A. C. & R. K. GRUEN. 1985. Mechanisms of appetite modulation by drugs. Fed. Proc. Fed. Am. Soc. Exp. Biol. 44: 139–144.
79. GARATTINI, S., W. BUCZKO, A. JORI & R. SAMANIN. 1975. On the mechanism of action of fenfluramine. Postgrad. Med. J. 51, Suppl. 1: 27–35.
80. GOUDIE, A. J., E. W. THORNTON & T. J. WHEELER. 1976. Effects of Lilly 110140, a specific inhibitor of 5-hydroxytryptamine uptake, on food intake and on 5-hydroxytryptophan-induced anorexia. Evidence for serotonergic inhibition of feeding. J. Pharm. Pharmacol. 28: 318–320.
81. YEN, T. T. & D. T. WONG. 1985. Oral activities of fluoxetine in normal and viable yellow obese mice. Int. J. Obesity 9: A110.
82. SIMPSON, R. J., D. J. LAWTON, M. H. WATT & B. TIPLADY. 1981. Effect of zimelidine, a new antidepressant, on appetite and body weight. Br. J. Clin. Pharmacol. 11: 96–98.
83. SMEDEGAARD, J., P. CHRISTIANSEN & B. SKRUMSAGER. 1981. Treatment of obesity by femoxetine, a selective 5 HT reuptake inhibitor. Int. J. Obesity 5: 377–378.
84. YEN, T. T., M. M. MCKEE & K. G. BEMIS. 1981. Ephedrine reduces weight of viable yellow obese mice (A^{vy}/a). Life Sci. 28: 119–128.
85. BUKOWIECKI, L., L. JAHJAH & N. FOLLEA. 1982. Ephedrine, a potential slimming drug, directly stimulates thermogenesis in brown adipocytes via β-adrenoceptors. Int. J. Obesity 6: 343–350.
86. ARCH, J. R. S., A. T. AINSWORTH & M. A. CAWTHORNE. 1982. Thermogenic and anorectic effects of ephedrine and congeners in mice and rats. Life Sci. 30: 1817–1826.
87. MALCHOW-MØLLER, A., S. LARSEN, H. HEY, K. H. STOKHOLM, E. JUHL & F. QUAADE. 1981. Ephedrine as an anorectic: the story of the 'Elsinore pill'. Int. J. Obesity 5: 183–187.
88. ASTRUP, A., J. MADSEN, J. J. HOLST & N. J. CHRISTENSEN. 1986. The effect of chronic ephedrine treatment on substrate utilization, the sympathoadrenal activity, and energy expenditure during glucose-induced thermogenesis in man. Metab. Clin. Exp. 35: 260–265.
89. COSCINA, D. V. & J. N. NOBREGA. 1984. Anorectic potency of inhibiting GABA transaminase in brain: studies of hypothalamic, dietary and genetic obesities. Int. J. Obesity 8, Suppl. 1: 191–200.
90. MANDENOFF, A., F. FUMERON, M. APFELBAUM & D. L. MARGULES. 1982. Endogenous opiates and energy balance. Science 215: 1536–1538.
91. SHIMOMURA, Y., J. OKU, Z. GLICK & G. A. BRAY. 1982. Opiate receptors, food intake and obesity. Physiol. Behav. 28: 441–445.
92. MORLEY, J. E., A. S. LEVINE, B. A. GOSNELL, J. KNEIP & M. GRACE. 1983. The kappa-opioid receptor, ingestive behaviors and the obese mouse (ob/ob). Physiol. Behav. 31: 603–606.
93. ATKINSON, R ..., L. K. BERKE, C. R. DRAKE, M. L. BIBBS, F. L. WILLIAMS & D. L. KAISER. 1985. Effects of long-term therapy with naltrexone on body weight in obesity. Clin. Pharmacol. Ther. 38: 419–422.
94. MALCOLM, R., P. M. O'NEIL, J. D. SEXAUER, F. E. RIDDLE, H. S. CURREY & C. COUNTS. 1985. A controlled trial of naltrexone in obese humans. Int. J. Obesity 9: 347–353.
95. ARCH, J. R. S., A. T. AINSWORTH, M. A. CAWTHORNE, V. PIERCY, M. V. SENNITT, V. E. THODY, C. WILSON & S. WILSON. 1984. Atypical β-adrenoceptor on brown adipocytes as target for anti-obesity drugs. Nature (London) 309: 163–165.
96. LEVIN, B. E. & A. C. SULLIVAN. 1986. Beta-1 receptor is the predominant beta-adrenoreceptor on rat brown adipose tissue. J. Pharmacol. Exp. Ther. 236: 681–688.

Dietary Treatments That Affect Brain Neurotransmitters

Effects on Calorie and Nutrient Intake[a]

RICHARD J. WURTMAN

Department of Brain and Cognitive Sciences
and
The Clinical Research Center
Massachusetts Institute of Technology
Cambridge, Massachusetts 02139

Consumption of a meal or snack, or the administration of particular nutrients that happen to be the precursors for monoamine neurotransmitters, can affect the nervous system in important ways: It can, like the administration of many drugs, change the rates at which neurons synthesize and release these neurotransmitters.[1,2] The foods or nutrients act by modifying the composition of the plasma. Carbohydrates and proteins, for example, tend to decrease and increase the plasma concentrations of most of the large neutral amino acids (LNAA).[3,4] Dietary choline or lecithin, phosphatidylcholine (PC), increase plasma choline levels.[5,6] These changes in plasma composition lead to parallel alterations in brain amino acid and choline[9] levels, which in turn, can affect the rates at which individual neurons convert tryptophan,[10] tyrosine,[11] and choline[6,12] to serotonin, the catecholamine neurotransmitters, and acetylcholine, respectively.[1,6,13]

This ability of a meal, depending on its composition, to increase or decrease the production of the brain chemicals that mediate communications across synapses continues to seem very strange. It is almost as though one had the option of increasing testosterone or estradiol production at will by eating a food rich in cholesterol, or of enhancing thyroxine production in euthyroid individuals by eating more fish. Its existence invites speculation as to how it could be advantageous to the body to couple the outputs of certain neurons to postprandial changes in plasma composition, and specifically, as to how disturbances in this process might contribute to abnormalities in eating behaviors or in other brain functions that could be involved in obesity. This article focuses on one such possible advantage: the ability it confers on the brain to use the metabolic changes that a meal or a snack produces in making decisions as to what to eat at subsequent meals or snacks. The brain's responses to foods and nutrients also provide the physician with a novel strategy, based on using supplemental nutrients as though they were drugs, for attempting to treat disorders involving precursor-dependent neurotransmitters. Brain responses also provide the researcher with novel hypotheses for explaining how metabolic disturbances that modify plasma composition can also cause neurologic and behavioral symptoms.

[a] Some of the studies described in this review were supported by research Grants from the National Institutes of Health (NS-21231), the National Institute of Mental Health (MH-28783), the U.S. Air Force (AFOSR 830366), and the National Aeronautics and Space Administration (NAG-2-210), and by a National Institutes of Health Grant to the M.I.T. Clinical Research Center (RR00088-24).

179

DIET COMPOSITION AND BRAIN SEROTONIN SYNTHESIS

The initial suggestion that food consumption normally causes short-term changes in neurotransmitter synthesis was based on studies performed on rats in 1971.[10] Animals were allowed to eat a test diet that contained carbohydrates and fat but lacked protein. Soon after the start of the meal, brain levels of the essential (and scarce) amino acid tryptophan were found to rise, increasing the substrate-saturation of the enzyme, tryptophan hydroxylase, which determines the rate at which serotonin is synthesized. The resulting increase in brain serotonin levels was found also to be associated with an elevation in serotonin's metabolite 5-hydroxyindole acetic acid (5-HIAA), suggesting that the release of serotonin had also increased.

The rise in brain tryptophan levels after the carbohydrate-rich meal was accompanied, in rats but not in humans, by a small increase in plasma tryptophan levels. Both of these changes had been unanticipated, because the insulin secretion elicited by dietary carbohydrates was known to lower plasma levels of most amino acids (cf reference 3). (Tryptophan's responses to insulin had apparently not been examined). The failure of plasma tryptophan levels to decline after insulin secretion or administration was soon thereafter recognized[14] as resulting from another of this amino acid's unusual properties: its propensity to bind loosely to circulating albumin. Insulin causes nonesterified fatty acid (NEFA) molecules to dissociate themselves from albumin and enter adipocytes; this dissociation increases the protein's capacity to bind tryptophan. Hence, whatever reduction insulin produces in free plasma tryptophan usually is compensated by a rise in the albumin-bound moiety, yielding, in humans, no significant change in total plasma tryptophan levels. (Because this binding to albumin is of low affinity, the tryptophan thus bound is almost as accessible as free tryptophan for uptake into the brain.[15])

Much more difficult to explain were data subsequently obtained on the changes in brain tryptophan and serotonin levels that occurred after rats consumed a meal rich in protein. Although plasma tryptophan levels rose, reflecting the contribution of some of the tryptophan molecules in the protein, brain levels of tryptophan and serotonin either failed to rise or, if the meal contained sufficient protein, actually fell.[7] The explanation for this paradox was found to reside in the kinetic properties of the transport systems that carry tryptophan across the blood-brain barrier[16] and into neurons.[17,18] The endothelial cells that line the brain's capillaries contain macromolecules that shuttle specific nutrients or their metabolites between the blood and the brain's extracellular space.[16] One such macromolecule mediates the transcapillary flux (by facilitated diffusion) of tryptophan and other LNAA; others move choline, basic or acidic amino acids, hexoses, monocarboxylic acids, adenosine, and adenine. The macromolecule transporting tryptophan and other LNAA has a poor affinity for its ligands, and thus is relatively unsaturated at normal plasma LNAA concentrations; hence a meal-induced rise in a particular plasma LNAA can, by suddenly increasing the macromolecule's saturation, rapidly increase its transport into the brain. Moreover, LNAA transport is competitive, such that the ability of circulating tryptophan molecules to enter the brain is increased when plasma levels of the other LNAA fall (as occurs after insulin is secreted[19]) and diminished when the other LNAA rise. Because all dietary proteins are considerably richer in the other competing LNAA than in tryptophan (which generally comprises only 1.0–1.5% of proteins), consumption of a protein-rich meal causes a decline in the plasma tryptophan ratio (the ratio of the plasma tryptophan concentration to the summed concentrations of its major circulating competitors for brain uptake: tyrosine; phenylalanine; the branched-chain amino acids leucine, isoleucine, and valine; and methionine). This decreases tryptophan's transport into the brain and slows its conversion to serotonin. (Similar competitive mechanisms mediate the fluxes of tryptophan and other LNAA between the brain's extracellular space and its neurons,[17,18] and similar plasma ratios predict brain levels of each of the other LNAA after treatments that modify plasma amino acid patterns.[8])

It seems counterintuitive that the meal that most effectively raises brain tryptophan levels is the one entirely lacking in tryptophan (that is, one containing carbohydrates but no proteins), whereas a protein-rich meal, which elevates blood tryptophan, has the opposite effect on the brain.

It requires only a small amount of a high-quality protein like casein in a rat's meal (about 5% of its calories) to block the effect of its carbohydrate content on brain tryptophan.[20] The ability of particular proteins to block the carbohydrate effect bears a relationship to their amino acid compositions; thus lactalbumin, a relatively good source of tryptophan, has little ability to block the carbohydrate-induced rise in brain tryptophan, whereas gelatin, which is poor in tryptophan, readily blocks it.[20] Perhaps the serotonin-releasing brain neurons serve primarily to distinguish between two categories of meals or snacks: those rich in carbohydrate and poor in protein, and all others.

Plasma tryptophan ratios in normal adult humans vary between about 0.065 and 0.160,[3,4] depending largely on the composition of the most recent meal or snack and on the interval that has elapsed since its ingestion. Such variations are capable, in rats, of causing sizeable differences in brain tryptophan and serotonin levels.[8,13] Subnormal plasma tryptophan ratios are often noted in obese people, reflecting elevated plasma levels of the branched-chain amino acids,[21] probably caused by insulin resistance; these ratios are further reduced if the subjects are put on a high-protein, low-carbohydrate diet.[21]

Obviously the extent to which any meal or snack raises or lowers the plasma tryptophan ratio depends on whether other foods are still present in the stomach at the time of its ingestion. The changes in this ratio are the result of two processes: insulin secretion and the intestinal absorption of amino acids in the dietary protein, which depend on the nutrient composition of the mixture entering the duodenum. This may be very different from that of the test meal itself, if that meal is diluted with previously eaten but undigested foods. It should be noted that the ability of a carbohydrate to increase brain serotonin, and thereby modify serotonin-dependent behaviors, is independent of its sweetness. A lunch containing 105 g of starch produces as much of an increase in the plasma tryptophan ratio as one containing even more (123 g) sucrose.[22]

The fact that giving pure tryptophan could increase brain serotonin synthesis,[23] and could thereby affect various serotonin-dependent brain functions (e.g., sleepiness and mood) had been known at least since 1968 (cf reference 24). What was novel and perhaps surprising about the above experiments was their demonstration that brain tryptophan levels, and serotonin synthesis, could normally exhibit important short-term variations, responding, for example, to the decision to eat a carbohydrate-rich versus a protein-rich breakfast. It remained possible, however, that mechanisms might exist outside the serotoninergic nerve terminal, which kept precursor-induced increases in serotonin's synthesis from causing parallel changes in the quantities of the neurotransmitter actually released into the synapses. Indeed, it was known that if rats were given very large doses of tryptophan, sufficient to raise brain tryptophan levels well beyond their normal range, the firing frequencies of their serotonin-releasing raphe neurons decreased markedly;[25] this was interpreted as reflecting the operation of a feedback system designed to keep serotonin-mediated neurotransmission from transcending its physiologic range. (Similar decreases in raphe firing had also been observed in animals given drugs, like monoamine oxidase (MAO) inhibitors[26] or serotonin-reuptake blockers, which cause persistent increases in intrasynaptic serotonin levels.) If rats were given small doses of tryptophan, however, sufficient to raise brain tryptophan levels, but not beyond their normal peaks,[27] or were allowed to raise brain tryptophan physiologically, by eating a carbohydrate-rich meal,[28] no decreases in raphe firing occurred. Hence, food-induced changes in serotonin synthesis are allowed to modulate the transmitter's release and, thereby, the output of information from serotoninergic neurons.

Although normal variations in brain tryptophan levels fail to affect raphe firing, the responses of the serotonin-releasing neurons to supplemental tryptophan is considerably enhanced when they happen to be firing frequently (unpublished observation). This coupling of a serotoninergic neuron's firing frequency to its precursor-responsiveness is similar in some ways to the relationships observed in catecholaminergic[13,29] or cholinergic[6,30] neurons. One important difference exists, however, between the precursor-responses of serotoninergic and other monoaminergic neurons: tryptophan administration (or carbohydrate consumption) invariably causes major increases in brain serotonin levels, whereas tyrosine has little effect on brain dopamine or norepinephrine levels (unless they have been depleted by persistent firing, as occurs in the locus coeruleus of stressed rats[31]), and choline or PC administration causes only small and inconstant increases in brain acetylcholine.[9] Apparently, serotonin synthesis is always coupled to tryptophan levels, whether or not the serotoninergic neuron happens to be active; by contrast, the extent to which each catecholamine or cholinergic neuron is affected by supplemental precursors varies with its physiological activity. The "open loop" and continuous dependence of serotonin synthesis on precursor (tryptophan) availability makes serotoninergic neurons ideal candidates to serve as sensors (i.e., of events, like eating, that change brain tryptophan levels).

TRYPTOPHAN, DIETARY CARBOHYDRATES, AND THE HUMAN BRAIN

The ability of supplemental tryptophan to enhance serotonin turnover within the human central nervous system (i.e., to elevate cerebrospinal fluid (CSF) 5-HIAA levels) was first shown in 1970;[32] apparently no neurochemical data are available concerning the human brain's responses to carbohydrate intake. Numerous behavioral effects (e.g. decreased sleep latency, pain sensitivity, and antidepressant activity) have been associated with tryptophan administration since Smith and Prockup's original observation that it caused drowsiness and euphoria.[33] Most of these effects have been reviewed extensively elsewhere,[24,34-37] and those unrelated to food intake are not further discussed here.

Only a few well-controlled studies have been published describing behavioral effects of dietary carbohydrates.[37] Some have involved administering a specific carbohydrate, sugar (sucrose), to hyperactive children whose parents or teachers believed it capable of exacerbating their behavioral problem. In general, the carbohydrate treatment has tended, if anything, to reduce activity,[37] similar to its (and tryptophan's) reported effect on normal individuals: a high-carbohydrate lunch increased sleepiness in women, calmness in men, and in subjects over 40, the tendency to commit errors in a standardized test of performance.[38] Apparently, hyperactive children consume larger quantities of sugar than control subjects,[39] when allowed the opportunity. This may reflect a greater need for energy, or conceivably, an unrecognized attempt at self-medication, similar to that postulated below for patients with the seasonal affective disorder syndrome (SAD) and for other groups of carbohydrate-cravers.[40] Perhaps their raphe neurons release inadequate quantities of serotonin, causing them to feel dysphoric; consumption of carbohydrates might then be expected to ameliorate their condition, if temporarily, by augmenting serotonin release. There is evidence that levels of serotonin or 5-HIAA are subnormal in CSF samples from violent psychiatric patients[24] and in brains of people who have died by suicide.[35,36] There is, apparently, no evidence about serotonin levels or turnover in brains of hyperactive children.

SEROTONIN, FOOD CHOICE, AND CARBOHYDRATE CRAVING

If rats are allowed to pick from among two food pans, present concurrently, which contain differing proportions of protein and carbohydrate, they choose among the two so as to obtain fairly constant (for each animal) amounts of these macronutrients.[41,42] If prior to "dinner," however, they receive either a carbohydrate-based "snack"[43] or a drug that facilitates serotoninergic neurotransmission,[41,44] they quickly modify their food choice, selectively diminishing their intake of carbohydrates. (A protein-rich premeal has the opposite effect.[42]) These observations support the hypothesis, proposed above, that the ability of serotoninergic neurons to derive information from food-induced changes in the plasma amino acid pattern allows them a special role, as "sensor," in the brain's mechanisms governing nutrient choice.[40] Perhaps they participate in a feedback loop through which the composition of "breakfast" (that is, its proportions of protein and carbohydrate) can, by increasing or decreasing brain serotonin levels, influence the choice of "lunch."[45] Interestingly, the proportions of protein and carbohydrate that adult animals choose per day, when they are allowed the choice, are those that cause brain serotonin levels neither to rise nor to fall, suggesting that these levels are somehow related to a set-point for macronutrient choice.[45] When rats were given a diet containing protein and fat, but lacking carbohydrate, for several days, and were than allowed to choose a meal from among two food pans whose contents differed in their proportions of carbohydrate, they overconsumed carbohydrates (in comparison with control animals). This overconsumption was independent of whether the test carbohydrate was a sugar or a starch,[43] indicating that the basis of the macronutrient's selection was metabolic and neurochemical, and not primarily gustatory, at least in the normal adult rat.

Similar mechanisms may operate to govern macronutrient choice in humans. Subjects housed in a research hospital were allowed to choose, at each meal, from six different isocaloric foods of varying protein and carbohydrate, but constant fat contents, taking as many small portions as they liked; they also had continuous access to a computer-driven vending machine, stocked with mixed carbohydrate-rich and protein-rich isocaloric snacks. It was observed[46,47] that the basic parameters of each person's food intake—total number of calories, grams of carbohydrate and protein, number and composition of snacks—tended to vary within only a narrow range, from day to day, and to be unaffected by placebo administration.

To assay the involvement of brain serotonin in maintaining this constancy of nutrient intake, pharmacologic studies were carried out on a particular population of subjects in whom the putative feedback mechanism might be impaired. These were obese people who claimed to suffer from carbohydrate craving, manifest as the tendency to consume large numbers of carbohydrate-rich snacks, usually at a characteristic time of day or evening.[47] As discussed in detail elsewhere in this volume, subjects were given fenfluramine, a widely-used drug that had been found[41] to decrease carbohydrate intake in normal rats, and which was known to cause weight-loss in obese people by a mechanism involving the release of brain serotonin. Administration of relatively low doses(15 mg of d-fenfluramine, twice daily), caused a major reduction in snack carbohydrate intake,[46,47] a smaller reduction in mealtime carbohydrates,[47] and no significant changes in mealtime protein intake.[47] (Too few protein-rich snacks were consumed by the subjects to allow assessment of the drug's effect on this source of calories.) Two other drugs thought to cause the selective enhancement of serotonin-mediated neurotransmission, the antidepressants zymelidine and fluoxetine, also have been found to cause weight loss; this contrasts with the weight gain (and carbohydrate craving) often associated with less chemically specific drugs like amitriptyline. It has not yet been determined whether these drugs also selectively suppress carbohydrate intake in humans. In studies on normal nonobese individuals, administration of one gram of tryptophan with a high-protein meal was shown to reduce subsequent carbohydrate intake,[48] whereas a tryptophan-deficient diet was found to suppress the subsequent intake of protein, but not of carbohydrate.[24] Administration of two or three grams of tryptophan forty-five minutes prior to a buffet-type luncheon decreased the intake of calories and especially of rolls and cookies by similar subjects.[49] Apparently, data are lacking on the effects of d-fenfluramine or of other serotoninergic drugs on macronutrient selection by normal nonobese individuals.

Severe carbohydrate-craving also is typical of patients suffering from SAD, a variant of clinical depression discussed at length elsewhere in this volume, which is associated with a November to January onset, a higher frequency in populations living far from the equator, and concurrent hypersomnia and weight-gain.[50,51] A reciprocal tendency of many obese people to suffer from affective disorders (usually depression) has also been noted.[51] Because serotoninergic neurons apparently are involved in the actions of both appetite-reducing and antidepressant drugs, they might constitute the link between a patient's appetitive and affective symptoms. Some patients with disturbed serotoninergic neurotransmission might present to their physicians with obesity, reflecting their overuse of dietary carbohydrates to treat their dysphoria. (The carbohydrates, by increasing intrasynaptic serotonin, would mimic the neurochemical actions of bona fide antidepressant drugs like the MAO inhibitors and tricyclic compounds). Other patients might present complaining of depression, and their carbohydrate craving and weight gain would be perceived as secondary problems. A third group of patients, the bulimics,[51] might seek medical assistance because of their concurrent appetitive and psychiatric problems. The participation of serotoninergic drugs in a large number of brain functions besides nutrient-choice regulation might have the effect of making these functions hostages to eating (seen in the sleepiness that can, for example, follow carbohydrate intake,[38] just as it could cause mood-disturbed individuals to consume large amounts of carbohydrates for reasons related neither to the nutritional value nor the taste of these foods).

FACTORS GENERALLY AFFECTING RESPONSES OF NEURONS TO NUTRIENT PRECURSORS

The coupling of brain serotonin synthesis to food-induced changes in plasma composition, and the perhaps-consequent involvement of serotonin in behavioral mechanisms governing nutrient choice, could be a unique property of this particular neurotransmitter. More likely, this will turn out not to be the case. As already mentioned, the syntheses of several other neurotransmitters, notably the catecholamines and acetylcholine, have already been shown to be affected (within physiologically active neurons) by increases in plasma and brain tyrosine and choline, and abundant evidence is already available from drug studies that these neurotransmitters are also involved in normal or pathologic appetitive mechanisms. Hence, even though most of the information currently available about feedback loops, involving protein versus carbohydrate choice, plasma amino acid composition, brain neurotransmission, and subsequent food choice, concerns serotonin, it is important to consider the possibility that additional loops also exist involving other nutrients (e.g. fats), other plasma indices besides the plasma tryptophan ratio, and other neurotransmitters besides serotonin.

On the basis of the tryptophan-serotonin relationship, one can formulate a list[1] of biochemical processes that would have to occur in order for any nutrient to affect the synthesis of its neurotransmitter product, and the additional steps that would be required for the nutrient to modulate neurotransmitter release. This type of list might help in identifying other brain neurotransmitters affected by (or affecting) the diet:

(1) Plasma levels of the precursor, and of other circulating compounds that affect its availability to the brain, must be allowed to increase after its administration (or after its consumption as a constituent of foods). That is, plasma levels of tryptophan or the other LNAA, or of choline, cannot be under tight homeostatic control (like, for example, plasma calcium or osmolarity). In actuality, their plasma levels do vary severalfold after the consumption of normal foods,[3,4,35] and those of many amino acids may vary as much as four- or sixfold.[3,4]

(2) Brain levels of the precursor must be dependent upon its plasma levels, that is, there must not be an absolute blood-brain barrier for circulating tryptophan (nor for tyrosine, nor choline).[16] Rather, facilitated diffusion mechanisms exist allowing these compounds (as well as basic amino acids, adenine, adenosine and other purines, and glucose) to enter the brain.

(3) The mechanism that allows brain levels of these compounds to be modified by some parameter of plasma composition (the plasma tryptophan ratio, the plasma tyrosine ratio, and plasma choline concentrations) must be unsaturated, such that a change in plasma composition can, by enhancing its saturation, rapidly accelerate the precursor's entry into the brain. As described above,[16] the brain capillary macromolecules that mediate the bidirectional fluxes of LNAA and choline across the blood-brain barrier are, in fact, highly unsaturated with their ligands (as are those mediating the fluxes of basic amino acids, adenine, adenosine, and glucose. It should be noted, however, that glucose flux into the brain apparently is not rate-limiting in glucose's utilization, except when plasma glucose levels are very low.[16])

(4) The rate-limiting enzyme, within presynaptic terminals, which initiates the conversion of the precursor to its neurotransmitter product, must, similarly, be highly unsaturated with this substrate so that, when presented with more tryptophan, tyrosine, or choline, it will immediately accelerate synthesis of the neurotransmitter. (Tryptophan hydroxylase[7] and choline acetyltransferase [CAT][1,9] do indeed have very poor affinities for their substrates tryptophan and choline. Tyrosine hydroxylase activity becomes tyrosine-limited when neurons containing the enzyme have been activated and the enzyme has been phosphorylated.[52-54]

(5) The activity of this enzyme cannot be subject to local end-product inhibition; that is, the products of tryptophan's hydroxylation, 5-hydroxytryptophan

and serotonin itself, may not appreciably suppress tryptophan hydroxylase activity. (Nor, for that matter, can acetylcholine levels within cholinergic nerve terminals affect CAT activity. Tyrosine hydroxylase activity may be subject to some end-product inhibition when the enzyme protein is in its nonphosphorylated state; once it is allosterically modified, however, the enzyme apparently is freed from this constraint).[54]

Available evidence suggests that only some of the neurotransmitters present in the human brain are likely to be subject to such precursor control, principally the monoamines mentioned above (serotonin; the catecholamines; dopamine; norepinephrine and epinephrine; and acetylcholine) and, possibly, histidine and glycine. Pharmacologic doses of the amino acid histidine do elevate histamine levels within nerve terminals,[55] and the administration of threonine, a substrate for the enzyme that normally forms glycine from serine, can elevate glycine levels within spinal cord neurons.[56] One very large family of neurotransmitters, the peptides, are almost certainly not subject to precursor control. Their brain levels have never been shown to be affected by experimental variations in brain amino acid levels; moreover, there are sound theoretical reasons why it is unlikely that their syntheses would be thus influenced. The immediate precursor for a brain protein or peptide is not an amino acid, per se, as is the case for some of the monoamine neurotransmitters, but the amino acid molecule attached to its particular species of tRNA. In brain tissue, the tRNA-charging enzymes, characterized to date, have very high affinities for their amino acid substrates,[57] such that their ability to operate at full capacity, in vivo, is probably unaffected by amino acid levels (except, possibly, in pathologic states, like phenylketonuria, associated with major disruptions in brain amino acid patterns).

Little information is available concerning the possible precursor control of the nonessential amino acids, like glutamate, aspartate, and gamma-aminobutyric acid (GABA), which are probably the most abundant neurotransmitters in the brain, for the reason that is is very difficult to do experiments on these relationships. Even though glutamate and aspartate can be formed, somewhere in the body, by way of a number of biochemical pathways, the precise pathways that synthesize these compounds within the terminals of neurons that use them as their neurotransmitters are not well established (and may turn out to be surprising); there is even evidence that ornithine, a basic amino acid, can serve in neurons as the precursor for the acidic amino acid glutamate.[58] In the case of GABA, although its precursor, glutamate, is well-established, brain levels of that amino acid apparently cannot be raised without sorely disrupting normal brain functions. The macromolecule that transports acidic amino acids like glutamate and aspartate across the blood-brain barrier is unidirectional, functioning to secrete these compounds, by an active transport mechanism, from the brain into the blood.[16] Hence, the administration of even an enormous dose of monosodium glutamate will not affect brain glutamate levels unless they elevate plasma osmolarity to the point of disrupting the blood-brain barrier.[59]

If, indeed, the monoaminergic neurotransmitters turn out to be the only ones subject to nutritional control, this will still provide the physician and the neuroscientist with a number of interesting mechanisms to explore and exploit. These same neurotransmitters are critically important in a large number of physiologic mechanisms and pathophysiologic states and are thought to mediate the actions of many neuropharmacologic agents. Moreover, they include a number of compounds besides serotonin that could be involved in normal appetitive-control mechanisms and in the pathogenesis of obesity.

CONCLUSIONS

It appears well-established that certain foods and pure nutrients can have important effects on nervous function, effectively modulating the neurotransmission mediated by serotonin, the catecholamines, and acetylcholine. Brain serotonin synthesis is directly controlled by the proportion of carbohydrate to protein in meals and snacks; these foods increase or decrease brain tryptophan levels, thereby changing the substrate-saturation of tryptophan hydroxylase and the rate of serotonin synthesis. The release of the catecholamine neurotransmitters, dopamine, norepinephrine, and epinephrine, from physiologically active brain neurons and sympathoadrenal cells is enhanced by tyrosine administration and diminished by the other LNAA, which compete with tyrosine for transport across the blood-brain barrier and neuronal membranes. Acetylcholine synthesis and release can likewise be amplified, in physiologically active neurons, by consumption of PC-rich foods.

The ability of serotoninergic neurons to have their output coupled to dietary macronutrients allows them to function as sensors of peripheral metabolism, and to subserve an important role in the control of appetite. It also, however, makes the other numerous functions mediated by these neurons (e.g. sleepiness and mood) vulnerable to food intake, and may explain why some obese and/or depressed people overconsume dietary carbohydrates, perhaps using these foods for their nonnutritional or gustatory effects.

REFERENCES

1. WURTMAN, R. J., F. HEFTI & E. MELAMED. 1980. Precursor control of neurotransmitter synthesis. Pharmacol. Rev. 32: 315–335.
2. WURTMAN, R. J. 1982. Nutrients that modify brain function. Sci. Am. 243: 42–51.
3. FERNSTROM, J. D., R. J. WURTMAN, B. HAMMARSTROM-WIKLUND, W. M. RAND, H. N. MUNRO & C. S. DAVIDSON. 1979. Diurnal variations in plasma concentrations of tryptophan, tyrosine, and other neutral amino acids: effect of dietary protein intake. Am. J. Clin. Nutr. 32: 1912–1922.
4. MAHER, T. J., B. S. GLAESER & R. J. WURTMAN. 1984. Diurnal variations in plasma concentrations of basic and neutral amino acids and in red cell concentrations of aspartate and glutamate: Effects of dietary protein intake. Am. J. Clin. Nutr. 39: 722–729.
5. WURTMAN, R. J., M. J. HIRSCH & J. GROWDON. 1977. Lecithin consumption raises serum free choline levels. Lancet 11: 68–69.
6. BLUSZTAJN, J. K. & R. J. WURTMAN. 1983. Choline and cholinergic neurons. Science 221: 614–620.
7. FERNSTROM, J. D. & R. J. WURTMAN. 1972. Brain serotonin content: Physiological regulation by plasma neutral amino acids. Science 178: 414–416.
8. FERNSTROM, J. D. & D. V. FALLER. 1978. Neutral amino acids in the brain: Changes in response to food ingestion. J. Neurochem. 30: 1531–1538.
9. HAUBRICH, D. R., N. H. GERBER & A. B. PFLUEGER. 1979. Choline availability: the synthesis of acetylcholine. In Choline and Lecithin in Brain Disorders. A. Barbeau, J. H. Growdon & R. J. Wurtman, Eds.: 1: 57–71. Raven Press. New York.
10. FERNSTROM, J. D. & R. J. WURTMAN. 1971. Brain serotonin content: Physiological dependence on plasma tryptophan levels. Science 173: 149–152.
11. WURTMAN, R. J., F. LARIN, S. MOSTAFAPOUR & J. D. FERNSTROM. 1974. Brain catechol synthesis: Control of brain tyrosine concentration. Science 185: 183–184.
12. MAIRE, J. C. & R. J. WURTMAN. 1985. Effects of electrical stimulation and choline availability on release and contents of acetylcholine and choline in superfused slices from rat striatum. J. Physiol. (Paris) 80: 189–195.

13. SVED, A. F. 1983. Precursor control of the function of monoaminergic neurons. *In* Nutrition and the Brain. R. J. Wurtman & J. J. Wurtman, Eds.: **6:** 223–275. Raven Press. New York.
14. MADRAS, B. K., E. L. COHEN, R. MESSING, H. N. MUNRO & R. J. WURTMAN. 1974. Relevance of serum free tryptophan to tissue tryptophan concentrations. Metab. Clin. Exp. **23:** 1107–1116.
15. YUWILER, A., W. H. OLDENDORF, E. GELLER & L. BRAUN. 1977. Effect of albumin binding and amino acid concentration on tryptophan uptake into brain. J. Neurochem. **28:** 1015–1023.
16. PARDRIDGE, W. M. 1977. Regulation of amino acid availability to the brain. *In* Nutrition and the Brain. R. J. Wurtman & J. J. Wurtman, Eds.: **7:** 141–204. Raven Press. New York.
17. LAJTHA, A. 1974. Amino acid transport in the brain *in vivo* and *in vitro*. *In* Ciba Foundation Symposium **22:** 25–41. Elsevier. London.
18. MORRE, M. C. & R. J. WURTMAN. 1981. Characteristics of synaptosomal tyrosine uptake: Relation to brain regions and to presence of other amino acids. Life Sci. **28:** 65–75.
19. MARTIN-DU-PAN, R., C. MAURON, B. GLAESER & R. J. WURTMAN. 1982. Effect of increasing oral glucose doses on plasma neutral amino acid levels. Metab. Clin. Exp. **31:** 937–943.
20. YOKOGOSHI, H. & R. J. WURTMAN. 1986. Meal composition and plasma amino acid ratios: Effect of various proteins on carbohydrate, and of various protein concentrations. Metab. Clin. Exp. **35:** 837–842.
21. HERAIEF, E., P. BURCKHARDT, C. MAURON, J. WURTMAN & R. J. WURTMAN. 1983. The treatment of obesity by carbohydrate deprivation suppresses plasma tryptophan and its ratio to other large amino acids. J. Neural Transm. **57:** 187–195.
22. LIEBERMAN, H. R., B. CABALLERO & N. FINER. 1986. The composition of lunch determines afternoon plasma tryptophan ratios in humans. J. Neural Transm. **65:** 211–217.
23. ASHCROFT, G. W., D. ECCLESTON & T. B. B. CRAWFORD. 1965. 5-Hydroxyindole metabolism in rat brain: A study of intermediate metabolism using the techniques of tryptophan loading. J. Neurochem. **12:** 483–492.
24. YOUNG, S. 1985. The clinical psychopharmacology of tryptophan. *In* Nutrition and the Brain. R. J. Wurtman & J. J. Wurtman, Eds.: **7:** 49–88. Raven Press. New York.
25. GALLAGER, D. W. & G. K. AGHAJANIAN. 1976. Inhibition of firing of raphe neurons by tryptophan and 5-hydroxytryptopha: Blockade by inhibiting serotonin synthesis with R04-4602. Neuropharmacology **15:** 149–158.
26. AGHAJANIAN, G. K., A. W. GRAHAM & M. H. SHEARD. 1970. Serotonin-containing neurons in brain: Depression of firing by monoamine ocidase inhibitors. Science **169:** 1100–1102.
27. BRAMWELL, G. J. 1974. Factors affecting the activity of 5-HT-containing neurons. Brain Res. **79:** 515–519.
28. TRULSON, M. E. 1985. Dietary tryptophan does not alter the function of brain serotonin neurons. Life Sci. **37:** 1067–1072.
29. MILNER, J. D. & R. J. WURTMAN. 1985. Tyrosine availability determines stimulus-evoked dopamine release from rat striatal slices. Neurosci. Lett. **59:** 215–220.
30. BIERKAMPER, G. G. & A. M. GOLDBERG. 1980. Release of acetylcholine from the vascular perfused rat phrenic nerve-hemidiaphragm. Brain Res. **202:** 234–237.
31. LEHNERT, H., D. K. REINSTEIN, B. W. STROWBRIDGE & R. J. WURTMAN. 1984. Neurochemical and behavioral consequences of acute, uncontrollable stress: Effect of dietary tyrosine. Brain Res. **303:** 215–223.
32. ECCLESTON, D., G. W. ASHCROFT, T. B. B. CRAWFORD, J. B. STANTON, D. WOOD & P. H. McTURK. 1970. Effect of tryptophan administration of 5-HIAA in cerebrospinal fluid in man. J. Neurol. Neurosurg. Psychiatry **33:** 269–272.
33. SMITH, B. & D. J. PROCKUP. 1962. Central-nervous-system effects of ingestion of L-tryptophan by normal subjects. N. Engl. J. Med. **267:** 1338–1341.

34. HARTMANN, E. & D. GREENWALD. 1984. Tryptophan and human sleep: An analysis of 43 studies. *In* Progress in Tryptophan and Serotonin Research. W. Schlossberg, B. Kochen, B. Linzen & H. Steinhart, Eds.: **1:** 297–304. Walter de Gruyter. Berlin.
35. GROWDON, J. H. 1979. Neurotransmitter precursors in the diet: Their use in the treatment of brain disease. *In* Nutrition and the Brain. R. J. Wurtman & J. J. Wurtman, Eds.: **3:** 117–181. Raven Press. New York.
36. VAN PRAAG, H. M. & C. LEMUS. 1985. Monoamine precursors in the treatment of psychiatric disorders. *In* Nutrition and the Brain. R. J. Wurtman & J. J. Wurtman, Eds.: **7:** 89–138. Raven Press. New York.
37. SPRING, B. 1985. Effects of foods and nutrients on the behavior of normal individuals. *In* Nutrition and the Brain. R. J. Wurtman & J. J. Wurtman, Eds.: **7:** 1–47. Raven Press. New York.
38. SPRING, B., O. MALLER, J. J. WURTMAN, L. DIGMAN & L. COZOLINO. 1983. Effects of protein and carbohydrate meals on mood and performance: Interactions with sex and age. J. Psychiatr. Res. **17:** 155–167.
39. PRINZ, R. J., W. A. ROBERTS & E. HANTMAN. 1980. Dietary correlates of hyperactive behavior in children. J. Consult. Clin. Psychol. **48:** 760–769.
40. WURTMAN, R. J. 1983. Behavioural effects of nutrients. Lancet **1:** 145–147.
41. WURTMAN, J. J. & R. J. WURTMAN. 1979. Drugs that enhance central serotoninergic transmission diminish elective carbohydrate consumption by rats. Life Sci. **24:** 895–904.
42. LI, E. T. & G. H. ADERNSON. 1983. Amino acids in the regulation of food intake. Nutr. Abstr. Rev. Clin. Nutr. **53:** 169–181.
43. WURTMAN, J. J., P. L. MOSES & R. J. WURTMAN. 1983. Prior carbohydrate consumption affects the amount of carbohydrate that rats choose to eat. J. Nutr. **113:** 70–78.
44. MOSES, P. L. & R. J. WURTMAN. 1984. The ability of certain anorexic drugs to suppress meal consumption depends on the nutrient content of the test diet. Life Sci. **35:** 1297–1300.
45. THEALL, C. L., J. J. WURTMAN & R. J. WURTMAN. 1984. Self-selection and regulation of protein-carbohydrate ratio in foods adult rats eat. J. Nutr. **114:** 711–718.
46. WURTMAN, J. J., R. J. WURTMAN, J. H. GROWDON, P. HENRY, A. LIPSCOMB & S. H. ZEISEL. 1981. Carbohydrate craving in obese people: Suppression by treatments affecting serotoninergic transmission. Int. J. Eating Disorders **1:** 2–15.
47. WURTMAN, J. J., R. J. WURTMAN, S. MARK, R. TSAY, W. GILBERT & J. GROWDON. 1985. D-fenfluramine selectively suppresses carbohydrate snacking by obese subjects. Int. J. Eating Disorders **4:** 89–99.
48. BLUNDELL, J. E., V. MAUJEE, C. J. WILLIAMS & A. H. HILL. 1986. Interactive effect of tryptophan and macronutrients on hunger notification and dietary preferences. Abstract, Amino Acids in Health and Disease: New Perspectives. UCLA/Searle Symposium. Keystone, Colorado, May 30–June 2.
49. HRBOTICKY, N., C. A. LEITER & G. H. ANDERSON. 1985. Effects of L-tryptophan on short term food intake in lean men. Nutr. Res. **5:** 595–607.
50. ROSENTHAL, N. E. & D. A. SACK, C. J. CARPENTER, B. L. PARRY, W. B. MENDELSON & T. A. WEHR. 1985. Antidepressant effects of light in seasonal affective disorder. Am. J. Psychiatry **142**(2): 163–170.
51. ROSENTHAL, N. E., M. M. HEFFERMAN. 1986. Bulimia, carbohydrate craving, and depression: a central connection? *In* Nutrition and the Brain. R. J. Wurtman & J. J. Wurtman, Eds.: **7:** 139–166. Raven Press. New York.
52. EL MESTIKAWAY, S., J. GLOWINSKI & M. HAMON. 1983. Tyrosine hydroxylase activation in depolarized dopaminergic terminals; involvement of calcium. Nature (London) **302:** 830–832.
53. MILNER, J. D. & R. J. WURTMAN. 1986. Catecholamine synthesis: Physiological coupling to precursor supply. Biochem. Pharmacol. **35:** 875–881.
54. LOVENBERG, W., M. M. AMES & P. LERNER. 1978. Mechanism of short-term regulation of tyrosine hydroxylase. *In* Psychopharmacology: A generation of progress. **1:** 247–259. Raven Press. New York.

55. SCHWARZ, J. C., C. LAMPART & C. ROSE. 1972. Histamine formation in rat brain *in vivo:* Effects of histidine loads. J. Neurochem. **19:** 801–810.
56. MAHER, T. J. & R. J. WURTMAN. 1980. L-threonine administration increases glycine concentrations in the rat central nervous system. Life Sci. **26:** 1283–1286.
57. BARRA, H. S., L. E. UNATES, M. S. SAYAVEDRA & R. CAPPUTO. 1972. Capacities of binding amino acids by tRNAs from rat brain and their changes during development. J. Neurochem. **19:** 2289–2297.
58. WROBLEWSKI, J. T., W. D. BLAKER & J. L. MEED. 1985. Ornithine as a precursor of neurotransmitter glutamate: Effect of canaline on ornithine aminotransferase activity and glutamate content in the septum of rat brain. Brain Res. **329:** 161–168.
59. MCCALL, A., B. S. GLAESER, W. MILLINGTON & R. J. WURTMAN. 1979. Monosodium glutamate neurotoxicity, hyperosmolarity, and blood-brain barrier dysfunction. Neurobehav. Toxicol. **1:** 279–283.

Regulation of Food Intake During Pregnancy and Lactation

PEDRO ROSSO

Department of Pediatrics
School of Medicine
Catholic University
Santiago, Chile

INTRODUCTION

Pregnancy and lactation determine an increase in food intake, which is limited to the duration of these periods and whose relative magnitude varies in different species. In general, species with large litters increase food intake proportionally more than those with small litters. For example, the rat increases its nonpregnant food consumption 100 percent during pregnancy and approximately 450 percent during lactation.[1] By contrast, a woman needs to increase food intake only 10–15 percent during pregnancy and 20–25 percent during lactation[2] (FIGURE 1). It is generally assumed that the greater food consumption during pregnancy and lactation reflects maternal adaptation to the nutrient drain caused by the fetus and later by milk production. Apparently the obviousness of the situation has discouraged researchers from investigating the mechanisms involved. In fact, the number of studies on this subject is surprisingly low considering that pregnancy and lactation are states of physiological hyperphagia and, as such, they offer the unique possibility of exploring mechanisms of food intake control in the absence of experimental manipulation.

Most of the experimental data on food intake regulation during pregnancy and lactation derives from studies conducted in rats. In this species, greater food consumption begins early in pregnancy, reaches a peak during midgestation, and decreases somewhat near term.[1] Food intake increases progressively during lactation, and near weaning, values are usually 2.5 times those observed during pregnancy.[1] After weaning, there is a sudden drop in food intake, which returns to prepregnancy levels. This pattern of changes is similar to that observed in humans, but as mentioned earlier, proportionally much greater. In this respect, it is important to point out the present scarcity of information regarding food intake during pregnancy and lactation in well-fed healthy women. The available studies have major limitations, such as reduced sample size and/or the possibility that intake was influenced by cultural and economic factors.

APPETITE CONTROL DURING PREGNANCY

Besides changes in food intake, pregnancy also induces changes in food preferences, at least in humans, the only mammalian species where the phenomenom has been observed. A study in a middle-income American population[3] found that foods frequently craved were ice cream, sweets and candy, fruits, and fish. Aversions focused on red meat, poultry, and certain sauces. The single most important

191

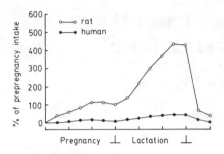

FIGURE 1. Changes in food intake during pregnancy and lactation in humans and rats. Values represent percent change over prepregnancy levels. Data on pregnant women adopted from various sources and pregnant rats.[1]

change was a substantial increase in milk consumption, whereas coffee consumption was drastically reduced. Somewhat similar changes seem to occur in other populations and countries, although, in general, national and ethnic food habits strongly influence the types of food preferred or averted.[4–6]

The causes of the changes in food preferences are unknown. The most accepted theory is that they reflect a reduction in taste acuity, a phenomenom that has been known for many decades[7] but that has never been adequately explored.

Pica, which is a craving for nonnutritional substances, is also more common among pregnant women. In the United States the consumption of laundry starch (amylophagia) has been described in low-income black women.[8,9] Studies have investigated, with inconclusive results, a possible link between this type of pica and the existence of iron deficiency.[10,11]

The mechanisms responsible for increased appetite during pregnancy remain unknown. Comparisons between changes in maternal food intake and fetal growth suggest that nutrient drain by the fetus has little, if any, influence on maternal appetite. As shown in FIGURE 2, maternal food intake begins to increase shortly after week 12 of gestation, when fetal body mass is too small to determine significant nutrient demands. Later on, between weeks 20 and 40 of gestation, daily caloric intake begins to fall off while fetal body weight and, presumably, nutrient requirements are increasing linearly. Similarly, maternal metabolic rate, reflected by oxygen consumption, increases linearly throughout gestation;[12] thus, the pattern of change seems unrelated to the changes in maternal food consumption.

Little is known about maternal physical activity during the course of pregnancy, except that it declines during the second half. Because daily physical activity is an important determinant of caloric needs, it seems logical to attribute the decline in maternal food intake observed at this stage to reduced physical activity.

The estimated pattern of maternal fat deposition during gestation closely resembles that of maternal food consumption (reference 13, p. 356). The most obvious explanation is a causal relationship between these two variables. Early in gestation, when maternal food intake is greater than fetal needs, the extra calories are deposited as fat. Later on, when maternal caloric intake decreases and fetal needs are greater, the rate of fat deposition decreases proportionally. It has been proposed, however,[14,15] that in certain physiological situations, including reproductive states, metabolic changes favoring fat deposition may precede changes in food intake.

As a whole, the data mentioned above suggest that factors other than fetal and maternal metabolic needs are influencing the increase in appetite. Landau has proposed that progesterone could be such a factor.[16]

Progesterone is secreted in large quantities by the placenta. Plasma levels of this hormone increase throughout pregnancy reaching, near term, concentrations considerably higher than those observed in the luteal phase of the menstrual cycle.[17] Plasma levels of estrogen, which antagonizes the effect of progesterone in various target tissues, also increase during gestation.[17]

The gestational increase of progesterone occurs earlier than that of estrogen. For this reason the first half of gestation is considered to be under the influence of progesterone, whereas during the second half, estrogen neutralizes some of the progesterone effects. Both hormones have been linked to the changes in appetite observed during the menstrual cycle. A double blind study conducted in a group of nutrition students found that daily caloric intake was 10–20 percent below average during the postmenstrual days when progesterone levels were lowest.[18]

The influence of ovarian hormones on food intake is well-known. Virgin rats injected with progesterone increase their food intake and, concomitantly, body fat.[19] Progesterone treatment does not cause these changes in male rats.

Female monkeys decrease food intake nearing ovulation, a time when estrogen levels are highest.[20] Similarly, rats decrease caloric intake during the proestrus phase.[21] This decrease reflects a reduced meal size not fully compensated by an increased meal frequency. A reduced meal size suggests increased sensitivity to satiety factors. The experimental data indicate that estrogen inhibits food intake and that in situations of high estrogen levels a decreased caloric intake should be expected. Conversely, when estrogen levels are low, caloric intake increases. Thus, the effect of progesterone on appetite would be mediated by the estrogen-antagonism of this hormone. Ovariectomized rats increase their caloric intake by increasing meal size and reducing meal frequency.[21] This is a transient change, however, because after a few days the animals return to previous intake levels by reducing meal frequency. Estradiol benzoate administration to long-term ovariectomized rats decreases meal size and, thus, reduces caloric intake.[21] Again, this is a transient effect for which the animals compensate by increasing meal frequency.

Research on the effects of estrogen and progesterone on the endogenous opioid system have lent further support to the role of these hormones in appetite. In the rat, estradiol administration decreases sensitivity to naloxone, a specific

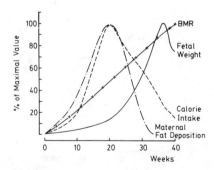

FIGURE 2. Changes in maternal calorie intake, maternal fat deposition, fetal weight and basal metabolic rate (BMR) during pregnancy. Values are expressed as percent of maximal change. Data on calorie intake adopted from V. Beal.[23] Maternal fat deposition, BMR, and fetal weight was adopted from Hytten,[13] p. 415.

opiate receptor antagonist that has been observed to decrease food intake under a variety of circumstances.[22] The decrease in receptor response has been interpreted as one of the mechanisms by which estradiol treatment decreases food intake. The other possible mechanisms would involve a reduction in endogenous opioid peptides.

Estradiol administration in the rat also decreases the response to ketocyclazocine, a kappa agonist that stimulates feeding.[22] Progesterone treatment reduces the estradiol effect on ketocyclazocine, thus providing further evidence of the interaction between these two hormones on appetite control. As previously mentioned, the idea of a "progesterone phase" and an "estrogen phase" of pregnancy, determined by the changing proportion in the plasma levels of these two hormones, fits well with the pattern of changes in food intake. During the first half of gestation, maternal food intake would increase because of the antagonistic effect of this hormone on estrogen. During the second half, the inhibition effect of estrogen would prevail. It would be overly simplistic, however, to attribute the gestational changes in food intake solely to estrogen/progesterone interactions (FIGURE 3). The levels of other hormones known to influence food intake, such as insulin and glucagon, are also affected by pregnancy.

APPETITE CONTROL DURING LACTATION

The mechanisms responsible for the increased food intake observed in lactating animals have been explored in some detail in the rat.[25] The following possibilities have been considered: 1) nipple stimulation may convey signals into the hypothalamus capable of influencing hunger-satiety centers, and 2) the metabolic consequences of milk production may produce a nutrient drain.

Ergocornine is an ergot alkaloid that inhibits prolactin secretion, hence lactation, without disrupting maternal behavior. When injected into lactating rats, ergocornine causes a marked drop in food intake despite continuous suckling by the pups. This substance also decreases food intake in nonlactating rats, but the drop is minimal compared with that observed in lactating rats (FIGURE 4). Thus, the data suggest that milk production *per se*, rather than nipple stimulation, is an important determinant of food intake in the rat. This conclusion is supported by

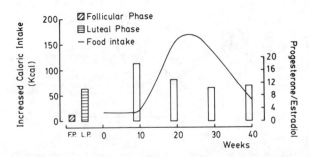

FIGURE 3. Changes in maternal calorie intake and progesterone/estradiol ratio during the course of pregnancy. Data on calorie intake adopted from V. Beal.[23] Data on plasma hormone levels during the menstrual cycle and pregnancy adopted from Tulchinsky and Ryan.[24]

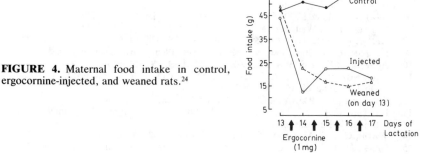

FIGURE 4. Maternal food intake in control, ergocornine-injected, and weaned rats.[24]

the effect of galactophore ligation, which also inhibits milk production without interfering with suckling. After this operation, lactating rats reduce their food intake although less than after ergocornine injection.

Hormones seem to play no role in food intake during lactation. Prolactin administration alone or combined with hydrocortisone and oxytocin had no effect on the food intake of rats that had lactated for 7 days and then weaned for 10 days.[25] Similarly, the effect of ovarian steroids also have to be ruled out.

The mechanisms by which the metabolic effect of milk production ultimately influences the hunger-satiety mechanisms are unknown. There are observations suggesting that lactating rats may have a reduced sensitivity to satiety factors.[26] For example, a comparison of the effects of cholecystokinin injection in lactating and nonlactating Zucker rats has revealed that this hormone, which causes a marked drop in food intake in virgin rats, does not alter food intake in lactating animals.

An increase in daily food intake can be accomplished by increasing meal frequencies, increasing meal size, or both. Increases in meal size reflect reduced sensitivity to satiety factors. During lactation, rats increase their daily food consumption by increasing meal size, rather than meal frequency. A similar phenomenon has been observed in the obese Zucker rat.

In summary, little is known about the mechanisms regulating food intake during pregnancy and lactation. The fragmentary information now available suggests that during pregnancy, placental steroids may play an important role, but this possibility has not been experimentally tested. These steroids may affect appetite by interacting with the endogenous opioid system.

During lactation, the main determinant of greater food consumption seems to be the nutrient drain imposed by milk production. In contrast with pregnancy, hormones do not play a significant role. The metabolic or hormonal mediators that modulate these food intake changes are unknown, but they seem to reduce sensitivity to satiety factors. Overall, pregnancy and lactation appear to be two unique models of physiological hyperphagia, which, so far, have been neglected.

REFERENCES

1. Cripps, A. W. & V. J. Williams. 1975. Br. J. Nutr. **33:** 17–32.
2. Recommended Dietary Allowances. 1980. National Academy of Sciences, Washington, D.C. 1980.
3. Hook, E. B. 1978. Am. J. Clin. Nutr. **31:** 1355–1362.

4. DICKENS, G. & W. H. TRETHOWAN. 1971. J. Psychosom. Res. **15:** 259–268.
5. HUNT, S. 1977. J. Hum. Nutr. **31:** 245–248.
6. BRUHN, C.Ms & R. M. PANGBORN. 1971. J. Am. Diet. Assoc. **59:** 347–355.
7. HANSEN, R. & W. LANGER. 1935. Klin. Wochenschr. **14:** 1173–1177.
8. KEITH, L., H. EVENHOUSE & A. WEBSTER. 1968. Obstet. Gynecol. Surv. **32:** 415–418.
9. PAYTON, E., E. P. CRUMP & C. P. HORTON. 1960. J. Am. Diet. Assoc. **37:** 129–136.
10. ANSELL, J. E. & S. WHEBY. 1972. Va. Med. Q. **99:** 951–954.
11. TALKINGTON, K. M., N. F. GANT, D. E. SCOTT & J. A. PRICHARD. 1970. Am. J.
    Obstet. Gynecol. **108:** 262–267.
12. WIDLUND, G. 1945. Acta Obstet. Gynecol. Scand. 25. Suppl. I.
13. HYTTEN, F. E. & I. LEITCH. 1971. The Physiology of Human Pregnancy. Blackwell
    Scientific Publications. Oxford.
14. WADE, G. & J. M. GRAY. 1979. Physiol. Behav. **22:** 583–594.
15. GRAY, J. M. & M. R. C. GREENWOOD. 1982. Am. J. Physiol. **243:** E407–E412.
16. LANDAU, R. L. 1983. JAMA **250:** 3323.
17. TULCHINSKY D. & C. J. HOBEL. 1973. Am. J. Obster. Gynecol. **17:** 884–893.
18. DALVIT, S. P. 1981. Am. J. Clin. Nutr. **34:** 1811–1815.
19. HERVEY, E. & G. R. HERVEY. 1967. J. Endocr. **37:** 361–384.
20. CZAJA, J. A. 1975. Physiol. Behav. **14:** 579–588.
21. BLAUSTEIN, J. D. & G. N. WADE. 1976. Physiol. Behav. **17:** 201–208.
22. MORLEY, J. E., A. S. LEVINE, M. GRACE, J. KNEIP & B. A. GOSNELL. 1984. Physiol.
    Behav. **33:** 237–241.
23. BEAL, V. 1971. J. Am. Diet. Assoc. **58:** 321.
24. TULCHINSKY, D. & K. J. RYAN. 1980. Maternal-fetal endocrinology. W. B. Saunders.
    Philadelphia.
25. FLEMING, A. S. 1976. Physiol. Behav. **17:** 841–846.
26. MCLAUGHLIN, C. L., C. A. BAILE & S. R. PEIKIN. 1983. Am. J. Physiol. **244:** E61–
    E65.

Disorders of Food Intake

Excessive Carbohydrate Snack Intake among a Class of Obese People

JUDITH J. WURTMAN

Department of Brain and Cognitive Science
Massachusetts Institute of Technology
Cambridge, Massachusetts 02139

The excessive calorie intake that characterizes the obesity of many individuals has been explained as an inability to regulate energy intake in accordance with energy needs. It has been assumed that the types of foods overeaten are randomly selected and if there is any tendency to consume excessive amounts of any particular type of food, it is due to the ready availability, inexpensive, or preferred taste of such foods.

Although these factors may account in part for the overeating that some obese individuals demonstrate, recent studies on patterns of food intake among the obese and those who suffer from a mild depression called seasonal affective disorder (SAD) are beginning to suggest that a subgroup of obese individuals may be consuming too many calories from one particular type of food, carbohydrates, and that they are doing so because eating such foods is associated with positive changes in their mood following carbohydrate intake. These people appear to be overeating not because of inability to control energy intake *per se* but because of a possible disturbance in the regulation of mood that generates a desire to overeat foods, that is, carbohydrates, which will improve their mood. Because the foods selected are often also high in fat, their consumption does increase the total daily calorie intake to levels that maintain an excessive weight or cause rapid weight gain, often after a period of weight loss or weight stability. Treatment of such individuals requires identifying this mood-related increased carbohydrate intake as the major cause of sustained obesity or rapid weight gain and use of therapies that address the problem of mood regulation as well as the regulation of food intake.

Our interest in whether some types of obesity may be associated with a disturbance in the regulation of nutrient intake was generated by observations made several years ago that carbohydrate intake is regulated independently of calorie intake.[1] The synthesis and activity of the brain neurotransmitter, serotonin, was shown to be enhanced following the consumption of a carbohydrate-rich, protein poor meal, due to the increased uptake into the brain of serotonin's precursor, tryptophan.[2,3] Conversely, the consumption of protein or a combination of protein and carbohydrate prevented this increase in serotonin synthesis, as the amino acids that normally competed with tryptophan for uptake into the brain were increased following protein consumption.[2,3] Because carbohydrate consumption was so directly related to serotonin synthesis, we became interested in whether brain serotonin was involved in regulating the consumption of carbohydrate intake. We carried out a series of animal experiments that demonstrated a separate regulation for energy intake and carbohydrate intake; when animals were treated

197

with drugs that increased serotoninergic neurotransmission, they decreased their intake only of high carbohydrate foods.[1] Moreover, when animals were given a meal sufficiently high in carbohydrate to increase serotonin synthesis, they subsequently consumed significantly more protein and less carbohydrate than animals prefed a meal containing both protein and carbohydrate.[4]

Subsequently, we began a series of clinical studies to learn whether carbohydrate intake is also regulated in people, and if so, whether its regulation involves brain serotonin. We were interested in whether some individuals might show a tendency to eat large amounts of carbohydrate alone, either at meals or as snacks, and whether this appetite for carbohydrate might be altered after treatment with drugs affecting serotoninergic neurotransmission.

In a preliminary study carried out on an outpatient basis with normal volunteers, we found that subjects who claimed to have a tendency to snack chose over 60% of their snacks as carbohydrate-rich foods. When they were treated with dl-fenfluramine, a drug known to increase serotoninergic neurotransmission, the consumption of carbohydrate-rich snacks decreased significantly.[5]

We followed this study with several inpatient studies to measure patterns of calorie, protein, and carbohydrate intakes from meals and as snacks. Initially, we examined the pattern of snack choice among obese individuals who claimed to have an excessive appetite for carbohydrate-rich snack foods. It was possible that their snack choices were influenced by the convenience or inexpense of carbohydrate-rich snack foods rather than by an excessive appetite for such foods. To distinguish between these possibilities, subjects were provided at all times with an assortment of both protein-rich and carbohydrate-rich snack foods. They were given a choice of 10 snacks; 5 high in carbohydrate and five high in protein. The snacks were isocaloric and contained the same amount of fat; thus the basis of snack choice was neither their calorie or fat contents. Snacks were dispensed in a refrigerated vending machine interfaced with a microcomputer that recorded the identity of the subject, the time a snack was removed from the vending machine, and the type of snack taken. In the first of these studies, subjects did not have a choice of meal foods but instead had to consume a study diet that met their daily nutrient needs and contained about 1000 calories. We found that despite the similar accessibility of both protein snacks and carbohydrate snacks, few protein snacks were consumed on a regular basis. Subjects consumed an average of 4.5 carbohydrate snacks a day and an average of 0.8 protein snacks a day. Subjects also exhibited a pattern of snacking behavior that was characteristic for each individual. Although the group as a whole tended to snack in the afternoon and evening, each individual was most likely to snack at only one of those times.[6] Serotonin appeared to be involved in this consumption of carbohydrate-rich foods because treatment with dl-fenfluramine decreased carbohydrate snack intake by 40 percent.[6] Subsequently we extended our observations on the patterns of food intake of obese snackers to measurements of calorie and nutrient choices from meals as well as snacks. We wanted to determine whether the excessive appetite for carbohydrate-rich foods was confined to snacks alone or might also be demonstrated in the nutrient choices made at meals. In two separate studies, subjects were allowed to choose their snack and meal foods from a variety of isocaloric items that were either high in carbohydrate or high in protein (TABLE 1). We found in both studies that the calorie intake from meals was moderate (about 2000 calories) as was consumption of both protein and carbohydrate foods from meals.[7,8] As in the first study, however, the subjects tended to choose most of their snacks as carbohydrate-rich foods (TABLE 2), and calorie intake from these carbohydrate snacks contributed an additional 700–800 calories to their daily calorie consumption. Moreover, in these as in the previous study, the snack intake of an individual was limited to a particular one- or two-hour period either in the afternoon or evening. The subjects in both studies were treated with d-fenfluramine, and such treatment resulted in a 40% decrease in carbohydrate snack consumption. Carbohydrate intake from meals was decreased following d-fenfluramine treatment to a lesser extent (by 22%), and protein intake was not decreased in the first study and by about 18% in the second.[7,9]

These results suggested that the appetite for carbohydrate-rich foods demonstrated by these subjects, whom we called carbohydrate cravers, was restricted to snack intake; at such time they consumed excessive amounts of carbohydrates, and their desire for these foods was markedly decreased by treatment with a drug that enhanced serotoninergic activity. They did not consume large amounts of

TABLE 1. Foods Offered at Meals and Snacks[a]

	High Carbohydrate	Low Carbohydrate
Breakfast	butter, crescent roll	canadian bacon
	chocolate-coated doughnut	cottage cheese
	granola bar	egg-cheese omelet
Lunch	corn souffle	tunafish salad
	peperoni pizza	sliced ham
	mixed vegetables (New England style) in sauce	chicken-cheese balls
Dinner	butterflake dinner roll	meatloaf
	rice pilaf	kielbasa and turkey plate
	chicken-flavored stuffing	crabmeat salad
Snacks	miniature goldfish	barbecued chicken wings
	date-nut granola cookies	ham/cheese rollup
	peanut cream patties	mozzarella cheese with honey loaf
	pecan sandie	lean cornbeef filled with cream cheese
	snickers bar (miniature)	

[a] This table lists the meal and snack foods offered in the final study on meal and snack intakes of obese carbohydrate cravers.[8,9] All breakfast items contained approximately 130 cal and 14–15 g of carbohydrate or protein; all lunch and dinner items contained approximately 150 calories and 15–16 g of carbohydrate or protein. Snacks were dispensed in a refrigerated vending machine and were available at all times except during meals. Each snack contained between 100 and 110 calories and 11–12 g of carbohydrate or protein.

carbohydrate at meals and did not restrict their choice of meal foods to carbohydrates but rather consumed protein along with carbohydrate at mealtime.

We were interested in learning whether the consumption of carbohydrate snack foods might be associated with changes in mood that followed such eating behavior. Anecdotal reports from our subjects indicated that they tended to experience positive changes in their mood following carbohydrate snacking. Because serotonin synthesis and activity is increased following the ingestion of carbohydrate, and because serotonin has been implicated in a variety of mood states including feeling of calmness, sleepiness, and decrease in pain perception, it was possible that our subjects were seeking to self-medicate themselves by eating carbohydrate-rich foods.

We measured changes in mood among obese carbohydrate cravers, following the consumption of a high carbohydrate lunch. Subjects were asked to consume a

TABLE 2. Meal and Snack Intakes among Obese Carbohydrate Cravers[a]

| Study | Subjects | Meals | | | Snacks | | |
		Kilocalories	Protein(g)	Carbohydrates(g)	Kilocalories	Protein(No.)	Carbohydrates(No.)
I	20	1940 ± 94	104 ± 6.1	121 ± 8.4	707 ± 97	0.7 ± 0.2	7.0 ± 0.4
II	51	1906 ± 41[b]	87 ± 2.5	143 ± 3.5	860 ± 34	0.9 ± 0.1	7.0 ± 0.4

[a] Calorie and nutrient intakes from meals and snacks were measured over a three day period. Subjects had access to six isocaloric foods at every meal; three were high in carbohydrate and three high in protein. At all times other than meals, subjects had access to 10 isocaloric snacks, five high in protein and five high in carbohydrate, dispensed in a computer-drive refrigerated vending machine.

TABLE 3. Seasonal Changes in Food Intake among Subjects with SAD[a]

| Season | Meals | | | Snacks | | |
	Kilocalories	Protein(g)	Carbohydrates(g)	Kilocalories	Protein(No.)	Carbohydrates(No.)
Fall/Winter	1734 ± 223	91 ± 12	131 ± 18	1173 ± 193	3.1 ± 1.0	9.0 ± 1.4
Spring/Summer	1333 ± 184[b]	86 ± 16	91 ± 16[c]	471 ± 150	1.8 ± 6.4	6.4 ± 1.5[c]

[a] These data represent average daily intake of calorie and nutrients from meals and snacks made in November and May. Subjects were given access to a variety of six isocaloric foods, three high in carbohydrate and three high in protein, at every meal, and eight isocaloric snack foods, four high in carbohydrate and four high in protein, at all times other than during meals. Measurements were made for 48 hrs during the fall and spring. Nine subjects participated in the study.
[b] Data are expressed as means and SEM p < 0.001.
[c] p < 0.005 decrease as compared to fall measurements.

large carbohydrate meal (104 g CHO) and to fill out standardized self reports on their mood 15 minutes prior to the meal and 2 hr following its completion. Their responses were compared with those of another subgroup of obese subjects (non-carbohydrate cravers) who also tended to consume an excessive number of their daily calories as snack foods,[8,9] but whose snack choices almost always included protein as well as carbohydrate foods. We found significant differences in the mood responses of these two groups of obese snackers.[8] The carbohydrate cravers felt significantly more vigorous, alert, less tired, and less depressed after the carbohydrate meal compared with the noncarbohydrate cravers. This remarkable difference in moods seen after carbohydrate ingestion among these two groups of obese snackers suggested that preference for or avoidance of carbohydrate snacks is associated with changes in moods experienced after such snack consumption. By ingesting carbohydrate-rich foods alone (without protein), the carbohydrate cravers would presumably increase serotonin synthesis and release and its concomitant effect on mood. By eating protein along with the carbohydrate, the noncarbohydrate cravers would prevent these changes in serotonin levels and activity and thus presumably avoid the resulting changes in mood (which in this group were experienced as unpleasant). Although we do not at this time have any explanation for the differences in mood seen between the two types of obese snackers, these results on the effects on mood of carbohydrate ingestion strongly suggest a disturbance in mood regulation in generating the type of eating behavior seen in these individuals.

Evidence that excessive consumption of carbohydrate may be associated with mood disorders has been provided recently by studies on SAD, a mild depression that is triggered by the short days of the fall and winter and relieved by the longer days of the spring and summer.[10] This mood disorder is reported to be associated with an excessive intake of carbohydrate-rich foods and weight gain.[10,11] We have measured patterns of calorie and nutrient intake among individuals suffering from SAD during the fall and the following spring. Measurements were made using methods similar to those described for the obese snackers. Calorie intake from meals and snacks was significantly lower in the spring as compared with the fall (TABLE 3). Subjects consumed substantially less carbohydrate from meals and as snacks; however, the most marked change was seen with snack intake. Over 1000 calories a day were consumed as snacks during the fall measurement period, and this was reduced to under 500 during the spring measurement period. The reduction in snack intake came almost exclusively from a decreased consumption of carbohydrate-rich foods. Although these results were obtained on a small sample of subjects,[9] they confirm earlier findings of Rosenthal et al. who described, based on self-reports, an excessive intake of carbohydrate-rich foods among individuals suffering from SAD. Although two of the nine were obese the increase in carbohydrate intake was not limited to these subjects; all the individuals participating in the study demonstrated similar increases in carbohydrate intake in the fall and reduction in the spring.

We treated these subjects with d-fenfluramine to see whether serotonin might also be involved in this depression-associated carbohydrate craving. Although the subject population was too small to allow definitive conclusions, we found a marked reduction in depression and, simultaneously, in carbohydrate intake.[12]

These results indicate that disturbances of mood regulation may be associated with disorders of food intake either chronically, as with our carbohydrate cravers, or periodically, as with individuals who suffer from SAD. Producing significant and lasting weight loss among obese individuals who consume excessive amounts of carbohydrate-rich foods might be accomplished by substituting low-calorie, high-carbohydrate snacks for the higher calorie ones typically consumed by such individuals, thus satisfying their need to ingest large amounts of carbohydrate without sacrificing caloric control. Both these individuals, however, as well as those suffering from SAD may also benefit from treatment with drugs that affect serotoninergic neurotransmission, because brain serotonin seems to be involved not only in the appetite for large amounts of carbohydrate foods, but also in the dysphoria that is associated with this carbohydrate craving. Moreover, if the disorders of mood and associated overeating reoccur on a predictable basis such as in SAD, such treatments may have to be used yearly in order to prevent weight gain and to sustain the weight loss that occurred during the previous seasons.

REFERENCES

1. WURTMAN, J. J. & R. J. WURTMAN. 1979. Drugs that enhance central serotoninergic transmission diminish elective carbohydrate consumption by rats. Life Sci 24: 895–904.
2. FERNSTROM, J. D. & R. J. WURTMAN. 1972. Brain serotonin content: Increase following ingestion of carbohydrate diet. Science 173: 1023–1025.
3. FERNSTROM, J. D., R. J. WURTMAN, B. HAMMERSTROM-WIKLUND, W. J. RAND, H. N. MUNRO & C. S. DAVIDSON. 1979. Diurnal variations in plasma concentrations of tryptophan, tyrosine and other neutral amino acids: effect of dietary protein intake. Am. J. Clin. Nutr. 32: 1911–1922.
4. WURTMAN, J. J., P. MOSES & R. J. WURTMAN. 1983. Prior carbohydrate consumption affects the amount of carbohydrate that rats choose to eat. J. Nutr. 113: 70–78.
5. WURTMAN, J. J. & R. J. WURTMAN. 1981. Suppression of carbohydrate consumption as snacks and at mealtimes by dl-fenfluramine or tryptophan. In Anorectic Agents: Mechanisms of Actions and of Tolerance. S. Garattini, Ed.: 169–192. Raven Press. New York.
6. WURTMAN, J. J., R. J. WURTMAN, J. GROWDON, P. HENRY, A. LIPSCOMB & S. ZEISEL. 1981. Carbohydrate craving in obese people: suppression by treatments affecting serotoninergic transmission. Int. J. Eating Disorders 1: 2–11.
7. WURTMAN, J. J., R. J. WURTMAN, S. MARK, R. TSAY, W. GILBERT & J. GROWDON. 1985. d-Fenfluramine selectively suppresses carbohydrate snacking among obese carbohydrate craving subjects. Int. J. Eating Disorders 4: 89–99.
8. LIEBERMAN, H. R., J. J. WURTMAN & B. CHEW. 1986. Changes in mood after carbohydrate consumption may influence snack choices of obese individuals. Am. J. of Clin. Nutr. 44: 772–778.
9. WURTMAN, J. J., R. J. WURTMAN, S. REYNOLD, R. TSAY & B. CHEW. d-Fenfluramine suppress food intake more effectively among carbohydrate cravers than among non-carbohydrate cravers. Int. J. Eating Disorders. In press.
10. ROSENTHAL, N., D. SACK, J. GILLIN, A. LEWY, F. GOODWIN, Y. DAVENPORT, P. MUELLER, D. NEWSOM & T. WEHR. 1984. Seasonal affective disorder: a description of the syndrome and preliminary findings with light therapy. Arch. Gen. Psychiatry 41: 72–80.
11. ROSENTHAL, N., D. SACK, C. CARPENTER, B. PARRY, W. MENDELSON & T. WEHR. 1985. Antidepressant effects of light in seasonal affective disorder. Am. J. Psychiatry 142: 163–170.
12. O'ROURKE, D., J. WURTMAN, A. BREZEZINSKI, T. ABOU-NADER, P. MARCHANT & R. WURTMAN. 1986. Treatment of seasonal affective disorder with d-fenfluramine. N.Y. Acad. Sci. This volume.

Induction of Obesity by Psychotropic Drugs

JERROLD G. BERNSTEIN

Clinical Research Center
Massachusetts Institute of Technology
Cambridge, Massachusetts 02142
and
Harvard Medical School
Massachusetts General Hospital
Boston, Massachusetts 02114

Many commonly prescribed medications have the capability of producing weight gain and, if the course of treatment is prolonged, may induce clinically significant obesity. The mechanisms, which have been invoked to explain drug-induced weight gain, include: stimulation of appetite, altered food preference, such as the production of specific carbohydrate cravings, and alterations in the metabolism of nutrients. Other significant mechanisms, which may account for drug-induced weight gain, include: impairment of metabolic processes as a result of suppression of thyroid gland function, fluid retention, and anabolic activity of steroids. Fortunately, many drugs, which induce weight gain, are primarily used either intermittently or for relatively short-term courses of therapy.

Stimulation of appetite and weight gain are commonly seen during treatment with cyproheptadine, a serotonin antagonist commonly used for allergic and pruritic symptoms.[1] Weight gain is also occasionally seen with other antihistaminic compounds, used in allergic disorders. Generally, such drugs are employed for brief courses of therapy, and, therefore, the extent of weight gain is limited. Another serotonin antagonist, methysergide, which is used in the prophylaxis of recurrent migraine headaches, may also, with prolonged use, induce weight gain.[1] Estrogen-containing oral contraceptives may produce weight gain, primarily through fluid retention. Androgenic hormones, prescribed for hypogonadism, lead to weight gain through their anabolic effect. Likewise, adrenal corticosteroids, widely prescribed for a variety of inflammatory, autoimmune, and neoplastic conditions, may be associated with considerable weight gain. Generally, steroids are prescribed for relatively short time intervals, and frequently, on an intermittent dosage regimen, which limits the extent of weight gain.[1]

Because a sizable proportion of patients receiving antipsychotic medications, antidepressants, and lithium will remain on medication for a year or, in some cases, many years, the potential of these drugs to effect food intake and weight gain is of great clinical significance.[2,3] Many patients discontinue medication too soon as a result of drug-induced side effects, including weight gain, thus giving rise to the potential recurrence of psychiatric symptoms.[2] It is common for patients receiving neuroleptic medications to gain ten to fifteen pounds in the course of one or more years of medication administration.[3] Tricyclic antidepressants may cause patients to gain twenty pounds during a year or more of treatment.[3] Lithium-treated patients may gain five to seven pounds during the first one or two months of treatment and often gain an additional five to ten pounds during the first year of lithium therapy.[3] Although the amount of weight gain is somewhat less after the

203

first year of psychotropic medication, many patients will continue to gain sizable amounts of weight for the duration of time that they remain on medication. Psychotropic drug-treated patients often have difficulty limiting their dietary intake and maintaining their pretreatment weight, presumably, because of specific pharmacological mechanisms of these medications, which contribute to changes in appetite, thirst, and body weight.[3]

The clinical literature has often underestimated both the frequency and seriousness of the potential development of obesity in psychotropic drug-treated patients. Animal models, which generally employ shorter periods of drug administration than those encountered in the clinical setting, have been less than satisfactory in providing clues to the mechanisms and management of psychotropic drug-induced weight gain.

This paper will examine some of the previously published observations on the association between psychotropic drugs and weight gain, as well as the author's own clinical experience with this phenomenon. Furthermore, attempts will be made to correlate clinical observations of the effects of these drugs on appetite and weight gain with their pharmacological actions on neurotransmitter reuptake mechanisms and receptor sites. The relative likelihood of weight gain, among different members of individual groups of psychotropic agents, will be explored, along with some practical approaches for reducing the risk of psychotropic drug-induced obesity.

ANTIPSYCHOTIC DRUGS

Chlorpromazine, introduced into clinical use in the mid-1950s, was the first effective antipsychotic agent. Weight gain was noted to occur with both short-term and long-term administration of this compound, although the mechanisms still remain uncertain. Advances in this area of therapeutics have given rise to a total of nearly twenty chemically different antipsychotic agents. These compounds all share in common the ability to block dopamine receptor sites within the central nervous system, and it is this action that is thought to be responsible for their clinical efficacy. The clinical potency of these drugs in alleviating psychotic symptoms, including hallucinations, delusions, and disordered thinking, directly parallels their affinity for dopamine receptor sites, as determined *in vitro*. Chlorpromazine, thioridazine, and mesoridazine, are considered low-potency neuroleptic compounds and must be used in larger milligram dosages than the high-potency neuroleptic drugs, such as piperazine phenothiazines, haloperidol, and molindone. The low-potency neuroleptic drugs appear clinically to have a greater appetite-stimulating and weight-promoting effect than do the high-potency compounds.[2,3]

In spite of the fact that the therapeutic action of neuroleptic drugs is linked to their ability to block dopamine receptors, these compounds have an affinity for a variety of receptors, including alpha adrenergic sites, histamine receptors, and acetylcholine receptors.[2,4] Some neuroleptic drugs inhibit serotonergic receptors and block reuptake mechanisms for norepinephrine, dopamine, and serotonin.[4,5] Molindone, the only neuroleptic whose use has been associated with a decrease in appetite and body weight, is interesting because of its unique indole structure reminiscent of the structure of serotonin.[2] Because serotonin has been implicated as a potential central mediator of appetite mechanisms and food choice, the possibility that differential actions of the various antipsychotic drugs in stimulating appetite mechanisms may be related to actions at the serotonin receptor site, is enticing.[6-8] Studies, using fenfluramine-induced facilitation of the hind limb withdrawal relex in spinal rats, indicate that chlorpromazine, thioridazine, and mesoridazine, exert potent inhibition of the serotonin receptor peripherally.[9] Using that experimental technique, trifluoperazine, haloperidol, pimozide, and molindone, all failed to block serotonin receptors.[9] It is intriguing to speculate on the possibility that the inhibitory effect of the low-potency neuroleptic drugs on serotonin receptor sites may correlate with their greater propensity to induce appetite stimulation and weight gain, and, furthermore, to relate the failure of molindone to block serotonin sites to its inability to stimulate appetite in patients.

The low-potency neuroleptic drugs, which are stronger appetite stimulants, also possess greater ability to block histamine receptor sites than do the higher potency neuroleptics.

Virtually all published studies of the obesity-inducing potential of antipsychotic drugs have cited chlorpromazine as the agent most likely to induce weight gain.[3] One study by Klett and Caffey[10] of male schizophrenic patients revealed a weight gain of eight to nine pounds over twelve weeks of chlorpromazine administration. Patients receiving other phenothiazines, including, promazine, mepazine, perphenazine, prochlorperazine, and triflupromazine, all experienced weight gain, but less than the chlorpromazine-treated patients. The greatest weight gain took place in the early weeks of treatment, and patients tended to return to premedication levels following discontinuation of medication. In that study, the investigators were unable to correlate changes in appetite with dosage of medication or the amount of weight increase.[11] A retrospective study of weight changes in male and female state hospital patients revealed an average weight increase of 15.9% of maximal ideal body weight in chlorpromazine-treated patients as compared to 8% in those taking perphenazine and 6.7% in those receiving clopenthixol.[11] In that study, there was a positive correlation of weight gain with chlorpromazine doses exceeding 400 mg per day. Patients in that study, who were switched from chlorpromazine to perphenazine in a therapeutically equivalent dosage, experienced, in 50% of cases, weight loss, which, in some cases, reached pretreatment body weight. Twenty-five percent of the patients, changing from chlorpromazine to perphenazine, continued gaining weight, and the remaining 25% remained at the increased body weight without any further gain or loss, following a change in medication.[11] Clinical experience with haloperidol, a high-potency butyrophenone neuroleptic agent in widespread clinical use for over twenty years, reveals a considerably lower potential of this drug to stimulate appetite and promote weight gain than that seen with chlorpromazine and other phenothiazine compounds.[2] Perhaps the failure of haloperidol to block central serotonergic receptors accounts for its lesser ability to stimulate appetite and weight gain.[2,9] Molindone, a structurally unique neuroleptic compound, as previously mentioned, is a clinically useful agent in the management of acute and chronic psychotic symptoms. This drug appears neither to stimulate appetite nor induce significant weight gain. In an eleven-week study, wherein molindone was compared with trifluoperazine, patients, receiving molindone, gained an average of 0.9 pounds, whereas those receiving trifluoperazine gained an average of 4.1 pounds.[12] Another study of twenty-three patients, treated with molindone for a period of six to nineteen months, revealed a mean weight loss of 6.5 pounds.[13] Five patients in that study, however, did gain some weight. Cole and Gardos studied nine chronically schizophrenic hospitalized patients and found a mean weight loss of 7.6 kilograms (range 0.9 to 16.8 kg) in a three-month course of treatment with molindone.[14] Following the course of molindone treatment, patients were returned to their previous neuroleptic therapy; some continued to lose weight, others resumed their pre-molindone pattern of weight gain.[14] The extent of weight loss reported with molindone in that latter study is dramatic, and may partially reflect the fact that patients had been receiving other neuroleptic medications just prior to starting the molindone study, and, therefore, the weight loss observed may have been a combination of discontinuation of the previous weight-promoting neuroleptic and the institution of molindone.

In addition to invoking a mechanism of serotonin antagonism to explain neuroleptic-induced appetite stimulation and weight gain, other mechanisms must also be considered. One of the most frequently seen side effects of psychotropic medication is the ability of both neuroleptics and tricyclic antidepressants to block acetylcholine receptors, both centrally and peripherally.[2] The peripheral anticholinergic effect gives rise to increased heart rate, decreased sweating, blurred vision, constipation, urinary retention, and dry mouth, with associated increased thirst.[2] It is very likely that the ability of psychotropic drugs to produce dry mouth and, thereby, stimulate thirst, plays a role in their ability to facilitate weight gain.[1,3] Patients with drug-induced dry mouth tend to consume large quantities of fluid in an attempt to quench their thirst. Consumption of large volumes of caloric soft drinks, as well as sweetened coffee and tea, can add considerably to the daily caloric intake of patients.[1] Certainly, patients who are psychiatrically ill and are being treated in a hospital setting are apt to have free access to such beverages and considerable time in which to consume them throughout the days and nights of their hospital stay. Also, psychiatric patients, who are not hospitalized, may be spending considerable amounts of time at home in close proximity to the foods and beverages in their kitchens.

Experimental studies in rats treated with phenothiazine compounds revealed increased food intake and greater utilization of calories.[15] Some studies, in both man and animals, have found a rise in serum glucose during chlorpromazine treatment.[16] One animal study found that chlorpromazine directly decreased glucose-induced insulin release from pancreatic beta cells in vitro and decreased glucose oxidation in the pentose-phosphate shunt and Embden-Meyerhof pathway in vitro.[17] A variety of endocrine changes have been found in patients receiving neuroleptic drugs, including increased serum prolactin levels and variable changes in serum cortisol concentration.[18] Although some investigators have attempted to link the neuroleptic-induced weight gain to changes in glucose metabolism and serum cortisol concentrations, there is little evidence to support this belief. Persistently abnormal serum glucose or insulin values are seldom seen, even in the course of long-term high-dose neuroleptic treatment. Likewise, chronic administration of neuroleptic drugs in several studies has failed to produce serum cortisol concentrations significantly different from those seen in normal controls.[18] Although a variety of metabolic changes may, on occasion, be seen in patients receiving neuroleptic medications, the tendency of these changes to be inconsistent and, indeed, to return toward normal with continuing long-term treatment, fails to support these as important mechanisms for neuroleptic-induced weight gain.[18]

Because increased consumption of high-calorie beverages is almost uniformly seen in patients experiencing dry mouth, secondary to psychotropic medications, it would be advisable, whenever possible, to prescribe those neuroleptic drugs with the lowest anticholinergic potency, and to minimize the long-term use of anticholinergically active antiparkinsonian medications in conjunction with prolonged neuroleptic therapy, because these compounds also increase thirst.[2]

Inasmuch as there appears to be a correlation between appetite stimulation, weight gain, and serotonin receptor-site blockade among neuroleptic drugs, conscious awareness of this phenomenon in the choice of the specific neuroleptic may minimize the amount of weight gain observed. Particularly, the use of molindone, in patients who are responsive to this agent, may be a desirable alternative to phenothiazines, because molindone has been documented to have the least ability to promote weight gain and, indeed, to have considerable ability to facilitate weight loss during treatment. In patients who are not responsive to molindone, but in whom the risk of weight gain is considered a high priority issue, treatment with haloperidol, which like molindone, fails to block serotonergic receptors, may be a desirable alternative, especially because clinical experience with haloperidol indicates its lesser propensity to facilitate appetite and weight gain. When neither of these agents can be employed, the third choice would be the use of a high-potency piperazine phenothiazine, such as perphenazine or trifluoperazine, which have weight promoting effects, but to a lesser degree than that seen with chlorpromazine and the low-potency neuroleptics.[2,3]

TRICYCLIC AND HETEROCYCLIC ANTIDEPRESSANTS

A wide variety of tricyclic antidepressant drugs have become well established as standard treatments for depressive disorders since the early 1960s. The most widely known of this group include amitriptyline, imipramine, desipramine, nortriptyline, and doxepin. The newest member of the tricyclic group of antidepressants is amoxapine, which exerts both antidepressant and neuroleptic effects, and possesses the unique characteristic of a rapid onset of antidepressant action.[2] Several newer antidepressant compounds, which possess a ring structure distinctly different from the tricyclic nucleus, have demonstrated efficacy in the management of depression, including maprotiline and trazodone. There are several investigational antidepressants, which are not structurally tricyclics, including fluvoxamine, and fluoxetine, which are soon to be released for marketing in the United States. Two other nontricyclic antidepressants, nomifensine and bupropion, were briefly marketed, but withdrawn because of potentially serious adverse effects. The term heterocyclic has been employed to include these structurally unique nontricyclic, non-monoamine oxidase inhibitor (MAOI) antidepressants. These compounds share in common an ability to inhibit nerve reuptake mechanisms for serotonin, norepinephrine, and dopamine.[2,4] Although the mechanism of the therapeutic action of these drugs is not incontrovertibly established, it is most likely that their inhibition of neurotransmitter reuptake with a consequent increase of neurotransmitters at active sites in the brain accounts for their therapeutic action.[2] In addition to the varying ability of these compounds to alter reuptake of neurotransmitters, they also possess a diversity of neurotransmitter receptor blocking activities, which may contribute both to their therapeutic effects and account for drug-induced side effects.[2,4,5] Chronic administration of antidepressant drugs produces variable down regulation of beta adrenergic and serotonin S_2 receptors.[19,20] These actions, may, at times, oppose the effects of reuptake inhibition. Most of the heterocyclic antidepressants antagonize histamine H_1 receptors and cholinergic receptors, and some antidepressants block dopamine and alpha adrenergic receptor sites.[20] Some of the heterocyclic antidepressants possess significant affinity for serotonin S_2 receptors.[20] Thus, the pharmacological action of the various heterocyclic antidepressants is considerably more complicated than is indicated by their ability to inhibit nerve reuptake mechanisms.

Most of the currently marketed tricyclic and heterocyclic antidepressants have an ability to stimulate appetite and create specific cravings for carbohydrate foods, both complex carbohydrates and sweets.[2,19] As a consequence of their effects on appetite, considerable weight gain is noted in association with prolonged use of these antidepressants. The anticholinergic action of these drugs produces dry mouth and increased thirst, which may lead to the frequent use of candy and chewing gum, and the consumption of large volumes of caloric beverages.[2] In clinical practice, patients being maintained on tricyclic antidepressants often report the consumption of prodigious amounts of fluid.

The problem of weight gain has been most prominently observed with amitriptyline, one of the oldest, most widely prescribed, and well-studied antidepressants. Paykel et al. investigated weight gain in 51 depressed women, who had responded favorably to initial treatment with amitriptyline.[21] Of those patients, 19 were maintained on the drug for nine months, whereas 32 were withdrawn from medication after three months.

During the first three months of treatment with amitriptyline, the 32 patients, who were to have their medication withdrawn at the three-month point in treatment, experienced a mean weight gain of 4.59 kg, whereas those 19 patients, who were to be maintained for an additional six months on active medication, experienced a mean weight gain of 3.33 kg.[21] During the subsequent six months on amitriptyline maintenance, patients gained a mean of 2.50 kg, while those patients, who were not maintained on active medication for the remaining six months of the study, gained a mean of 0.20 kg.[21] Eighty-seven percent of the maintenance amitriptyline patients reported persistent craving for carbohydrates, as compared to 29% of the nondrug maintained patients.[21] The extent of carbohydrate craving correlated with the dose of amitriptyline, although the amount of weight gain was not related significantly to drug dosage.[21]

Berken, Weinstein, and Stern examined the effects of amitriptyline, nortriptyline, and imipramine on appetite and weight gain in forty depressed outpatients. These investigators found a mean weight increase of 1.3 to 2.9 pounds per month during six months of treatment, yielding a total weight gain of 3 to 16 pounds over the period of the study.[22] The observed increase in weight paralleled the increased preference for sweets, and caused some patients to discontinue antidepressant drug treatment. Significant weight loss was observed following discontinuation of the medication. This latter investigation reported significant weight gains in patients receiving either amitriptyline or nortriptyline in daily doses of 25 mg or less per day and noted a more marked increase in weight among patients receiving higher doses, with patients on standard therapeutic dosage levels of amitriptyline gaining an average of four pounds per month.[22] Thirty-five percent of the patients in that study reported hyperphagia and 73% experienced carbohydrate craving and a preference for sweets.[22] Amitriptyline administration in a dose of 50 mg twice daily to six normal volunteers, over a period of twenty-eight days, failed to produce weight gain, although two subjects experienced an increase in appetite. In these normal volunteers, there were no significant abnormalities in glucose tolerance curves, or fasting or peak insulin levels, during the course of drug administration.[23] Likewise, in the group of 51 depressed women, previously mentioned, there were no abnormalities noted in fasting glucose, plasma insulin, or glucose tolerance. That study, however, did suggest that in patients on amitriptyline, greater carbohydrate craving was associated with a higher growth hormone response to exogenous insulin.[21]

Studies of the effects of amitriptyline on appetite and weight gain have generally observed an increase in both of these parameters to begin between the first and second month of drug treatment.[3,21] In clinical practice, a similar time course of the onset of appetite stimulation and weight gain is most commonly seen. Furthermore, in the clinical use of antidepressants, amitriptyline appears to be the drug most frequently associated with carbohydrate craving and weight gain. When patients experience these side effects during amitriptyline treatment and change to a different antidepressant, there is an almost invariable diminution in carbohydrate craving that will frequently slow down or arrest the otherwise continuous process of weight gain.

Clinically, doxepin, trimipramine, and imipramine stimulate appetite and weight gain slightly less than does amitriptyline, and occasionally changing treatment from the latter compound to one of the former compounds will reduce the rate and extent of weight gain somewhat. Nomifensine and bupropion both had minimal ability to increase appetite and facilitate weight gain, but are not currently available because of the occurrence of other unwanted adverse effects. Amoxapine clinically has much less ability to increase appetite and facilitate weight gain than does amitriptyline. Amoxapine has minimal effects on either serotonin reuptake or serotonin receptors.[2] It is conceivable that its lesser tendency to facilitate weight gain may be related to the fact that its antagonism of histamine H_1 and acetylcholine receptors is considerably weaker than many other commonly used antidepressants.[20] Because patients experience little anticholinergic effect and thirst while receiving amoxapine, this may account for lesser consumption of caloric beverages. Inasmuch as neuroleptic drugs may stimulate appetite and weight gain, it is likely that the weak neuroleptic effect of amoxapine contributes to its lesser effect on appetite. I have observed numerous patients who have gained considerable weight on either amitriptyline or imipramine, who, when changed to a regimen of amoxapine, experienced a decrease in appetite, carbohydrate craving, and weight gain. This antidepressant is worthy of serious consideration in patients for whom weight gain on antidepressant medications is a problem.

Desipramine has minimal antihistaminic, anticholinergic, and antiserotonin activity, and, primarily, exerts its antidepressant action by inhibiting nerve reuptake of norepinephrine, rather than serotonin.[2,20] Patients experience less dry mouth and thirst, while receiving desipramine, than with many other antidepressants and tend not to consume excessive amounts of fluids on this medication. Clinically, desipramine appears to have considerably less ability to stimulate appetite and encourage weight gain than do drugs such as amitriptyline. Indeed, many patients, who have received other tricyclic antidepressants, in the past, when switched to desipramine, will find less appetite stimulation, and a greater ability to diet and lose weight. Stern et al. recently reported on a study of desipramine in seventeen female and fourteen male depressed patients.[24] They found that, during a five-week period of treatment with desipramine, patients were able to lose a mean of just over two pounds, in contrast to the expectation that they might gain weight during an initial course of antidepressant therapy.[24] In that study, 24 of 31 patients lost weight, 6 patients gained some weight, and 1 patient experienced no weight change. Appetite and weight increases with psychotropic drugs seems very likely linked to actions at the serotonin receptor site. Compounds that increase serotonergic activity may decrease appetite and facilitate weight loss, whereas those that antagonize serotonin receptors may increase appetite and stimulate weight gain.[7] Desipramine is essentially devoid of both serotonergic and serotonin antagonist effects.[2] It thus seems that the mechanism involving anticholinergic-induced thirst, which is minimal with desipramine, may, at least partially, explain its lesser ability to produce weight gain.

Histamine antagonism by psychotropic drugs may be another mechanism by which these compounds increase appetite and weight, and thus the very weak histamine antagonism of desipramine may further explain its favorable profile from the standpoint of appetite and weight.[19,20]

Fluoxetine is a structurally unique antidepressant compound, whose primary mode of action appears to be its ability to block serotonin reuptake mechanisms.[7,8] This drug has minimal effects on either norepinephrine or dopamine reuptake.[20] Fluoxetine is essentially devoid of alpha adrenergic blocking activity, antihistaminic activity, and anticholinergic effect.[20] Because of its relative freedom from anticholinergic action, fluoxetine administration is not associated with anticholinergic side effects, which are so commonly seen with conventional antidepressant drug therapy. Most striking is the fact that numerous studies in both depressed and nondepressed individuals have documented an ability of fluoxetine to decrease appetite, to produce a specific reduction in carbohydrate craving, and to facilitate clinically significant weight loss.[7,25] This drug would appear to be a highly promising therapeutic agent in depressed patients who are either attempting to lose weight or attempting to avoid treatment-associated weight gain. Unfortunately, fluoxetine is not infrequently associated with some increase in anxiety and insomnia, the occurrence of which may require the coadministration of benzodiazepine-type antianxiety agents.[25]

Robinson et al. compared trazodone, amoxapine, and maprotiline in a multicenter study of 243 endogenously depressed outpatients.[26] In that four-week double-blind trial, they observed significantly smaller weight gains in trazodone-treated patients (0.90 pounds) than in amoxapine- (1.6 pounds) or maprotiline- (4.0 pounds) treated patients. In the treatment of depressed patients who have previously gained weight on antidepressant regimens, it would seem most reasonable to employ fluoxetine, trazodone, amoxapine, or desipramine, rather than amitriptyline or other tricyclic antidepressants, which are more likely to stimulate appetite and weight gain. Fundamentally, the choice of the appropriate antidepressant must be made on the basis of achievement of a satisfactory therapeutic response in the face of a tolerable range of side effects. Under most circumstances, patients must be given a therapeutic trial of two or more antidepressant drugs before an ideal match of therapeutic response and acceptable side effects is found for the individual patient.

MONOAMINE OXIDASE INHIBITOR ANTIDEPRESSANTS

Monoamine oxidase inhibitor (MAOI) type antidepressants became available for clinical use prior to the now more widely used tricyclic agents. Early studies of MAOI antidepressants, however, suggested that they were somewhat less effective than tricyclics, and because of their possible interaction with tyramine-rich foods and phenylethylamine-containing medications, the risk of hypertensive reactions with these drugs made them less desirable than alternative antidepressants.[2] More recent studies of MAOI-type antidepressants, using higher dosages and monitoring of platelet MAO levels, suggest that, in some subgroups of depressed patients, these compounds may be as effective or more effective than tricyclics.[2] Furthermore, MAOI antidepressants exert unique therapeutic benefits in patients with phobic and panic disorders. Careful instruction of patients regarding dietary and drug restrictions generally allows for the safe and beneficial use of these compounds, which have recently enjoyed increasing popularity. Monoamine oxidase inhibitors, like other antidepressants, may also facilitate weight gain, appetite stimulation, and carbohydrate craving. The two most widely used

MAOI antidepressants, phenelzine and tranylcypromine have somewhat different side effect profiles, pharmacological characteristics, and chemical structures. Phenelzine is a hydrazine compound, and thereby carries with it a slight risk of hepatotoxicity.[2] Furthermore, this compound occasionally induces fluid retention and peripheral edema; on rare instances, positive antinuclear antibodies and a lupus-like reaction have been reported with this drug. Tranylcypromine is a non-hydrazine compound, which has an amphetamine-like structure, and may, indeed, exert a direct stimulant effect in addition to its antidepressant action mediated through inhibition of monoamine oxidase.[2]

Phenelzine has not infrequently been associated with increased appetite, carbohydrate craving, and weight gain.[3] Its ability to stimulate appetite and weight gain is less than that seen with amitriptyline. Occasional, however, patients may gain considerable amounts of weight, and I have seen two individuals who have each gained approximately 30 pounds during a course of one year of treatment with this agent. Most often, weight increases with phenelzine are in the range of 5 to 10 pounds during a one-year course of treatment, whereas patients on amitriptyline, may not uncommonly gain 10 to 20 pounds during a one-year course of therapy.

Tranylcypromine has much less likelihood of stimulating appetite and weight gain and may be a useful alternative in patients who have previously been responsive to phenelzine, but who have experienced intolerable appetite stimulation and weight gain on this medication.[2] In several patients, whom I have changed from phenelzine to tranylcypromine, comparable levels of control of both depressive and panic symptoms have been maintained concurrently with a decrease in appetite, carbohydrate craving, and weight. Indeed, patients, who are overweight when they start an MAOI antidepressant or those who have previously gained weight on either tricyclic antidepressants or phenelzine, may best be treated with tranylcypromine. Although patients may generally be switched from a tricyclic to an MAO inhibitor without a drug-free interval, as was previously suggested some years in the past, changing therapy from phenelzine to tranylcypromine is best accomplished following a 7 to 14-day phenelzine-free period, because full levels of MAO inhibition, prior to instituting tranylcypromine, may predispose the patient to an initial hypertensive response to tranylcypromine, perhaps because of its amphetamine-like structure.[2]

Van Praag and Leijnse found a significant decline in fasting blood sugar following oral glucose tolerance tests in patients treated with hydrazine-type MAO inhibitors.[27] They suggested an association between reduced blood sugar and the hunger-stimulating effect of these agents.[27] Studies by Cooper and Ashcroft found that phenelzine increased insulin-induced hypoglycemia, whereas tranylcypromine did not.[28] Gander found that appetite stimulation, carbohydrate craving, and weight gain were greater in a series of patients receiving combined MAOI and tricyclic antidepressants.[29] In my experience with combined regimens, only one patient has had a striking enhancement of appetite, carbohydrate craving, and weight, in comparison to prior treatment on single antidepressant regimens.

One advantage of MAOI antidepressants is that they produce considerably less dry mouth and thirst than do tricyclic antidepressants, thus lessening the contribution of excessive fluid consumption as a potential source of weight gain.

LITHIUM

Lithium is of value as an adjunct in the treatment of acute mania and depression. It finds its primary area of usefulness, however, as a maintenance medication employed in the prophylaxis of both mania and depression in patients with bipolar affective illness.[30] Because lithium is generally employed over prolonged periods of time, its ability to stimulate appetite and weight gain is extremely important, inasmuch as repeated clinical studies and observations support an association between lithium maintenance and the development of considerable obesity.[31,32]

Vendsborg et al. found a mean weight gain of ten kg in 45 of 70 patients who had been receiving lithium for a period of two to six years.[31] Most of those patients experienced an increase in thirst, and there was a clear correlation between fluid intake and the extent of weight gain. That study also noted that when lithium was administered in conjunction with other psychotropic medications, enhanced weight gain was experienced. They found that patients who were overweight at the start of the study were more likely to experience weight gain during lithium treatment. O'Connell reported a mean weight gain of 8.9 pounds in 44 patients who received lithium over a thirty-month period.[33] Most studies of long-term lithium maintenance have found increased thirst in association with lithium and have attributed at least a portion of the weight gain to the continual consumption of high-calorie beverages.[32] Many lithium-treated patients complain of excessive hunger and food cravings, particularly for carbohydrates. The effects of lithium on brain serotonin are complex. Lithium increases brain concentrations of tryptophan, the precursor of serotonin, and also is capable of stimulating serotonin synthesis, although in some studies, lithium has been shown to either inhibit or have no effect on serotonin turnover.[30] Lithium has been demonstrated to reduce brain serotonin receptors in the rat.[34] It is conceivable that the reduction in brain serotonin receptors may, at least in part, account for appetite stimulation and weight gain associated with lithium therapy. The common thread of reduced serotonin receptor-site sensitivity in association with chronic administration of neuroleptic drugs, antidepressant drugs, and lithium may be a fruitful clue in explaining appetite stimulation, carbohydrate craving, and weight gain seen with this chemically diverse range of psychoactive substances.

Although some investigators have suggested changes in glucose tolerance to explain the influence of lithium on weight gain, studies in humans and animals have been inconsistent, and persistent changes in one direction or the other have not been demonstrated in association with short-term or long-term lithium treatment.[35] Some studies have also suggested that lithium-induced stimulation of glycogen synthesis and other metabolic effects may explain its weight-promoting action, though again, the data are neither consistent nor convincing for this mechanism.[36] Shortly after instituting lithium therapy, many patients experience an increase in fluid retention, and it is not uncommon to observe the occurrence of peripheral edema.[2,31] A significant number of lithium-maintained patients may retain as much as five to seven pounds of fluid as a result of lithium. In these individuals cautious use of diuretics, either thiazides or spironolactone, in conjunction with regularly measured serum electrolytes and lithium concentrations, may be a safe and effective means to minimize weight gain, secondary to fluid retention.[2,32]

In those patients whose affective illness requires maintenance treatment with lithium, but in whom weight gain is excessive, carbamazepine maintenance may be considered. Numerous studies have documented an acute antimanic effect of carbamazepine, and several investigators have found this compound to be useful in the prophylaxis against recurrent affective episodes.[2] Carbamazepine does not appear to stimulate appetite or weight gain and has been used by myself and other investigators successfully in the maintenance of patients who previously gained excessive amounts of weight during lithium therapy.[2]

Several published studies and extensive clinical experience indicate that in many patients lithium has a significant effect on thyroid function. Some degree of hypothyroidism is not uncommonly seen in patients maintained over prolonged periods of time with lithium.[30,32] Also, many patients maintain a clinically euthyroid state with normal blood thyroid indices, but develop goitrous enlargement of the thyroid gland during long-term lithium administration.[30,32] Decreased thyroid function or the development of a goiter may contribute to lithium-associated weight gain and may require the coadministration of thyroid hormone, along with continuing lithium therapy.[2]

Some patients are more susceptible to developing overweight problems during the course of psychotropic drug treatment. Numerous studies, with a variety of psychoactive drugs have indicated a correlation between pretreatment obesity problems and the risk of gaining weight during the course of medication treatment.[1] Patients who are more conscious of their weight at the outset of treatment and strictly limit food and beverage consumption can minimize weight gain.[1] On the other hand, some patients do not become conscious of the problem until they have gained considerable weight and experienced difficulties taking it off. Patients should be advised in advance regarding the risk of weight gain with psychotropic medications and should be engaged in the process of negotiation regarding the choice of the specific medication to be prescribed, keeping in mind the variation in the propensity of the various drugs to induce appetite increase and weight gain. Patients must be urged to consume water and other low calorie beverages and markedly limit their use of soft drinks, fruit juices, and sweetened coffee and tea, all of which can add significantly to the caloric load and the risk of obesity.

SUMMARY

Evidence from published studies and clinical experience indicates that neuroleptic drugs, tricyclic and heterocyclic antidepressants, monoamine oxidase inhibitor antidepressants, and lithium all possess varying abilities to increase appetite, stimulate carbohydrate craving, and cause weight gain over prolonged periods of administration. Sedatives and benzodiazepine-type antianxiety drugs fail to stimulate appetite or induce weight gain, and it is unlikely that the sedative or calming effects of other psychotropic drugs contribute significantly to changes in appetite or weight. Studies of the endocrine and metabolic aspects of psychotropic drugs suggest that these mechanisms do not contribute significantly to explaining the observed effects on appetite or weight.

Numerous studies indicate that a wide variety of compounds, including the serotonin precursor, tryptophan, the serotonin receptor stimulant, fenfluramine, and the serotonin reuptake inhibitor, fluoxetine, are all capable of decreasing carbohydrate hunger, reducing consumption of carbohydrate-rich foods, and inhibiting weight gain in humans and animals.[6,7] Widely divergent psychotropic drugs produce antagonistic effects at serotonin receptor sites, and it is likely that this action contributes to their ability to stimulate appetite, carbohydrate craving, and weight gain. Those psychotropic drugs that inhibit serotonin reuptake mechanisms, increasing serotonin activity within the central nervous system, either fail to stimulate carbohydrate hunger and weight gain or are actually capable of decreasing carbohydrate craving and facilitating weight loss.[6,7] Because many antidepressants, including trazodone and amitriptyline, the neuroleptic, chlorpromazine, and the mood stabilizer, lithium, may all, under some circumstances, inhibit serotonin reuptake mechanisms and may simultaneously block serotonin receptor sites, their effects on appetite and weight gain may represent a balance between serotonergic and antiserotonin activities. Monoamine oxidase inhibitors, which slow the metabolic degradation of monoamines, including serotonin and norepinephrine, allow for increased levels of these neurotransmitters within the brain. It is conceivable that the relative noradrenergic effect related to an amphetamine-like structure of tranylcypromine may explain its lesser ability to stimulate appetite and weight gain than the appetite and weight effects observed with phenelzine. Furthermore, the production of dry mouth and thirst by psychotropic drugs appears to contribute to weight gain, secondary to consumption of high-calorie beverages. In some cases, coadministration of fenfluramine, along with tricyclic antidepressants, may be useful, because the former serotonergic compound is capable of suppressing appetite and carbohydrate craving, which may accompany tricyclic antidepressant drug therapy. Likewise, fenfluramine may be useful in decreasing lithium-associated appetite stimulation and weight gain. Fenfluramine, however, is not applicable in the treatment of patients receiving monoamine oxidase inhibitors because of the potential of a drug interaction that may lead to hypertensive effects.

REFERENCES

1. KALUCY, R. S. 1980. Drug-induced weight gain. Drugs 19: 268–278.
2. BERNSTEIN, J. G. 1983. Handbook of Drug Therapy in Psychiatry. John Wright-PSG Inc. Boston, MA.
3. ROCKWELL, W. J. K., E. H. ELLINWOOD & D. W. TRADER. 1983. Psychotropic drugs promoting weight gain: health risks and treatment implications. South. Med. J. 76: 1407–1412.
4. RICHELSON, E. & M. PFENNING. 1984. Blockade by antidepressants and related compounds of biogenic amine uptake into rat brain synaptosomes: most antidepressants selectively block norepinephrine uptake. Eur. J. Pharmacol. 104: 277–286.
5. HALL, H. & S. O. OGREN. 1981. Effects of antidepressant drugs on different receptors in the brain. Eur. J. Pharmacol. 70: 393–407.
6. WURTMAN, J. J. & R. J. WURTMAN. 1984. d-Fenfluramine selectively decreases carbohydrate but not protein intake in obese subjects. Int. J. Obesity 8(Suppl. 1): 79–84.
7. FULLER, R. W. 1986. Pharmacologic modification of serotonergic function: drugs for the study and treatment of psychiatric and other disorders. J. Clin. Psychiatry 47(Suppl. 4): 4–8.
8. MURPHY, D. L., E. A. MUELLER, N. A. GARRICK & C. S. AULAKH. 1986. Use of serotonergic agents in the clinical assessment of central serotonin function. J. Clin. Psychiatry 47(Suppl. 4): 9–15.
9. WEIDLEY, E. F., P. E. SETLER & J. A. RUSH. 1980. The serotonin blocking properties of antipsychotic drugs. Pharmacologist 22: 279.
10. KLETT, C. J. & E. M. CAFFEY JR. 1960. Weight changes during treatment with phenothiazine derivatives. J. Neuropsychiatry 2: 102–108.
11. AMDISEN, A. 1964. Drug-produced obesity: experiences with chlorpromazine, perphenazine and clopenthixol. Dan. Med. Bull. 11: 182–189.
12. GALLANT, D. M. & M. P. BISHOP. 1968. Molindone: a controlled evaluation in chronic schizophrenic patients. Curr. Ther. Res. Clin. Exp. 10: 441–447.
13. KELLNER, R., R. T. RADA, A. EGELMAN et al. 1976. Long-term study of molindone hydrochloride in chronic schizophrenics. Curr. Ther. Res. Clin. Exp. 20: 686–693.
14. GARDOS, G. & J. O. COLE. 1977. Weight reduction in schizophrenics by molindone. Am. J. Psychiatry 134: 302–304.
15. GREENBERG, S. M., T. ELLISON & J. K. MATHUES. 1962. Comparative studies of growth stimulating properties of phenothiazine analogs in the rat. J. Nutr. 76: 302–309.

16. ERLE, G., M. BASSO, G. FEDERSPIL *et al.* 1977. Effect of chlorpromazine on blood glucose and plasma insulin in man. Eur. J. Clin. Pharmacol. **11:** 15–18.
17. AMMON, H. P. T., L. ORCI & J. STEINKE. 1973. Effect of chlorpromazine (CPZ) on insulin release *in vivo* and *in vitro* in the rat. J. Pharmacol. Exp. Ther. **187:** 423–429.
18. HIPPIUS, H., M. ACKENHEIL & F. MULLER-SPAHN. 1985. Neuroendorcinological and biochemical effects of chronic neuroleptic treatment. *In* Chronic Treatment in Neuropsychiatry. D. Kemali & G. Racagui, Eds. Raven Press. New York.
19. RICHARDSON, J. W. & E. RICHELSON. 1984. Antidepressants: a clinical update for medical practitioners. Mayo Clin. Proc. **59:** 330–337.
20. RICHELSON, E. & A. NELSON. 1984. Antagonism by antidepressants of neurotransmitter receptors of normal human brain *in vitro*. J. Pharmacol. Exp. Ther. **230:** 94–102.
21. PAYKEL, E. S., P. S. MUELLER & P. M. DE LA VERGNE. 1973. Amitriptyline, weight gain and carbohydrate craving: a side effect. Br. J. Psychiatry **123:** 501–507.
22. BERKEN, G. H., D. O. WEINSTEIN & W. C. STERN. 1984. Weight gain: a side effect of tricyclic antidepressants. J. Affective Dis. **7:** 133–138.
23. NAKRA, B. R. S., P. RUTLAND, S. VERMA & R. GAIND. 1977. Amitriptyline and weight gain: a biochemical and endrocrinological study. Current Med. Res. Opin. **4:** 602–606.
24. STERN, S. L., T. B. COOPER, M. JOHNSON *et al.* 1986. Desipramine does not cause weight gain. American Psychiatric Association, New Research Poster Presentation. Washington, DC. May 10–16, 1986.
25. ASBERG, M., B. ERIKSSON, B. MARTENSSON *et al.* 1986. Therapeutic effects of serotonin uptake inhibitors in depression. J. Clin. Psychiatry **47**(Suppl. 4): 23–35.
26. ROBINSON, D. S., J. CORCELLA, J. P. FEIGHNER *et al.* 1984. A comparison of trazodone, amoxapine, and maprotiline in the treatment of endogenous depression: results of a multicenter study. Curr. Ther. Res. Clin. Exp. **35:** 549–560.
27. VAN PRAAG, H. M. & B. LEIJNSE. 1963. The influence of some antidepressives of the hydrazine type on the glucose metabolism in depressed patients. Clin. Chim. Acta **8:** 466–475.
28. COOPER, A. J. & G. ASHCROFT. 1966. Potentiation of insulin hypoglycemia by MAOI antidepressant drugs. Lancet **1:** 407–409.
29. GANDER, D. R. 1966. The clinical value of monamine oxidase inhibitors and tricyclic antidepressants in combination. Amsterdam. Excerpta Medica. International Congress Series No. 122.
30. ORTIZ, A., M. DABBAGH & S. GERSHON. 1984. Lithium: clinical use, toxicology and mode of action. *In* Clinical Psychopharmacology. J. G. Bernstein, Ed.: 2nd edit.: 111–144. John Wright-PSG Inc. Boston, MA.
31. VENDSBORG, P. B., P. BECH & O. J. RAFAELSEN. 1976. Lithium treatment and weight gain. Acta Psychiat. Scand. **53:** 139–147.
32. VESTERGAARD, P., A. AMDISEN & M. SCHOU. 1980. Clinically significant side effects of lithium treatment. Acta Psychiat. Scand. **62:** 193–200.
33. O'CONNELL, R. A. 1971. Lithium's site of action: clues from side effects. Compr. Psychiatry **12:** 224–229.
34. TREISER, S. & K. J. KELLAR. 1980. Lithium: effects on serotonin receptors in rat brain. Eur. J. Pharmacol. **64:** 183–185.
35. SHOPSIN, B., S. STERN & S. GERSHON. 1972. Altered carbohydrate metabolism during treatment with lithium carbonate. Arch. Gen. Psychiatry **26:** 566–571.
36. PLENGE, P., E. T. MELLERUP & O. J. RAFAELSON. 1970. Lithium action on glycogen synthesis in rat brain, liver, and diaphragm. J. Psychiatr. Res. **8:** 29–36.

Disturbances of Appetite and Weight Regulation in Seasonal Affective Disorder

NORMAN E. ROSENTHAL, MICHAEL GENHART,
FREDERICK M. JACOBSEN, ROBERT G. SKWERER, AND
THOMAS A. WEHR

Unit of Outpatient Studies
Clinical Psychobiology Branch
National Institute of Mental Health
Bethesda, Maryland 20982

INTRODUCTION

For those species that live outside the tropics, the advent of winter represents a marked adaptational challenge, in that extremely cold temperatures occur at a time when food supplies are scarce. These environmental contraints have been termed the "ultimate factors," which have exerted evolutionary pressures for animals to develop mechanisms for conserving energy in order to survive.[1] Different species have evolved different mechanisms for conserving energy, some of which involve alterations in eating behavior and body weight. Thus hamsters, for example, store energy in the form of body fat and become obese in the winter.[2-4] Voles, on the other hand, actually conserve energy by losing weight, thus decreasing their energy requirements, and continue to forage during the winter months.[5,6] They compensate for the thermal insulation lost in becoming leaner by developing a long, winter pelage, which insulates their bodies as well as the fat they have lost.[6]

Although humans are not generally regarded as seasonal creatures, there is ample evidence from epidemiological data that seasonal rhythms occur in a variety of human phenomena including the rates of birth, growth, suicide, and death from natural causes.[7] There is also extensive evidence, dating back to the end of the last century and well reviewed by Attarzadeh,[8] of a seasonal variation in weight in humans, with a tendency to increase weight in the fall and winter and to lose it most easily in the spring and summer. This phenomenon can even be observed in growing children, despite the fact that growth in height occurs maximally in the spring and summer months. These observations have practical applications for the treatment of obesity. For example, a recently conducted Polish study showed that the best results in a weight loss program were observed in the spring and the worst during the winter.[9] Humans also reveal seasonal changes in food choice, which appear to be independent of the availability of different types of foods. Thus a study conducted in a cafeteria at the National Institutes of Health revealed that purchases of starchy foods and cooked vegetables declined significantly during the spring and summer months, at which time purchases of salads, cottage cheese, yogurt and skim milk rose. A reversal of this trend was seen in the fall. Sales of whole milk decreased significantly in the summer months, whereas sales of skim milk increased.[10]

Patients with seasonal affective disorder (SAD) show an exaggerated behavioral response to the seasons, which during the fall and winter months reaches such a degree of severity as to impair functioning both at work and in interpersonal relationships. These patients, most of whom are women, become anergic and unmotivated and tend to withdraw from others during the fall and winter months. By contrast, in the spring and summer their energy level, degree of motivation, and tendency to interact with others, are often even higher than normal. Their winter state frequently meets clinical criteria for depression, whereas their spring and summer state often meets criteria for hypomania.[12] The winter depression is generally accompanied by a tendency to oversleep, overeat, gain weight, and crave carbohydrates, though a significant minority of patients show the opposite symptoms of insomnia, anorexia, and weight loss.[11] The psychological symptoms of depression become particularly severe if patients experience demands, either from the outside world or from within, during their anergic winter states, They feel unable to rally and meet these demands and frequently experience sadness, anxiety, guilt, and feelings that life is not worth living at such times.

As part of their winter depressions many SAD patients suffer from a reversible form of obesity. This is of relevance to students of obesity because a percentage of obese patients will show particular difficulty with weight gain at certain times of

TABLE 1. Fall-Winter Changes in Eating, Weight and Carbohydrate Craving in SAD Patients (Seasonal Screening Questionnaire)

	Increase	Same	Decrease
Weight change	N = 130	N = 24	N = 21
(N = 175)	74%	14%	12%
Appetite change	N = 127	N = 15	N = 40
(N = 182)	70%	8%	22%

	Present	Absent
Carbohydrate craving	N = 109	N = 52
(N = 161)	68%	32%

the year, but perhaps more importantly because it provides a model studying reversible mechanisms that underlie the regulation of appetitive behavior and body weight.

CHANGES IN APPETITE AND WEIGHT IN SAD

On the initial screening of SAD patients, it is apparent that alterations in appetite and weight are cardinal symptoms of the condition (see TABLE 1). During their winter phase approximately three-quarters of patients report weight gain, whereas a minority (12%) report weight loss or no change in weight (14%). Appetite increases are reported by 70% of SAD patients, decreased appetite by 22%, and only 8% report no appetite changes at all. At the same time, approximately two-thirds of patients report carbohydrate craving. By analyzing data from a second questionnaire, the seasonal pattern assessment questionnaire (SPAQ), which can be administered to both normal and patient populations, it is apparent that normal subjects also report a history of seasonal changes in appetite, food preference, and weight. Although the pattern of seasonal changes in eating and weight in patients and normals are remarkably similar (see FIG. 1A and 1B), patients, as one would predict, report a far greater degree of seasonal changes than do normal subjects (see TABLES 2 and 3). Approximately the same percentage of normal subjects and SAD patients, however, report seasonal changes in food preference (see TABLE 4). Wurtman and colleagues analyzed the food records of 8 SAD patients during fall and spring and noted that patients chose many more carbohydrate snacks and calories during the fall (J. J. Wurtman, D. A. O'Rourke, R. J. Wurtman, unpublished observation, 1986). Their carbohydrate intake during meals was also increased but to a more modest degree than their snacking behavior. Although there was an overall increase in calorie intake during the fall, protein intake did not increase.

When patients' weights are measured longitudinally, the marked seasonal fluctuations they report are borne out. Whereas the patterns of weight change vary from patient to patient and within patients from one year to the next, the pattern of fall-winter weight gain and spring-summer weight loss is apparent in many

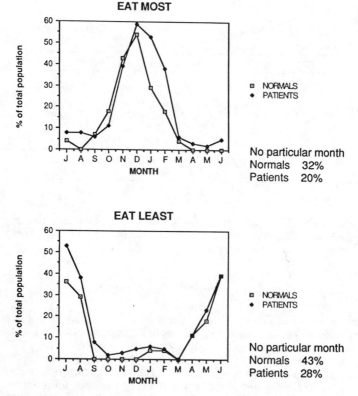

FIGURE 1A. Seasonal patterns of eating for SAD patients (N = 64) and normals (N = 28), as reported retrospectively by subjects in response to questions on the seasonal pattern assessment questionnaire (SPAQ), which inquires during what months of the year the subjects eat most and least.

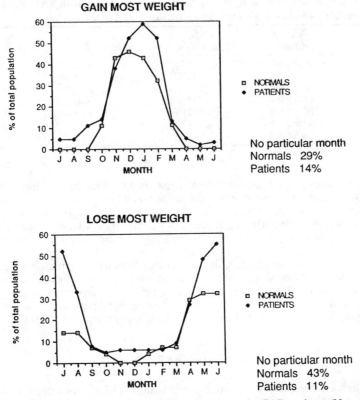

GAIN MOST WEIGHT

□ NORMALS
♦ PATIENTS

No particular month
Normals 29%
Patients 14%

LOSE MOST WEIGHT

□ NORMALS
♦ PATIENTS

No particular month
Normals 43%
Patients 11%

FIGURE 1B. Seasonal patterns of weight gain and loss for SAD patients (N = 64) and normals (N = 28), as reported retrospectively by subjects in response to questions on the seasonal pattern assessment questionnaire (SPAQ), which inquires during what months of the year the subjects lose and gain the most weight.

TABLE 2. Degree of Change in Appetite and Weight Experienced by SAD Patients (N = 64) and Normals (N = 28) (Seasonal Pattern Assessment Questionnaire)

	No Change	Slight	Moderate	Marked	Extreme
Weight					
Patients	3 (5%)	19 (30%)	20 (31%)	14 (22%)	7 (11%)
Normals	11 (39%)	11 (39%)	4 (14%)	0	0
Appetite					
Patients	9 (14%)	6 (9%)	22 (34%)	19 (30%)	4 (6%)
Normals	13 (46%)	11 (39%)	1 (4%)	2 (7%)	0

TABLE 3. Self-Reported Weight Fluctuation during the Year in SAD Patients and Normals (Seasonal Pattern Assessment Questionnaire)

Weight Change	Patients (N = 64)	Normals (N = 28)
0–3 lbs	5 (8%)	10 (36%)
4–7 lbs	15 (23%)	8 (29%)
8–11 lbs	20 (31%)	8 (29%)
12–15 lbs	7 (11%)	0
16–20 lbs	7 (11%)	1 (4%)
over 20 lbs	9 (14%)	0
not coded	1 (2%)	1 (4%)

cases, for example, the patient shown in FIGURE 2A. Some patients find it difficult in the spring and summer months to lose the weight they gained the previous fall and winter, which may result in chronic obesity (see FIG. 2B). The less frequent pattern of regular summer weight gain and winter weight loss, reported by certain patients on history, can be confirmed on longitudinal observation of these cases (see FIG. 2C).

As one would predict, the symptoms of weight gain and increased appetite are significantly correlated with one another as well as with carbohydrate craving. They are also significantly correlated with hypersomnia, however, suggesting that the regulation of the pattern of sleeping and eating in SAD may be coordinated by neurophysiological systems that vary seasonally in an interrelated way.

PHOTOTHERAPY IN SAD

Whereas extremes of temperature and scarcity of food have been termed the ultimate factors responsible for the evolutionary pressure to develop seasonal rhythms, it is clear that these factors come too late in the season to serve as effective triggers for initiating the seasonal energy conservation changes in weight and metabolism seen in certain animals. In fact, another set of environmental changes known as "proximate factors" have been recruited in the course of evolution to take on this direct triggering function of initiating seasonal behavior changes.[1] Of these proximate factors, photoperiod, the illuminated fraction of the 24-hour day, is by far the most important across the many types of seasonal rhythms studied.[13] It is understandable that this would be the case, because changes in daylength vary most predictably from year to year. Thus the winter weight gain observed in hamsters can be reproduced in the laboratory by artificially shortening the photoperiod,[2-4] as can the winter weight loss observed in voles.[5,6]

Humans, however, naturally increase the length of their photoperiod by the

TABLE 4. Changes in Food Preference during Different Seasons (Seasonal Pattern Assessment Questionnaire)

	Normals (N = 28)	Patients (N = 64)
No	7 (25%)	13 (20%)
Yes	19 (68%)	44 (69%)
not coded	2 (7%)	7 (11%)

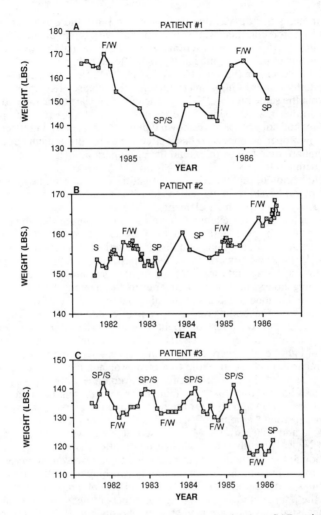

FIGURE 2. Patterns of weight change over time are shown for three SAD patients. Patient #1 (FIG. 2A) shows the most common pattern seen in this population, that is, weight gain in fall and winter and weight loss in spring and summer. Patient #2 (FIG. 2B) shows a similar pattern of seasonal weight change but fails during spring and summer to lose all the weight she has gained the previous fall and winter, thus developing a chronic weight problem. Patient #3 (FIG. 2C) shows a reverse pattern of seasonal weight change, showing weight loss in the fall and winter and weight gain in spring and summer.

use of artificial lighting. If the seasonal changes in eating and weight described above are influenced by photoperiod, how is it that they persist despite the use of artificial lighting? The first clue to resolving this paradox came from the observation of Lewy and colleagues, that whereas the nocturnal secretion of melatonin by the pineal could be suppressed by ordinary intensity artificial light in animals, it required light of far higher intensity (2500 lux) to suppress nocturnal melatonin secretion in humans.[14] It was this finding that inspired the treatment of patients with SAD by extending their winter photoperiod with bright artificial light.[11,15-17] Three studies performed by Rosenthal and colleagues have shown that bright (2500 lux) artificial light is significantly more effective than dim (300 lux or less) control light in reversing the symptoms of SAD.[11,16,17] This effect can be observed within two to four days of initiating treatment, and relapse of symptoms generally occurs within the same number of days. The effect appears to be mediated by way of the eyes rather than the skin.[18] It does not appear, however, to be photoperiodic, as Wehr and colleagues have shown that light treatments administered during the natural photoperiod appear to be as effective as light treatments of equivalent duration that are timed so as to extend the photoperiod.[19] This point is discussed in greater detail below.

It should be noted, that while all investigators who have studied the effects of phototherapy on SAD are in agreement that it is an effective treatment, there is some controversy as to which elements of the treatment are necessary. Wirz-Justice and colleagues, for example, have recently reported that lower intensity light (300 lux) may be as effective as light of higher intensity (2500 lux) in achieving a therapeutic effect, a finding that disagrees with the studies of Rosenthal and colleagues.[20] Lewy and coworkers have emphasized the importance of timing in phototherapy, stressing that for most patients, it is crucial to administer treatment in the morning hours, and that treatments in the evening hours may actually undermine the therapeutic effects of morning treatment.[21] This point of view is in disagreement with the findings of three separate studies. Thus James and coworkers showed that five hours of bright light administered in the evening were effective in treating 9 patients with SAD.[17] Hellekson and coworkers showed that two hours of light per day were effective in the treatment of 6 patients with SAD in Alaska regardless of whether the treatment was administered in the morning, the evening, or divided between morning and evening.[22] More recently, Jacobsen and colleagues have shown that two hours of bright light administered to 16 SAD patients between noon and 2:00 PM are as effective in reversing the symptoms of SAD as an equivalent amount of light administered in the early morning hours (between 6:30 and 9:00 AM), (F. M. Jacobsen, R. G. Skwerer, D. A. Sack, T. A. Wehr, and N. E. Rosenthal, unpublished observation, 1986).

Even though the above differences have yet to be resolved, such resolution is not critical to our present discussion. A more disturbing theoretical issue is raised by the findings that the antidepressant effects of phototherapy are not photoperiodic,[19] for the animal studies examining the effects of light on seasonal rhythms have all suggested that they are mediated by photoperiod.[23] Studies of reproductive rhythms in animals have clearly shown that timing is crucial for the seasonal effects of light;[23] a few seconds of light exposure at certain critical times are sufficient to modify seasonal rhythms of reproduction in hamsters, whereas light exposure outside this critical period, at times that fall within the winter photoperiod, do not have this effect.[24] In studies of seasonal rhythms in weight gain, the question of photoperiodicity has not been examined as closely as in the area of seasonal reproduction. It would be interesting to see whether bright light exposure during the normally illuminated fraction of the day would modify the winter pattern of eating and weight patterns in animals as it appears to do in patients with SAD.

Given that bright light treatment has generalized antidepressant effects in SAD, it is of relevance to this paper to inquire how the symptoms that pertain to eating behavior and weight are affected in relation to the other symptoms of SAD. TABLE 5 summarizes the results of bright light phototherapy in 47 patients treated in a variety of different study paradigms. In all cases, light was administered for five to six hours per day for a period of one to two weeks. The timing of light, however, differed in two of the different studies.[11,16,17,19] It is apparent that carbohydrate craving is the dietary symptom that responds most rapidly and dramatically to phototherapy (t = 4.02, p < .001), changing to a far greater extent than the symptoms of increased appetite and weight gain. When one considers the short

TABLE 5. Effect of Bright Light on Mood in SAD as Measured by 21-Item HRSD and Supplementary Items (N = 47)

	Baseline (x ± SEM)	Rx (x ± SEM)	t value	p	Percent Reduction
HRSD Symptoms					
depressed mood	2.20 ± .15	0.85 ± .15	−7.21	.0001	61
guilt	1.40 ± .13	0.60 ± .12	−4.05	.0002	57
suicide	1.00 ± .16	0.40 ± .12	−4.59	.0001	60
early insomnia	0.85 ± .13	0.81 ± .13	−0.60	ns	5
middle insomnia	1.20 ± .14	0.91 ± .14	7.55	.0001	24
late insomnia	0.81 ± .14	0.57 ± .10	−1.66	ns	27
low work functioning	2.90 ± .14	1.30 ± .19	−7.03	.0001	55
retardation	1.30 ± .10	0.64 ± .12	−4.82	.0001	51
agitation	0.97 ± .12	1.10 ± .13	0.40	ns	−4
anxiety psychic	2.10 ± .15	1.10 ± .15	−4.73	.0001	48
anxiety somatic	1.40 ± .18	0.68 ± .15	−3.48	.001	51
g.i. somatic	0.72 ± .11	0.34 ± .09	−3.49	.001	53
general somatic	1.60 ± .08	1.00 ± .12	−3.96	.0003	38
low sex drive	1.30 ± .12	0.60 ± .11	−5.05	.0001	54
hypochondriasis	0.74 ± .13	0.53 ± .13	−2.48	.02	28
weight loss	0.47 ± .13	0.53 ± .12	0.28	ns	−13
lack of insight	0.00 ± .00	0.03 ± .03	1.00	ns	
diurnal variation	1.40 ± .09	1.20 ± .12	−1.46	ns	14
diurnal severity	1.70 ± .09	1.30 ± .11	−2.38	.02	23
depersonalization	0.53 ± .12	0.25 ± .10	−2.00	.01	53
paranoia	0.48 ± .10	0.21 ± .07	−2.23	.03	56
obsessive-compulsive	0.55 ± .10	0.35 ± .09	−1.95	ns	36
Supplementary Symptoms					
increased appetite	0.81 ± .14	0.72 ± .13	−0.52	ns	11
carbohydrate craving	1.60 ± .18	0.81 ± .16	−4.02	.0002	49
weight gain	0.79 ± .14	0.49 ± .12	−1.71	ns	38
hypersomnia	1.30 ± .21	0.43 ± .11	−3.78	.0005	67
fatigue	3.10 ± .14	1.50 ± .21	−6.17	.0001	52
social withdrawal	2.70 ± .15	1.10 ± .20	−7.63	.0001	59

duration of treatment examined here, however, it is remarkable that the reports of weight gain should have decreased to the extent reported, that is, by 38 percent. One suspects that after prolonged phototherapy, one would observe a significant decrease in this symptom, especially because we have not observed the development of tolerance to this treatment modality. Unfortunately we do not have systematic data that speak to this point.

Whereas phototherapy has proven to be a highly effective treatment for SAD, it is important to remember that this treatment is not effective in all cases (in our experience, approximately 20% of patients do not respond to conventional photo-therapy), and even in those patients who do respond, the treatment frequently fails to reverse all the symptoms. This observation is reminiscent of studies of seasonal obesity in hamsters where environmental stimuli other than photoperiod have been shown to be important in modifying these rhythms. Thus Hoffman and colleagues have shown that reducing the environmental temperature can interact with shortening the photoperiod to produce seasonal obesity in golden hamsters,[2] and Bartness and Wade have reported that the content of dietary fat also contributes to the development of obesity in Syrian hamsters.[25] It would be interesting to see whether modifications of ambient temperature might enhance the antidepressant effects of phototherapy, especially in poor responders. It would also be logical to treat the obesity of patients with SAD with a combination of phototherapy and diet to maximize weight loss.

MECHANISMS INVOLVED IN SEASONAL RHYTHMS OF EATING BEHAVIOR AND WEIGHT

A consideration of the mechanisms involved in the disturbances in eating and weight regulation in SAD should take into account those environmental variables that may influence these behavior changes as well as the specific neurochemical and neurophysiological characteristics of this population that make them especially sensitive to these environmental changes. As discussed above, it appears as though increasing the intensity of environmental light, not necessarily by means of expanding the photoperiod, can decrease the severity of the symptoms of SAD. Thus far, no other environmental influences have been studied.

There are few studies that speak directly to the neurochemical and neurophysiological control of the seasonal changes in eating and body weight seen in humans. A discussion of possible abnormalities of this system, which would explain the exaggerated seasonal behaviors of SAD patients thus depends partly upon the few existing studies of direct relevance, but predominantly on speculation based on our knowledge of the neurophysiology of eating and weight regulation in animals. We shall discuss the two neurochemical modulators about which most information of relevance to this topic exists: melatonin and serotonin.

Melatonin

This indole derivative, secreted by the pineal gland nocturnally on a circadian basis, is an important neurochemical transducer of photoperiod in lower animals.[26] Photoperiodic information is conveyed by way of the retina, retinohypo-thalamic tract, suprachiasmatic nuclei, and superior cervical ganglia to the pineal gland, where it both suppresses and influences the timing of melatonin secretion. The resulting pattern of melatonin secretion, a product of both endogenous production and photoperiod, may influence the seasonal behavioral response. The role of melatonin in the regulation of seasonal rhythms has been established more clearly for reproductive behavior than for metabolism. Wade and Bartness,[27] however, have shown that in Syrian hamsters housed in long photoperiods, daily injections of melatonin in the late afternoon increase body weight and fat content, an effect that is also seen if the photoperiod is shortened. These authors, however, have also shown that the body weight increases induced by shortening the photoperiod occur even in pinealectomized animals, suggesting that there are multiple redundant mechanisms mediating the effects of photoperiod, which include gonadal hormones and dietary fat content. Hoffman and colleagues in their study of golden hamsters have shown that weight gain may be produced both by shortening the photoperiod and by reducing the ambient temperature to 10°C.[2] The effects of photoperiod were observed even when the animals were pinealectomized or blinded. When animals were both pinealectomized and blinded, however, the effects of photoperiod were lost. Based on these observations, the authors have also argued that multiple mechanisms are responsible for the photoperiodically mediated changes in weight and metabolism.

As discussed above, patients with SAD appear to experience a decrease in appetite, especially for carbohydrates, and to lose weight as part of a general antidepressant response to an increase in their environmental light. Inasmuch as this response is only found after the patients are exposed to bright light (2500 lux), a similar intensity to that required for the suppression of nocturnal human melatonin secretion, we postulated that the antidepressant response might be mediated by an influence on melatonin secretion.[28] We investigated this question in several ways. We measured plasma melatonin profiles in 6 SAD patients and 6 normal controls and found that the patients tended to secrete more melatonin in the late afternoon and early evening hours. We administered melatonin and placebo orally, in a double-blind crossover fashion, to 8 SAD patients, who had responded to phototherapy, while continuing to administer phototherapy in the morning and evening hours. There was no difference between the patients' responses to melatonin and placebo, as measured by the standard 21-item Hamilton Rating Scale for Depression (HRSD).[29] There was a significant difference, however, in a cluster of symptoms not measured by this scale, but measured by a supplementary scale developed specifically for use in SAD.[30] These symptoms, which include overeating, oversleeping, carbohydrate craving, and weight gain, were reported by patients to be significantly worse in the melatonin than on the placebo condition.

In another study, we treated 19 SAD patients with atenolol, a beta-adrenergic blocking agent, and placebo in a double-blind crossover study. Although we found that atenolol suppressed melatonin secretion, as measured by the 24-hour level of 6-hydroxymelatonin-sulphate, the major melatonin metabolite in the urine,[31] there was no overall difference in response between the melatonin and placebo conditions. Three of 19 patients, however, appeared to do exceptionally well on atenolol.

In a final study, we treated seven SAD patients, housed in dim rooms on our inpatient unit, with two different types of light treatment in a double-blind crossover design. The treatments, two different skeleton photoperiod conditions, were administered for 5 days each and were separated by a period of withdrawal from lights.[19] We predicted that one of the two conditions, the long skeleton photoperiod, in which two three-hour pulses of bright (2500 lux) environmental light were separated by 9 hours of dim light, would result in melatonin suppression, which, if melatonin were the neurochemical mediator of the phototherapeutic response, should result in an antidepressant effect. Conversely, according to this hypothesis, the short skeleton photoperiod, in which the same two light pulses were separated by only two hours of dim light, should not cause melatonin suppression and therefore should not have an antidepressant effect. In fact, we found that whereas only the long skeleton photoperiod suppressed melatonin, as measured by the 24-hour excretion of 6-hydroxymelatonin sulphate in the urine,[31] both conditions produced equivalent and significant antidepressant effects.

The results of all the above studies are compatible with melatonin having some role in the pathogenesis of some of the symptoms of SAD, notably those involving changes in eating and weight, and perhaps a more prominent role in the entire clinical picture in a small subset of SAD patients. It appears highly unlikely, however, that melatonin has a critical role in mediating the overall winter picture of SAD in most patients. These findings are reminiscent of the animal studies that suggest that seasonal changes in eating and weight are regulated by multiple mechanisms. Perhaps, in a similar fashion, the secretion of melatonin is just one of several mechanisms influencing seasonal energy regulation in SAD.

If melatonin is involved in the seasonal eating and weight changes seen in SAD, how might its effects be mediated? Although most animal studies on the effects of melatonin have examined its influence on reproduction, where it may have either an inhibitory or stimulatory effect, melatonin has also been shown to have a suppressant effect on thyroid function both in hamsters and in rats.[2,32-34] It is thus conceivable that melatonin might play a role in mediating the effects of winter climatic conditions, especially the shortened photoperiod, by means of its modulation of the thyroid axis. Several authors have described a seasonal variation of thyroid hormone levels in normal adults,[35-40] and reciprocal changes in serum concentrations of T_3 and reverse T_3 between summer and winter have been demonstrated.[41] Furthermore, hypothyroid patients treated with T_4 replacement have been found to have an exaggerated TSH response to TRH stimulation in the winter as compared with the summer.[42] Although patients with SAD have not thus far been shown to have any obvious abnormality of thyroid function,[11] systematic and sophisticated studies on large numbers of patients have not been performed to date. It would seem highly worthwhile to do so in view of the clinical evidence suggesting metabolic changes between summer and winter in this population.

The pineal gland has also been reported to have effects on growth hormone secretion in animal studies,[43-45] which might be involved in its modulation of seasonal rhythms of weight in animals and, conceivably, in SAD patients as well. A more recent study, however, has suggested that the previously reported inhibitory effects of melatonin on growth hormone might have been the result of stress, anesthesia, or both.[46]

Serotonin

There is considerable evidence that serotonergic systems vary seasonally. Wirz-Justice and Richter studied six normal subjects and found a significant annual rhythm in total platelet serotonin uptake,[47] a function reported to be abnormal in depressed patients,[48] with the highest levels in April, May, and June and the lowest levels in August and September. Swade and Coppen reported that active uptake of serotonin in platelets of depressed patients was significantly lower in May and June than in other months but found no seasonal variation of platelet serotonin uptake in normal controls.[49] More recently Arora and colleagues have described a seasonal rhythm in the number of platelet serotonin uptake sites in normal subjects, with the lowest values in April and June. They noted a similar trend in their depressed patients, but in patients the lowest values occurred in December.[50] Seasonal rhythms have also been described in platelet [³H]imipramine binding, which is thought to label serotonin uptake sites.[51,52] Of even greater interest are the findings of Carlsson and colleagues, who showed a significant seasonal rhythm of human hypothalamic serotonin content, with highest levels in the fall and lowest levels in the winter, in the postmortem specimens of subjects who had died of nonneurological, nonpsychiatric conditions.[53] More recently, Brewerton and colleagues examined the cerebrospinal fluid 5-hydrox-yindoleacetic acid, the major serotonin metabolite, in 25 normal subjects who underwent lumbar punctures at different times of the year, and showed a significant seasonal rhythm, with lowest levels occurring during the spring and the highest levels in the summer months (T. D. Brewerton, W. H. Berrettinin, J. I. Nurnberger, M. Linnoila, and E. S. Gershon, unpublished observation, 1986). It is difficult to reconcile all of these findings and explain them in terms of a single seasonal influence on serotonin metabolism. The finding of seasonal rhythms, however in such diverse parameters related to serotonin metabolism and by so many groups of investigators suggests that the serotonin system is markedly responsive to seasonal changes and that serotonin should be regarded as a likely modulator of some human seasonal behavior changes.

There has been a long-standing interest in serotonergic functioning both in depression, where it has been postulated to be depleted,[54] and in the eating disorders,[29] because of the well-established role of serotonin in the regulation of satiety.[55] Of particular relevance is the work of Wurtman and colleagues,[56,57] who have demonstrated in animal studies that dietary carbohydrates enhance serotonin synthesis in the brain. More recently they have speculated about the possibility of similar mechanisms existing in humans and have theorized that eating carbohydrates may be part of a complex behavioral-biochemical feedback loop for regulating serotonin homeostasis.[58] Thus the symptom of carbohydrate craving may reflect a depletion of brain serotonin, which is transiently corrected by the ingestion of large amounts of carbohydrates. Wurtman and colleagues have shown that the administration of the serotonin agonist, *d*-fenfluramine, is capable of selectively suppressing the intake of carbohydrate in obese patients who crave carbohydrates.[59] More recently they have shown in 12 patients with SAD that *d*-fenfluramine can similarly ameliorate the other winter depressive symptoms as well as the tendency to binge on carbohydrates (D. A. O'Rourke, J. J. Wurtman, J. Bernstein, and R. J. Wurtman, unpublished observation, 1986). A larger number of SAD patients, however, will have to be studied before the value of fenfluramine in this group is established. The strong seasonal changes in serotonin metabolism, as well as the importance of serotonin in the regulation of appetitive behavior and mood, would seem to make this area a promising one for further research efforts.

CONCLUSION

It is apparent that there are seasonal rhythms of eating behavior, weight gain, and metabolism (at least as reflected by thyroid function) in the general population. These rhythms are particularly marked in certain individuals, specifically patients with SAD, who also show marked seasonal rhythms in other behaviors. Supplementation of environmental lighting is capable of reversing to some extent these behavioral changes even over the course of a week. More prolonged treatment of this kind might have an even more marked effect on these behaviors. It is possible, however, that other environmental variables besides light, notably temperature, or endogenous factors that are not amenable to being reversed by environmental manipulations may also be involved in the development of these behaviors. An understanding of this form of overeating and obesity would be of considerable interest to students of obesity not only in order to help those individuals affected by these seasonal changes but also for the knowledge it is sure to yield about the interaction of environmental change and endogenous susceptibility in the regulation of eating and weight control in humans. Thus, patients with SAD provide an excellent model for the study of reversible obesity in humans.

REFERENCES

1. THOMSON, A. L. 1950. Factors determining the breeding seasons of birds: an introductory review. Ibis **92:** 173–184.
2. HOFFMAN, R. A., K. DAVIDSON & K. STEINBERG. 1982. Influence of photoperiod and temperature on weight gain, food consumption, fat pads and thyroxine in male golden hamsters. Growth **46:** 150–162.
3. CAMPBELL, C. S., J. TABOR & J. D. DAVIS. 1983. Small effect of brown adipose tissue and major effect of photoperiod on body weight in hamsters (*Mesocricetus auratus*). Physiol. Behav. **30:** 349–352.
4. WADE, G. N. 1983. Dietary obesity in golden hamsters: reversibility and effects of sex and photoperiod. Physiol. Behav. **30:** 131–137.
5. DARK, J., I. ZUCKER & G. N. WADE. 1983. Photoperiodic regulation of body mass, food intake, and reproduction in meadow voles. Am. J. Physiol. **245:** R334–R338.
6. DARK, J. & I. ZUCKER. 1985. Seasonal cycles in energy balance: regulation by light. *In* The Medical and Biological Effects of Light. R. J. Wurtman, M. J. Baum & J. T. Potts, Jr., Eds.: **453:** 170–181. Annals of the New York Academy of Sciences.
7. ASCHOFF, J. 1981. Annual rhythms in Man. *In* Biological Rhythms, Handbook of Behavioral Neurobiology. J. Aschoff, Ed.: **4:** 475–487. Plenum Press, New York.
8. ATTARZADEH, F. 1983. Seasonal variation in stature and body weight. Int. J. Orthodontics **21**(4): 3–12.
9. ZAHORSKA-MARKIEWICZ, B. 1980. Weight reduction and seasonal variation. Int. J. Obesity **4:** 139–143.
10. ZIFFERBLATT, S. M., C. S. CURTIS & J. L. PINSKY. 1980. Understanding food habits. J. Am. Diet. Assoc. **76:** 9–14.
11. ROSENTHAL, N. E., D. A. SACK, J. C. GILLIN, A. J. LEWY, F. K. GOODWIN, Y. DAVENPORT, P. S. MUELLER, D. A. NEWSOME & T. A. WEHR. 1984. Seasonal affective disorder: A description of the syndrome and preliminary findings with light therapy. Arch. Gen. Psychiatry **41:** 72–80.
12. SPITZER, R. L., J. ENDICOTT & E. ROBINS. 1978. Research diagnostic criteria: Rationale and reliability. Arch. Gen. Psychiatry **35:** 773–782.
13. IMMELMANN, K. 1973. Role of the environment in reproduction as source of "predictive" information. *In* Breeding Biology of Birds. D. S. Farner, Ed.: 121–147. National Academy of Sciences. Washington, D.C.
14. LEWY, A. J., T. A. WEHR, F. K. GOODWIN, D. A. NEWSOME & S. P. MARKEY. 1980. Light suppresses melatonin secretion in humans. Science **210:** 1267–1269.
15. LEWY, A. J., H. E. KERN, N. E. ROSENTHAL & T. A. WEHR. 1982. Bright artificial light treatment of a manic-depressive patient with a seasonal mood cycle. Am. J. Psychiatry **139:** 1496–1498.
16. ROSENTHAL, N. E., D. A. SACK, C. J. CARPENTER, B. L. PARRY, W. B. MENDELSON & T. A. WEHR. 1985. Antidepressant effects of light in seasonal affective disorder. Am. J. Psychiatry **142:** 606–608.
17. JAMES, S. P., B. L. PARRY, D. A. SACK, B. L. PARRY & N. E. ROSENTHAL. 1985. Treatment of seasonal affective disorder with light in the evening. Br. J. Psychiatry **147:** 424–428.
18. WEHR, T. A., R. G. SKWERER, F. M. JACOBSEN, D. A. SACK & N. E. ROSENTHAL. 1986. Eye- versus skin-phototherapy of seasonal affective disorder. Am J. Psychiatry. In press.
19. WEHR, T. A., F. M. JACOBSEN, D. A. SACK, J. ARENDT, L. TAMARKIN & N. E. ROSENTHAL. 1986. Timing of phototherapy and its effect on melatonin secretion do not appear to be critical for its antidepressant effect in seasonal affective disorder. Arch. Gen. Psychiatry **43:** 870–875.
20. WIRZ-JUSTICE, A., C. BUCHELI, P. GRAW, P. KIELHOLZ, H-U. FISCH & B. WOGGON.

1986. Light treatment of seasonal affective disorder in Switzerland. Acta Psychiatr. Scand. **74:** 193–204.

21. LEWY, A. J., R. L. SACK & C. M. SINGER. 1985. Melatonin, light and chronobiological disorders. In Photoperiodism, Melatonin and the Pineal. D. Evered & S. Clark, Eds.: 231–252. Pitman. London.

22. HELLEKSON, C. J., J. A. KLINE & N. E. ROSENTHAL. 1986. Phototherapy for seasonal affective disorder in Alaska. Am. J. Psychiatry **143:** 1035–1037.

23. HOFFMAN, K. 1981. Photoperiodism in vertebrates. Handbook of Behavioral Neurobiology. J. Aschoff, Ed.: **4:** 449–473. New York. Plenum Press.

24. ELLIOTT, J. A. 1976. Circadian rhythms and photoperiodic time measurement in mammals. Fed. Proc. Fed. Am. Soc. Exp. Biol. **35:** 2339–2346.

25. BARTNESS, T. J. & G. N. WADE. 1984. Photoperiodic control of body weight and energy metabolism in Syrian hamsters (Mesocricetus auratus): role of pineal gland, melatonin, gonads, and diet. Endocrinology **114:** 492–498.

26. TAMARKIN, L., C. J. BAIRD & O. F. X. ALMEIDA. 1985. Melatonin: a coordinating signal for mammalian reproduction? Science **227:** 714–720.

27. WADE, G. N. & T. J. BARTNESS. 1984. Seasonal obesity in Syrian hamsters: effects of age, diet, photoperiod, and melatonin. Am. J. Physiol. **16:** R328–334.

28. ROSENTHAL, N. E., D. A. SACK, F. M. JACOBSEN, S. P. JAMES, B. L. PARRY, J. ARENDT, L. TAMARKIN & T. A. WEHR. 1986. Melatonin in seasonal affective disorder and phototherapy. J. Neural Transm (Suppl.) **21:** 257–267.

29. HAMILTON, M. 1967. Development of a rating scale for primary depressive illness. Br. J. Soc. Clin. Psychol. **6:** 278–296.

30. ROSENTHAL, N. E. & M. M. HEFFERNAN. 1986. Bulimia, carbohydrate craving and depression: a central connection? In Nutrition and the Brain. R. J. Wurtman & J. J. Wurtman, Eds,: **7:** 139–166. Raven Press. New York.

31. ARENDT, J., C. BOJKOWSKI, C. FRANEY, J. WRIGHT & V. MARKS. 1984. Immunoassay of 6-hydroxymelatonin sulfate in human plasma and urine: abolition of the urinary 24-hour rhythm with atenolol. J. Clin. Endocrinol. Metab. **60(6):** 1166–1173.

32. VRIEND, J. & R. J. REITER. 1977. Free thyroxin index in normal, melatonin treated and blind hamsters. Horm. Metab. Res. **9:** 231–234.

33. VRIEND, J., B. A. RICHARDSON, M. K. VAUGHAN, L. Y. JOHNSON & R. J. REITER. 1982. Effects of melatonin on thyroid physiology of female hamsters. Neuroendocrinology **35:** 79–85.

34. VAUGHAN, G. M., M. K. VAUGHAN, L. G. SERAILLE & R. J. REITER. 1982. Thyroid hormones in male hamsters with activated pineals or melatonin treatment. Prog. Clin. Biol. Res. **92:** 187–196.

35. OSIBA, S. 1957. The seasonal variation of basal metabolism and activity of thyroid gland in man. Jpn. J. Physiol. **7:** 355–365.

36. DURUISSEAU, J. P. 1965. Seasonal variation of PBI in healthy Montrealers. J. Clin. Endocrinol. Metab. **25:** 1513–1515.

37. SMALS, A. G. H., H. A. ROSS & P. W. C. KLOPPENBORG. 1977. Seasonal variation in serum T_3 and T_4 levels in man. J. Clin. Endocrinol. Metab. **44:** 998–1001.

38. NAGATA, H., T. IZUMIYAMA, K. KAMATA, S. KONO, Y. YUKIMURA, M. TAWATA, T. AIZAWA & T. YAMADA. 1976. An increase of plasma triiodothyronine concentration in man in a cold environment. J. Clin. Endocrinol. Metab. **43:** 1153–1156.

39. KONNO, N. 1976. Comparison between the thyrotropin response to thyrotropin-releasing hormone in summer and that in winter in normal subjects. Endocrinol. Jpn. **25:** 635–640.

40. PASQUALI, R., G. BARALDI, F. CASIMIRRI, L. MATTIOLI, M. CAPELLI, N. MELCHIONDA, F. CAPANI & G. LABO. 1984. Seasonal variations of total and free thyroid hormones in healthy men: a chronobiological study. Acta Endocrinol. **107:** 42–48.

41. KONNO, N. 1980. Reciprocal changes in serum concentrations of triiodothyronine and reverse triiodothyronine between summer and winter in normal adult men. Endocrinol. Jpn. **27:** 471–476.

42. KONNO, N. & K. MORIKAWA. Seasonal variation of serum thyrotropin concentration and thyrotropin response to thyrotropin-releasing hormone in patients with primary hypothyroidism on constant replacement dosage of thyroxine. J. Clin. Endocrinol. Metab. **54:** 1118–1124.

43. SORRENTINO, JR., S., R. J. REITER & D. S. SCHALCH. 1971. Pineal regulation of growth hormone synthesis and release in blinded and blinded-anosmic male rats. Neuroendocrinology 7: 210–218.
44. SORRENTINO, JR., S., R. J. REITER, D. S. SCHALCH & R. J. DONOFRIO. 1971. Role of the pineal gland in growth restraint of adult male rats by light and smell deprivation. Neuroendocrinology 8: 116–124.
45. RELKIN, R. 1972. Effects of pinealectomy, constant light and darkness on growth hormone in the pituitary and plasma of the rat. J. Endocrinol. 53: 289–293.
46. RØNNELKEIV, O. K. & S. M. MCCANN. 1978. Growth hormone release in conscious pinealectomized and sham-operated male rats. Endocrinology 102: 1694–1701.
47. WIRZ-JUSTICE, A. & R. RICHTER. 1979. Seasonality in biochemical determinations: A source of variance and a clue to the temporal incidence of affective illness. Psychiatry Res. 1: 53–60.
48. COPPEN, A., C. SWADE, & K. WOOD. 1978. Platelet 5-hydroxytryptamine accumulation in depressive illness. Clin. Chem. Acta 87(1): 165–168.
49. SWADE, C. & A. COPPEN. Seasonal variations in biochemical factors related to depressive illness. J. Affective Dis. 2: 249–255.
50. ARORA, R. C., L. KREGEL & H. Y. MELTZER. 1984. Seasonal variation of serotonin uptake in normal controls and depressed patients. Biol. Psychiatry 19: 795–804.
51. WHITAKER, P. M., J. J. K. WARSH, H. C. STANCER, E. PERSAD & C.K. VINT. 1984. Seasonal variation in platelet ³H-imipramine binding: comparable values in control and depressed populations. Psychiatry Res. 11: 127–131.
52. MENDLEWICZ, J. 1984. Seasonal variation in platelet ³H-imipramine binding in man. Psychiatry Res. 12: 179.
53. CARLSSON, A., L. SVENNERHOLM & B. WINBLAD. 1980. Seasonal and circadian monoamine variations in human brains examined post-mortem. Acta Psychiat Scand, 61(Suppl 280): 75–85.
54. MURPHY, D. L., I. CAMPBELL & J. L. COSTA. 1978. Current status of indoleamine hypothesis of the affective disorders. In Psychopharmacology: A Generation of Progress. M. A. Lipton, A. KiMascio & K. E. Killam, Eds.: 1235–1247. Raven Press. New York.
55. BLUNDELL, J. E. 1983. Problems and processes underlying the control of food selection and nutrient intake. In Nutrition and the Brain, Vol 6. R. J. Wurtman & J. J. Wurtman, Eds.: 163–222. Raven Press. New York.
56. FERNSTROM, J. D. & R. J. WURTMAN. 1972. Brain serotonin content: Physiological regulation by plasma neutral amino acids. Science 178: 414–416.
57. WURTMAN, R. J. & J. J. WURTMAN. 1984. Nutritional control of central neurotransmitters. In The Psychobiology of Anorexia Nervosa. K. M. Pirke & D. Ploog, Eds.: 4–11. Springer-Verlag. Berlin.
58. WURTMAN, J. J., R. J. WURTMAN, J. H. GROWDON, P. HENRY, A. LIPSCOMB & S. H. ZEISEL. Carbohydrate craving in obese people: Suppression by treatments affecting serotoninergic transmission. Int. J. Eating. Disord., 1: 2–15.
59. WURTMAN, J. J., R. J. WURTMAN, S. MARK, R. TSAY, W. GILBERT & J. GROWDON. 1985. D-fenfluramine selectively suppresses carbohydrate snacking by obese subjects. Int. J. Eating Disorders 4: 89–99.

Food Intake and Mood in Anorexia Nervosa and Bulimia[a]

B. TIMOTHY WALSH, MADELINE GLADIS, AND
STEVEN P. ROOSE

The New York State Psychiatric Institute
and
The Department of Psychiatry
College of Physicians and Surgeons
Columbia University
New York, New York 10032

INTRODUCTION

The syndrome of anorexia nervosa was first identified almost 300 years ago, and the salient feature of bulimia, uncontrollable binge eating, has probably also been recognized for centuries. It is only in the last several years, however, that investigators have focused on disturbances of mood accompanying these eating disorders and have attempted to understand the relationship of food intake and mood in anorexia nervosa and bulimia. In this chapter, we will briefly review the clinical characteristics of anorexia nervosa and bulimia, discuss the nature of the mood disturbance commonly seen in these disorders, and, finally, consider how pathological eating behavior may be related to the pathology of mood.

CLINICAL CHARACTERISTICS OF ANOREXIA NERVOSA AND BULIMIA

Anorexia nervosa is an illness in which individuals, in a relentless pursuit of thinness, lose substantial amounts of weight through rigorous dieting and strenuous exercise. Even though significantly malnourished, they are intensely afraid of becoming fat and often do not acknowledge the serious medical implications of their weight loss. Anorexia nervosa is a serious illness with a mortality on long-term follow-up in the range of 10 percent.

Bulimia is a syndrome characterized by recurrent episodes of binge eating, during which individuals feel unable to control their eating. Typically, they binge-eat alone, and, upon completing a binge, induce vomiting to avoid absorption of the calories they have consumed. Although bulimia was virtually unknown a decade ago, some recent surveys have suggested that several percent of college women may currently have this syndrome.

There is good reason to believe that anorexia nervosa and bulimia are related illnesses. Though most patients presenting to clinics with bulimia are of normal body weight, about one-third have past histories of anorexia nervosa. Conversely, about one-half of patients admitted to a hospital for treatment of anorexia nervosa

[a] This work was supported in part by NIH Grants AM-28150 and MH-00383, and by the Communities Foundation of Texas, Inc.

also have bulimia. Both illnesses primarily affect women in their late teens and early 20s and are characterized by an intense preoccupation with body shape and weight.

PHENOMENOLOGY OF MOOD DISTURBANCE IN ANOREXIA NERVOSA AND BULIMIA

In what is thought to be the first written description of a case of anorexia nervosa, Richard Morton, in 1689, noted that his patient suffered from a "multitude of cares and passions of her mind."[1] Until recently, most clinicians, although noting mood disturbance among patients with anorexia nervosa, did not focus great attention on its characteristics or significance. The last twenty years have witnessed the development of phenomenologically based criteria for psychiatric diagnoses and the evolution of semistructured interviews that permit the reliable collection of symptoms and signs of psychiatric illness. When these interviewing methods and diagnostic criteria have been applied to patients with anorexia nervosa and bulimia, the results have consistently documented that many patients with eating disorders meet diagnostic criteria for major depressive illness.[2-7] This finding has led to the hypothesis that some, or perhaps many, patients with anorexia nervosa and bulimia have unusual forms of typical depressive illness, and that their pathological eating behaviors may be symptoms of depression. Investigators have attempted to evaluate this hypothesis by determining whether other characteristics of typical major depression occur in patients with eating disorders.

BIOLOGICAL SIMILARITIES BETWEEN EATING DISORDERS AND MAJOR DEPRESSIVE ILLNESS

There has been great excitement in the last decade concerning the presence of biological abnormalities in patients with depressive illness. It is now well-established that patients with typical major depressive illness are prone to exhibit characteristic abnormalities of adrenal activity and of sleep. For example, about half of patients with major depression show evidence of increased adrenal activity, such as elevated levels of plasma cortisol and inadequate suppression of cortisol secretion following dexamethasone administration. If patients with eating disorders have a similar form of major depressive illness, then one would expect to find similar abnormalities of adrenal activity.

Disturbances of adrenal activity do, in fact, occur in anorexia nervosa, and, in many ways, these disturbances resemble those found in major depressive illness. Patients with anorexia nervosa have elevated levels of plasma cortisol and inadequate responses to dexamethasone suppression as do patients with major depression.[8] In addition, Gold and his colleagues at the National Institute of Mental Health recently demonstrated that patients with anorexia nervosa and patients with major depression exhibit a diminished ACTH response to corticotropin-releasing hormone, suggesting the presence of a similar hypothalamic disturbance in both illnesses.[9]

The serious weight loss characteristic of anorexia nervosa, however, clouds the interpretation of this biological similarity. Patients with nonpsychologically motivated forms of malnutrition develop increased levels of plasma cortisol and inadequate responses to dexamethasone suppression, as do patients with anorexia nervosa.[8] Furthermore, the adrenal abnormalities of anorexia nervosa correct rapidly with relatively small amounts of weight gain.[10,11] These data suggest that weight loss and malnutrition may be critical determinants of the adrenal disturbances in anorexia nervosa.

Initial studies of adrenal activity in bulimic patients of normal weight examined the response of plasma cortisol to dexamethasone suppression. Several research groups reported a higher than expected frequency of positive dexamethasone suppression tests in patients with bulimia.[12-17] Because the patients studied were generally at normal weight, the influence of malnutrition on adrenal activity could be excluded. These results suggested an increase in adrenal activity in bulimia similar to that associated with major depression.

We have recently reported that bulimic patients of normal weight tend to achieve lower levels of plasma dexamethasone following a standard 1 mg dexamethasone suppression test than do age- and sex-matched controls.[18] These data suggest that the abnormal dexamethasone suppression test in bulimia cannot be definitely interpreted as evidence of increased adrenal activity. In addition, we found that the 24-hour pattern of cortisol secretion in 12 women with bulimia was entirely normal.[19] Similarly, Gold and his colleagues found that the ACTH response to corticotropin-releasing hormone in normal weight bulimics was also normal.[9] Thus, although the initial interpretation of the dexamethasone suppression test in bulimia suggested increased adrenal activity, more direct measures of adrenal function do not appear to support this conclusion.

In short, patients with anorexia nervosa have adrenal disturbances similar to those of patients with classic major depressive illness, but the presence of malnutrition in patients with anorexia nervosa clouds the significance of this similarity. Although fewer data are available concerning adrenal activity in normal weight patients with bulimia, it appears that such individuals do not generally exhibit increased adrenal activity. Thus, studies of adrenal activity in patients with eating disorders do not provide convincing evidence of a biological similarity to major depressive illness.

SLEEP DISTURBANCES

Patients with major depressive illness frequently complain of insomnia. Using all-night EEG monitoring, it has been possible to demonstrate the presence of characteristic sleep-EEG abnormalities in depression, including shortened REM latency, increased REM density, and reduced slow wave sleep. Patients with anorexia nervosa also frequently complain of sleep problems, and several studies using EEG monitoring have documented sleep abnormalities, particularly disruptions of the continuity of sleep. A few patients with anorexia nervosa have been found to have very short REM sleep latencies, but, in general, the EEG-monitored characteristics of the sleep of most patients with anorexia nervosa do not resemble those of major depressive illness.[20,21] Three groups have presented data on EEG sleep measures in normal weight patients with bulimia, and all three groups have found that the sleep of bulimic patients was quite similar to that of control subjects.[20-22]

At present, then, the studies of adrenal activity and of sleep in patients with eating disorders do not support a strong biological resemblance between these eating disorders and classic major depressive illness. There is, however, at least one caveat about the use of these biological markers of major depressive illness. There are indications that the increase in adrenal activity and the abnormalities in EEG-monitored sleep are more frequently observed in older depressed patients. Although these abnormalities have been reported in younger patients, they may not be a sensitive indicator of major depression in patients with eating disorders who are usually in their twenties.

FAMILY STUDIES

One of the striking characteristics of typical depressive illness is its tendency to run in families. An increased frequency of mood disturbance among the relatives of patients with eating disorders would be strong evidence of some form of relationship between these two illnesses. To date there have been only two studies of the frequency of depression among the relatives of normal weight patients with bulimia, and, unfortunately, these two studies arrived at different conclusions. Hudson et al.[23] found an increased frequency of depressive diagnoses among the relatives of bulimic patients compared to the relatives of patients with borderline personality or with schizophrenia. On the other hand, Stern et al.[24] were unable to document an increased prevalence of depression in the families of bulimic individuals compared to controls.

By contrast, all studies that have examined the frequency of psychiatric illness among the relatives of patients with anorexia nervosa have concluded that there is an increased frequency of depression.[6,23,25-29] This finding is one of the most persuasive pieces of evidence for an association between major depressive illness and anorexia nervosa. It should be noted, however, that the interpretation of these data is not straightforward. First, an increased familial frequency does not demonstrate a genetic link. Second, as we have already noted, many patients with anorexia nervosa themselves have mood disturbances. Thus, the finding of an increased frequency of mood disturbance in the relatives of patients with anorexia nervosa may simply document that mood disturbance runs in families. Finally, there are no reports of an increased frequency of anorexia nervosa among relatives of depressed patients that one would expect if anorexia nervosa were simply a form of familial depressive illness.

TREATMENT RESPONSE

One of the exciting developments in the last decade in the study of anorexia nervosa and bulimia is the finding that some patients with these eating disorders appear to respond to treatment with antidepressants. Unfortunately, the response in patients with anorexia nervosa does not appear to be robust. For example, though Halmi et al.[30] were recently able to document that the antidepressant amitriptyline was superior to placebo in the treatment of patients hospitalized for anorexia nervosa, the magnitude of the effect was relatively small.

The results of the treatment of patients with bulimia have been more encouraging. Four of five double-blind, placebo-controlled trials have found that standard antidepressant agents (tricyclic antidepressants or monoamine oxidase inhibitors) are significantly more effective than placebo in reducing binge frequency among patients with bulimia.[31-35] Curiously, in none of these studies has the response to antidepressants been linked to the presence of pretreatment depression. That is, even bulimic patients who are not depressed respond to medication.

Certainly the response of some eating disorder patients to treatment with antidepressant medication is suggestive of a link between depression and eating disorders. It should be noted, however, that not all that responds to antidepressant medication is depression. For example, tricyclic antidepressants are potent suppressors of cardiac arrhythmias, an activity that is not thought to bear any direct connection to their effects on mood.

In summary, although patients with eating disorders frequently have significant mood disturbances, it seems premature to conclude that eating disorders are simply variants of more classic forms of depression. The biological disturbances characteristic of major depression do not occur frequently in normal weight patients with bulimia, and when they do occur in patients with anorexia nervosa, their significance is obscured by serious weight loss. Though there appears to be an increased prevalence of depression among the relatives of patients with anorexia nervosa, the meaning of this observation is uncertain. Finally, although some patients with eating disorders do respond to antidepressant medication, this does not, in itself, demonstrate that these eating disorders are a form of depressive illness.

ABNORMAL EATING AS A RESPONSE TO EMOTIONAL DISTURBANCE

Thus, the idea that the abnormal eating behaviors of patients with anorexia nervosa and bulimia are simply atypical symptoms of classic depressive illness does not seem compelling on the basis of currently available data. An alternative and intriguing possibility is that in patients with eating disorders, particularly patients with bulimia, manipulations of eating behavior are attempts to cope with mood disturbances. A number of investigators have noted that dysphoric emotional states, particularly anxiety, are frequent precipitants of binge eating. In a series of structured interviews of 32 patients with bulimia, Abraham and Beumont[36] found that 91% cited "tension" as the most frequent precipitant of a binge. Similarly, Mitchell *et al.*[37] found that 83% of 229 bulimic patients gave feeling "tense" and "anxious" as the reason for their binge eating.

There is also evidence suggesting that the binge eating itself provides some degree of relief from the emotional state that preceded it. Thirty-four percent of the patients interviewed by Abraham and Beumont[36] described relief from anxiety during the binge, and 66% felt free of anxious feelings after the binge had concluded. Kaye and his colleagues at NIMH[38] asked 12 women with bulimia to binge eat in a laboratory setting and to rate their emotional states before and after the binge. Eight of the 12 patients reported a substantial decrease in anxiety following the binge, whereas only 4 of 12 had a substantial decrease in depression. These kinds of reports have suggested to several authors that the binge-purge cycle in some patients with bulimia may be perpetuated by the emotional relief it provides.

How might binge eating produce an alteration in emotional state? One possibility, based on Wurtman's work, is that patients with bulimia consume a large carbohydrate load and, by doing so, produce a rise in brain serotonin, which in turn leads to a change in mental state. In support of this hypothesis is the common impression of most patients who binge eat that their binges consist mostly of junk food, which are high in sugar.

The meager data available on the nutritional contents of binges, however, suggest that this anecdotal impression may not be entirely accurate. At least three groups have asked patients to binge in a laboratory setting and, in doing so, have obtained information on the nutritional contents of binges.[38-40] The results of these studies have been surprisingly similar. The caloric content of binges varies greatly among patients but averages between 3500 and 4500 kcals in each study. The average nutritional composition of a binge was also similar between studies: approximately 50% carbohydrate, 40% fat, and 10% protein. Certainly, this is a large amount of carbohydrate consumption, on the order of 2000 kcals in less than an hour. Yet, the nutritional composition of a binge rather closely resembles that of freely selected human diets.[41] In other words, patients with bulimia do consume large amounts of carbohydrate while bingeing, but they do not exclusively consume carbohydrate, suggesting that factors other than carbohydrate craving play a role in the selection of binge foods. It is possible that patients with bulimia are using other psychological and physiological satiety signals in the service of altering their emotional states.

SUMMARY

It is clear that patients with anorexia nervosa and bulimia have disturbances of mood, and it is likely that the mood disturbances bear an important relationship to the disturbances of eating behavior. We have as many questions, however, about the relationship between mood and eating behavior in these syndromes as we have answers. Although patients with anorexia nervosa and bulimia are frequently depressed, they fail to exhibit many of the biological characteristics of typical depressive illness, suggesting that these eating disorders are probably not simply variants of depression. Patients with bulimia appear to binge in response to dysphoric emotional states and to derive some transient relief from their bingeing. But it is unclear what facet or facets of the binge produce the alteration in emotional state, and thereby may serve to reinforce the behavior. A more detailed examination of this issue may significantly advance our understanding of the relationship between mood and food in eating disorders.

REFERENCES

1. MORTON, R. 1689. Phthisiologica: or a Treatise of Consumptions. London.
2. STROBER, M. 1981. The significance of bulimia in juvenile anorexia nervosa: an exploration of possible etiologic factors. Int. J. Eating Disorders 1: 28–43.
3. HUDSON, J. I., H. G. POPE, J. M. JONAS & D. YURGELUN-TODD. 1983. Phenomenologic relationship of eating disorders to major affective disorder. Psychiatry Res. 9: 345–354.
4. BIEDERMAN, J., T. M. RIVINUS, D. B. HERZOG, R. A. FERBER, G. P. HARPER, P. J. ORSULAK, J. S. HARMATZ & J. J. SCHILDKRAUT. 1984. Platelet MAO activity in anorexia nervosa patients with and without a major depressive disorder. Am. J. Psychiatry 141: 1244–1247.
5. HERZOG, D. B. 1984. Are anorexic and bulimic patients depressed? Am. J. Psychiatry 141: 1594–1597.
6. PIRAN, N., S. KENNEDY, P. E. GARFINKEL & M. OWENS. 1985. Affective disturbance in eating disorders. J. Nerv. Ment. Dis. 173: 395–400.
7. WALSH, B. T., S. P. ROOSE, A. H. GLASSMAN, M. GLADIS & C. SADIK. 1985. Bulimia and depression. Psychosom. Med. 47: 123–131.
8. WALSH, B. T., J. L. KATZ, J. LEVIN, J. KREAM, D. K. FUKUSHIMA, L. D. HELLMAN, H. WEINER & B. ZUMOFF. 1978. Adrenal activity in anorexia nervosa. Psychosom. Med. 40: 499–506.

9. GOLD, P. W., H. GWIRTSMAN, P. C. AVGERINOS, L. K. NIEMAN, W. T. GALLUCCI, W. KAYE, D. JIMERSON, M. EBERT, R. RITTMASTER, D. L. LORIAUX & G. P. CHROUSOS. 1986. Abnormal hypothalamic-pituitary-adrenal function in anorexia nervosa. N. Engl. J. Med. **314:** 1335–1342.
10. DOERR, P., M. FICHTER, K. M. PIRKE & R. LUND. 1980. Relationship between weight gain and hypothalamic pituitary adrenal function in patients with anorexia nervosa. J. Steroid Biochem. **13:** 529–537.
11. WALSH, B. T., J. L. KATZ, J. LEVIN, J. KREAM, D. K. FUKUSHIMA, H. WEINER & B. ZUMOFF. 1981. The production rate of cortisol declines during recovery from anorexia nervosa. J. Clin. Endocrinol. Metab. **53:** 203–205.
12. HUDSON, J. I., P. S. LAFFER & H. G. POPE. 1982. Bulimia related to affective disorder by family history and response to the dexamethasone suppression test. Am. J. Psychiatry **139:** 685–687.
13. GWIRTSMAN, H. E., P. ROY-BYRNE, J. YAGER & R. M. GERNER. 1983. Neuroendocrine abnormalities in bulimia. Am. J. Psychiatry **140:** 559–563.
14. HUDSON, J. I., H. G. POPE, J. M. JONAS, P. S. LAFFER, M. S. HUDSON & J. C. MELBY. 1983. Hypothalamic-pituitary-adrenal axis hyperactivity in bulimia. Psychiatry Res. **8:** 111–117.
15. MITCHELL, J. E., R. L. PYLE, D. HATSUKAWI & L. I. BONTACOFF. 1984. The dexamethasone suppression test in patients with bulimia. J. Clin. Psychiatry **45:** 508–511.
16. MUSISI, S. & P. GARFINKEL. 1985. Comparative dexamethasone suppression test measurements in bulimia, depression, and normal controls. Can. J. Psychiatry **30:** 190–194.
17. LINDY, D. C., B. T. WALSH, S. P. ROOSE, M. GLADIS & A. H. GLASSMAN. 1985. The dexamethasone suppression test in bulimia. Am. J. Psychiatry **142:** 1375–1376.
18. WALSH, B. T., E. S. LO, T. COOPER, D. C. LINDY, S. P. ROOSE, M. GLADIS & A. H. GLASSMAN. 1986. The DST and plasma dexamethasone levels in bulimia. Arch Gen. Psychiatry. In press.
19. WALSH, B. T., S. P. ROOSE, J. L. KATZ, I. DYRENFURTH, L. WRIGHT, R. VANDE WIELE & A. H. GLASSMAN. 1986. Hypothalamic-pituitary-adrenal activity in anorexia nervosa and bulimia. Psychoneuroendocrinology. In press.
20. WALSH, B. T., R. R. GOETZ, S. P. ROOSE, S. FINGEROTH & A. H. GLASSMAN. 1985. EEG-monitored sleep in anorexia nervosa and bulimia. Biol. Psychiatry **20:** 947–956.
21. LEVY, A. B., K. N. DIXON & H. S. SCHMIDT. 1986. Sleep architecture in eating disorder patients. Presented at the Annual Meeting, American Psychiatric Association. May, 1986.
22. HUDSON, J. I., J. M. JONAS, H. G. POPE & V. GROCHOCHINSKI. 1985. Sleep EEG in bulimia. Presented at the Annual Meeting, American Psychiatry Association. May, 1985.
23. HUDSON, J. I., H. G. POPE JR., J. M. JONAS & D. YURGELIN-TODD. 1983. Family history study of anorexia nervosa and bulimia. Br. J. Psychiatry **142:** 133–138.
24. STERN, S. L., K. N. DIXON, E. NEMZER, M. D. LAKE, R. A. SANSONE, D. J. SMELTZER, S. LANTZ & S. S. SCHRIER. 1984. Affective disorder in the families of women with normal weight bulimia. Am. J. Psychiatry **141:** 12224–1227.
25. CANTWELL, D. P., S. STURZENBERGER, J. BURROUGHS, B. SALKIN & J. K. GREEN. 1977. Anorexia nervosa. An affective disorder? Arch. Gen. Psychiatry **34:** 1087–1093.
26. WINOKUR, A., V. MARCH & J. MENDELS. 1980. Primary affective disorder in relatives of patients with anorexia nervosa. Am. J. Psychiatry **137:** 695–698.
27. STROBER, M., B. SALKIN, J. BURROUGHS et al. 1982. Validity of the bulimic-restrictor distinction in anorexia nervosa: parental personality characteristics and family psychiatric morbidity. J. Nerv. Ment. Dis. **170:** 345–351.
28. GERSHON, E. S., J. R. HAMOVIT, J. L. SCHREIBER et al. 1983. Anorexia nervosa and major affective disorders associated in families: a preliminary report. In Childhood Psychopathology and Development. S. B. Guze, F. J. Earls & J. E. Barrett, Eds.: 279–286. Raven Press. New York.

29. RIVINUS, T. M., J. BIEDERMAN, D. B. HERZOG, K. KEMPER, G. P. HARPER, J. S. HARMATZ & S. HOUSEWORTH. 1984. Anorexia nervosa and affective disorders: a controlled family history study. Am. J. Psychiatry **141:** 1414–1418.
30. HALMI, K. A., E. ECKERT, T. J. LADU & J. COHEN. 1986. Anorexia nervosa: Treatment efficacy of cyproheptadine and amitriptyline. Arch. Gen. Psychiatry **43:** 177–181.
31. POPE JR., H. G., J. I. HUDSON, J. M. JONAS & D. YURGELIN-TODD. 1983. Bulimia treated with imipramine: a placebo-controlled, double-blind study. Am. J. Psychiatry **140:** 554–558.
32. WALSH, B. T., J. W. STEWART, S. P. ROOSE, M. GLADIS & A. H. GLASSMAN. 1984. Treatment of bulimia with phenelzine: A double-blind, placebo-controlled study. Arch. Gen. Psychiatry **41:** 1105–1109.
33. HUGHES, P. L., L. A. WELLS, C. J. CUNNINGHAM & D. M. ILSTRUP. 1986. Treating bulimia with desipramine. Arch. Gen. Psychiatry **43:** 182–186.
34. MITCHELL, J. E. & R. GROAT. 1984. A placebo-controlled, double-blind trial of amitriptyline in bulimia. J. Clin. Psychopharmacol. **4:** 186–193.
35. KENNEDY, S., N. PIRAN, P. E. GARFINKEL, E. HENDERSON, P. PRENDERGAST, B. WILKES, C. WHYNOT & C. BROUILLETTE. 1986. Isocarboxazid (Marplan)—a double-blind trial in the treatment of bulimia. Presented at the 2nd International Conference on Eating Disorders. New York. April, 1986.
36. ABRAHAM, S. F. & P. J. V. BEUMONT. 1982. How patients describe bulimia or binge eating. Psychol. Med. **12:** 625–635.
37. MITCHELL, J. E., D. HATSUKAMI, E. D. ECKERT & R. L. PYLE. 1985. Characteristics of 275 patients with bulimia. Am. J. Psychiatry **142:** 482–485.
38. KAYE, W. H., H. E. GWIRTSMAN, D. T. GEORGE, S. R. WEISS & D. C. JIMERSON. 1986. Relationship of mood alterations to bingeing behaviour in bulimia. Br. J. Psychiatry **149:** 479–485.
39. MITCHELL, J. E. & D. C. LAINE. 1985. Monitored binge-eating behavior in patients with bulimia. Int. J. Eating Disorders **4:** 177–184.
40. KISSILEFF, H. R., B. T. WALSH, J. G. KRAL & S. CASSIDY. 1986. Laboratory studies of eating behavior in women with bulimia. Physiol. Behav. **38:** 563–570.
41. KISSILEFF, H. R. & T. B. VAN ITALLIE. 1982. Physiology of the control of food intake. Annu. Rev. Nutr. **2:** 371–418.

Alcoholism: Is It a Model for the Study of Disorders of Mood and Consummatory Behavior?[a]

TING-KAI LI, LAWRENCE LUMENG, WILLIAM J. McBRIDE, AND JAMES M. MURPHY

Indiana University School of Medicine
and
Veterans Administration Medical Center
Indianapolis, Indiana 46223

INTRODUCTION

This presentation on alcoholism, more specifically an animal model of alcoholism, has been included in this volume on obesity because disorders of drinking, eating, and mood appear to share some sociocultural, behavioral, metabolic, and neurobiological concomitants. Alcohol is used in modern society primarily for its drug-related properties. Its effect on mood and behavior is biphasic. At low blood alcohol concentrations (BACs), it is disinhibitory, thereby facilitating spontaneous behavior, but at high BACs, its effects are sedative-hypnotic. Ethanol is also a good source of calories. It is oxidized first to acetaldehyde and then to acetate in the liver. Acetate is further oxidized to carbon dioxide and water principally in the extrahepatic tissues. The conversion of one gram of ethanol to carbon dioxide and water yields 7 kcals of energy. One drink of most kinds of alcoholic beverages, therefore, provides approximately 70 kcals from ethanol.[1]

Clinicians have long recognized an association of alcoholism with depression and with eating disorders. Primary alcoholics frequently become depressed and suicidal in the course of their illness, and patients with primary depression often become alcoholic secondarily from that illness. There is, however, no evidence at this time in support of a genetic link between the major affective disorders and alcoholism.[2] An association between alcoholism and anorexia nervosa, bulimia, and compulsive eating has been reported, with eating disorders occurring before the onset of alcohol abuse.[3] In view of the high prevalence of both types of disorders in the general population, it cannot be ruled out at this time that the discovered association is chance occurrence. On the other hand, clinicians who treat alcoholics have noted that many newly abstinent patients develop carbohydrate craving. The fellowship of Alcoholics Anonymous traditionally advises new members to carry candies with them to help suppress the urge to drink. A recent study of the relationship of dietary choice and abstinence in treated alcoholic patients showed that those who stayed sober longer consumed more carbohydrates in their diet and used substantially more sugar in their beverages.[4]

[a] This work was supported in part by a Grant from the Public Health Service: AA-03243.

239

ALCOHOLISM AND ANIMAL MODELS FOR THE STUDY OF ALCOHOLISM

Research in the last 20 years has shown convincingly that expression of the disorder, alcoholism, is influenced both by genetic predisposition and by environmental provocation.[5,6] The precise nature of these risk factors is still unknown, but all of them are expressed through a final common behavioral path, which is alcohol self-administration or alcohol-seeking behavior. In this context, alcoholism can be defined as a disorder of abnormally intense alcohol-seeking behavior, which over time leads to loss of control over drinking and tolerance. Psychological dependence (increased salience of this behavior or compulsion to drink), and physical dependence are also created. The degree or extent of the abnormality in alcohol-seeking behavior embodied in this definition contains all the essential elements of the alcohol-dependence syndrome posited by Edwards and Gross,[7] which forms the conceptual framework for the ICD 9 classification of alcoholism developed by the World Health Organization in 1981.[8]

Irrespective of etiologies, it is clear that the understanding of the neurobiological substrates of alcoholism must come from studies in experimental animals. Over the years, various investigators interested in the experimental analysis of alcoholism have attempted to develop suitable animal models for alcoholism research. In a recent review,[9] the kinds of criteria that an animal model of alcoholism should ideally satisfy were discussed, and the limitations of the animal models then extant were evaluated. With the realization that the sociocultural and psychosocial variables that influence drinking behavior in humans cannot be incorporated into an animal model, the following criteria were proposed: (1) The animal must self-administer ethanol in pharmacologically significant amounts. Specifically, the following conditions must be met: ethanol should be self-administered by oral intake; ethanol should be preferentially consumed when there is a choice between it and another equally palatable fluid or water; consumption should give rise to pharmacologically meaningful BACs; voluntary intake should be based on its pharmacological effects, not because of its caloric value, taste, or smell. (2) Tolerance to ethanol should be demonstrable following a period of continuous consumption. Specifically, animals should be less affected in performance by the same dose of ethanol and BAC after a period of chronic exposure. (3) Physical and psychological dependence on ethanol should also develop after a period of continuous consumption. Physical dependence is measured by characteristic behavioral and physiological signs during acute ethanol withdrawal. Although psychological or behavioral dependence in the human sense of the term cannot be elicited from an animal, its operant behavior to ethanol as a reinforcer can provide a measure of abuse liability or reinforcing efficacy of the substance for that animal. When ethanol is able to maintain operant responding, some degree of behavioral dependence can be assumed to have occurred; the degree to which it has occurred may be equated with the degree of reinforcing efficacy that ethanol has displayed in that animal.

Most species of laboratory animals thus far examined do not exhibit a liking for unadulterated aqueous solutions containing moderate to high concentrations of ethanol. An obvious reason is that most animals do not like the taste of moderately concentrated alcoholic solutions, despite its potentially reinforcing properties. Actually, most humans do not particularly enjoy the taste of unflavored 10 percent ethanol at room temperature either, inasmuch they have gone to great lengths to disguise the taste of alcohol in alcoholic beverages.

A number of approaches to increasing oral consumption of ethanol in experimental animals have been explored;[10] the most successful of these has been genetic. McClearn and Rodgers[11] first showed that inbred strains of mice differed widely in their preference for a 10% solution of ethanol versus water. Differences among inbred strains in a trait may be regarded as prima facie evidence of a genetic influence on that trait. Capitalizing on this genetic potential, a number of rat lines that differ in alcohol preference have been selectively bred from genetically heterogeneous outbred stocks of rats that displayed a wide range of variation in alcohol preference. Selective breeding systematically mates individuals that exhibit the most extreme levels of a chosen phenotype (*e.g.*, high and low voluntary alcohol consumption). Over many generations, the selected lines would have a high or low frequency of the genes that impact on that trait, whereas the frequency of the genes not affecting that trait should remain randomly distributed. These pharmacogenetically different animal lines provide useful tools for investigating mechanisms, because associated traits are likely to share common mechanisms through common gene action (pleiotropy). On the other hand, phenotypic associations in inbred strains may be entirely fortuitous, because fixation of genes is entirely random.

There currently exist three pairs (high and low) of rat lines that differ in alcohol preference, developed through selective breeding from different foundation stocks. The first of these, the UChA (low preference) and the UChB (high preference) lines were developed by Mardones and coworkers in Chile.[12] Subsequently, the high preference (AA) and low preference (ANA) lines were established in Findland,[13] and the high preference (P) and the low preference (NP) lines were raised in this country.[14] The P line of rats has now been systematically characterized with regard to the criteria of an animal model of alcoholism. Furthermore, a number of phenotypic associations of alcohol drinking preference have been discovered by comparing the P and NP lines. These have potential importance to our understanding of the physiological and neurochemical basis of alcohol-seeking behavior. A study of the effect of dietary composition of carbohydrates on alcohol drinking has also been performed. The remainder of this paper summarizes those findings already published and describes other findings not yet published in greater detail.

THE P LINE OF RATS AS AN ANIMAL MODEL OF ALCOHOLISM

The P and NP lines were developed by mass selection for high and low alcohol preference from a foundation stock of Wistar rats.[14,15] Testing was performed with an unflavored 10% (v/v) solution of ethanol made continuously available in a Richter tube to individually housed animals. Water in an identical Richter tube as an alternate source of fluid and solid food were provided *ad libitum*. The amounts of 10% ethanol, water, and food consumed daily were measured for 3 weeks, and those animals exhibiting the highest and lowest consumption scores (g ethanol/kg body weight/d) were mated to initiate subsequent generations of P and NP lines, respectively. After 20 generations, the consumption scores (g/kg/d; mean $\pm$ SD) were P males, 5.5 $\pm$ 1.2; P females, 7.3 $\pm$ 1.7; NP males, 1.1 $\pm$ 0.6; and NP females 1.0 $\pm$ 0.9. The P and NP animals in the current S30 generations display similar characteristics. The P rats on test consume between 20–30% of the total calories as ethanol, and substitute the ethanol calories for a part of the food calories. Weight gain is the same as control animals not given the ethanol solution as a fluid choice.[16]

The P rats drink about 70% of the ethanol in the dark, when they also eat most of the food. Drinking occurs in bursts at irregularly spaced intervals,[17] and some animals consume as much as 2–3 g ethanol/kg body weight in a single drinking episode. When blood is sampled at regular intervals, for example, at the 3d and 11th hours of the dark cycle, BACs ranging from 2 to 160 mg% have been obtained; mean values are about 65 mg%.[14,18] At one hour after observed drinking epidsodes, BACs are 42–218 mg%; mean is 87 mg%.[19] Clearly, these animals are attaining systemic alcohol concentrations that are pharmacologically active, at least for humans. Studies have also been performed to determine what BACs coincide with cessation of voluntary drinking and whether BACs produced by intravenous infusion would lead to curtailment of oral intake.[19,20] It was found that on the average, 50 to 70 mg% would do both. It appears, therefore, that the reinforcing action of ethanol for these animals may be at concentrations below 100 mg% and that the higher BACs attained with oral intake represent overshoot, caused by delayed gastrointestinal absorption.

With chronic free-choice drinking of 10% ethanol, with food and water available at all times, the P rats develop behavioral or neuronal tolerance as assessed with a jumping test. This test measures the degree of motor impairment produced by moderate to high doses of ethanol and the course of recovery.[21] The time it takes for the animals to recover jumping to a criterion height (e.g., 70% of control) and the BAC at this time point can be employed to assess tolerance development. It was found that after 14 days of free-choice drinking, the P rats exhibited neuronal tolerance as judged by the significantly shorter time for them to recover to criterion performance and by the significantly higher BACs at time of recovery.[22] In separate experiments, the P rats were also shown to develop metabolic tolerance with chronic free-choice drinking of 10% ethanol. After 6 weeks, the ethanol elimination rate of the ethanol-consuming animals was 15% higher than that of the control animals.[18] Weight gain and total caloric intake of the animals were identical in the two groups.

It has also been demonstrated that chronic free-choice drinking by the P rats produces physical dependence.[17] Experimental animals were given constant access to 10% ethanol and water for 20 weeks, while control animals received only water. Food was available ad libitum. After 20 weeks, the ethanol solution was taken away from the experimental animals and, in the first 24 hours following removal of ethanol, 18 of the 19 ethanol-exposed animals exhibited signs of withdrawal that abated within 72 hours. As expected, none of the control animals showed withdrawal signs.

We showed very early on in our studies that the P rats will work to obtain ethanol through operant responding.[23] In fact, response rates of over 1000 bar-presses/24 hours were obtained in each of the animals tested. Inasmuch as food and water were freely available to the animals, it seemed unlikely that the P animals found the ethanol solutions rewarding because of caloric needs or thirst. In sharp contrast, rats unselected for ethanol preference would not bar-press for ethanol as reward unless they had been weight-reduced and restricted in caloric intake.[24] In a recent study, we compared the oral ethanol self-administration behavior of the P and NP rats with different concentrations of ethanol in a two-lever operant design. The animals were trained to bar-press for reward at a response to reinforcement ratio of 5. They were then given the choice of two levers, the pressing of one produced water in a dipper and the pressing of the other, an alcohol solution. Food was available at all times. Both P and NP rats exhibited preference for the 2 and 5 percent ethanol solutions over water. The amounts of ethanol self-administered, however, were less than 2 g/kg body wt/day for both the P and NP rats. With 10% and higher concentrations of ethanol, the P rats continued to self-administer more of the ethanol solution than water (average ethanol intake now 5.2 g/kg per day), whereas the NP rats essentially stopped the ethanol self-administration. With 15% and 20% ethanol, the P rats self-administered between 8.5 and 9.5 g ethanol/kg per day. These amounts are higher than what they would normally drink out of Richter tubes at these ethanol concentrations.[16] The difference in behavior between the P and NP rats indicates that ethanol, 10% and higher in concentration, is aversive to the NP animals (probably because of taste in most animals), whereas it remains reinforcing for the P rats. The data also show that work increases the salience of ethanol as a reinforcer for the P rats.

The above studies could not distinguish whether the reinforcing properties of ethanol for the P rats arise from its systemic actions or its taste and smell. To demonstrate that the postingestive effects of ethanol are reinforcing to the P rats, intragastric ethanol self-administration experiments were performed, using the experimental design reported by Deutsch and coworkers.[25,26] It was found that with food freely available throughout the experiment, the P rats consistently self-infused greater volumes of the ethanol solution and lesser volumes of the water than did the NP rats, regardless of whether the concentration of infused ethanol was 10, 20, 30, or 40 percent.[27] The amount of ethanol infused by the NP rats was less than 1 g/kg/d at all concentrations of ethanol tested. By contrast, the amount of ethanol infused by the P rats increased from 3.0 ± 0.3 g/kg/d with 10% ethanol to 9.4 ± 1.7 g/kg/d with 40% ethanol. The BACs of animals measured 30 minutes after observed episodes of ethanol self-infusion of 20% ethanol were 100–400 mg percent. All animals repeatedly showed signs of intoxication. The BACs attained with intragastric self-administration were considerably higher than those observed in the P rats with free-choice drinking, suggesting that orosensory cues may be an important modulator of ethanol drinking.

It is important to note that Deutsch and Eisner[28] were able to demonstrate intragastric self-administration of large amounts of ethanol in rats unselected for ethanol preference only if the rats had been first made physically dependent by the prior, forcible administration of ethanol. Ethanol self-administration behavior was quickly extinguished in unselected animals not made ethanol-dependent, as was observed also in this study with the NP rats. By contrast, the P animals in this study had not been made dependent on ethanol and, in fact, were ethanol-free for at least a month before these experiments. Clearly, the innate ethanol preference of experimental animals is an important if not crucial variable in studies of ethanol self-administration, as well as in efforts to establish an oral consumption animal model of alcoholism. Conversely, differences between animals in sensitivity to the postingestional effects of ethanol can also affect drinking behavior. As we found in a recent study, ethanol, 1 g/kg given intraperitoneally, induced a much stronger conditioned taste aversion to saccharin in the NP rats than in the P rats.[29]

RELATION BETWEEN CARBOHYDRATE CONTENT OF DIET AND VOLUNTARY ETHANOL CONSUMPTION

Past studies have shown that the composition of diets can influence voluntary ethanol consumption. For example, diets deficient in vitamins, high in fat, low in carbohydrate and high in protein have been reported to increase intake.[30–32] By

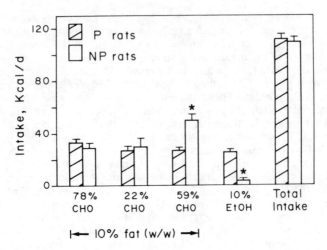

FIGURE 1. Free-choice consumption of 10% (v/v) ethanol, water, and three solid diets with different carbohydrate (CHO) contents by P and NP rats.

contrast, a recent paper showed that a 1:1 (by weight) mixture of sucrose and powdered regular diet or powdered regular diet mixed with Crisco dramatically decreased the ethanol intake of C57B1 mice. It was concluded that this elasticity in ethanol intake is an indication of a nutritional need to drink alcohol and not because of drug-seeking behavior in the normally alcohol-preferring C57B1 mice.[33]

We have studied the influence of dietary cabohydrate and protein content on ethanol consumption in the P and NP rats. In the first experiment, three powdered diets with different carbohydrate contents, water, and a 10% ethanol were made available to the animals *ad libitum*. All the diets contained 4.34 kcal/g and 10% fat

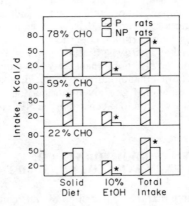

FIGURE 2. Free-choice consumption of 10% (v/v) ethanol, water, and one of three solid diets with different carbohydrate (CHO) contents by P and NP rats.

(w/w) as vegetable oil. The carbohydrate content (w/w as corn starch) of the three diets was 78%, 59% (normal diet), and 22 percent. Protein content was 12%, 31%, and 68% (casein), respectively. In the second experiment the three diets were presented individually to the P and NP rats, together with water and 10% ethanol, *ad libitum*. As shown in FIGURES 1 and 2, the alcohol consumption of the P rats was inelastic to dietary manipulation. Furthermore, under all test conditions, the P rats ate less solid food than the NP rats, because they substituted ethanol calories for the solid food calories. The P rats appeared to like all three diets equally well, but consumed more solid diet when all three were available (FIGURE 1) than when they were presented individually (FIGURE 2). On the other hand, the NP rats appeared to like the diet with the normal carbohydrate content (59%) better than the others. The diets with lesser palatability, however, did not induce the NP rats to drink ethanol because of the caloric need. The results demonstrate, therefore, that the ethanol preference of the P (high) and NP (low) rats are relatively inelastic.

DIFFERENCES IN RESPONSE TO LOW AND HIGH DOSE ETHANOL BETWEEN THE P AND NP RATS

The findings summarized above indicate that the P line of selectively bred rats should be a useful animal model for elucidating the biology of alcohol-seeking behavior and for exploring conditions and agents that lessen this kind of behavior. Furthermore, they suggest that ethanol at concentrations below 100 mg% in blood is reinforcing to the P rats and that ethanol at high concentrations may be more aversive to the NP rats than to the P rats. A number of studies have been performed to examine these relationships further.

The P rats are innately more active than the NP rats,[14] and they exhibit increased spontaneous motor activity (SMA) following the intraperitoneal injection of ethanol, 0.07 to 0.5 g/kg body weight. BACs achieved with these doses are about 15–75 mg percent. By contrast, the NP rats do not manifest stimulation at all. The increase in SMA in the P rats is as much as 50% with repeated daily injections of ethanol, 0.25 g/kg. No tolerance or reverse tolerance was observed over seven days.[34]

With sedative-hypnotic doses of ethanol, striking differences in response are also observed between the P and the NP lines. Whereas the P and the NP rats do not differ in CNS sensitivity to the sedative-hypnotic actions of ethanol, as measured by the loss of the aerial righting reflex following the intraperitoneal injection of 3 g ethanol/kg body weight, the P rats regain their righting reflex in a shorter period of time than the NP rats. The BAC at the time when this occurs is higher in the P than in the NP rats. Thus the P rats develop acute tolerance more quickly than do NP rats, and this conclusion has been confirmed by BAC measurements in studies using the jumping-descending platform test.[35,36] Even more interestingly, we recently found that acute tolerance developed in the P rats to a single dose of ethanol can persist for as long as 10 days, whereas tolerance was dissipated within 3 days in the NP rats.[37] It is of interest that the most robust association of high voluntary alcohol consumption thus far discovered in animal studies has been acute tolerance development. In addition to the P and NP rats, this association has been seen in the alcohol-preferring C57B1 and the alcohol-nonpreferring DBA mouse strains,[38,39] in the HS/Ibg (heterogeneous stock) mice,[40] and in the selectively bred alcohol-preferring AA and the alcohol-nonpreferring ANA rats.[41]

The combination of low-dose stimulation by ethanol and the rapid development of acute tolerance to the high-dose effects and its persistence offers an
attractive hypothesis for an underlying mechanism of biological propensity for
alcohol abuse. This hypothesis assumes that the low-dose stimulation observed in
the P rats is a reflection of the positively reinforcing or rewarding features of
ethanol consumption, whereas the high-dose depressant effect is aversive and
inhibits drinking. As tolerance to the high-dose effects of ethanol develops, the
rewarding actions of ethanol become progressively extended into the higher blood
alcohol concentration range, leading to increased consumption. We are currently
testing this hypothesis in the P line of rats and looking at neurohumoral concomitants of these effects.

NEUROCHEMICAL DIFFERENCES BETWEEN ETHANOL-NAIVE P AND NP RATS

Studies have been performed to discern whether there are neurochemical
differences between the P and the NP rats. A major discovered difference is in the
regional brain content of serotonin (5-HT). Ethanol-naive P rats consistently have
lower levels of serotonin in the cerebral cortex, corpus striatum, thalamus, hypothalamus, and hippocampus, and lower levels of 5-hydroxyindole acetic acid (5-
HIAA) in the cerebral cortex and hippocampus, than do ethanol-naive NP rats.[42]
Less consistently, a lower content of norepinephrine (NE) and dopamine (DA)
has been found in certain brain regions of P than of NP rats, for example, NE in
cortex and pons-medulla and DA in cortex. Differences in gamma-aminobutyric
acid (GABA) and other putative amino acid neurotransmitters, for example, Glu,
Asp, Ala, and Gly, have not been observed between the ethanol-naive P and NP
animals. We have also measured the regional brain monoamine content of alcohol-preferring and alcohol-nonpreferring animals in the N/Nih heterogeneous
stock rats. The principal finding was a lowered content of 5-HT and 5-HIAA in the
thalamus and hypothalamus of the alcohol-preferring animals and a lowered content of DA and NE in the thalamus.[43] These observations strengthen the relevance
of the association between brain 5-HT and alcohol drinking behavior.
    Further support of this relation has come from neuropharmacological studies.
Serotonin and norepinephrine reuptake inhibitors have been found to be effective
in reducing voluntary ethanol consumption in rats.[44] These drugs display a similar
action in the P rats, both on the 24-hour free-choice oral consumption schedule,
and with intragastric ethanol self-administration.[45,46] Clearly, we are interested in
the specificity of this kind of response in relationship to the postulated roles of
serotonin and/or norepinephrine in the reinforcing actions of ethanol.

SUMMARY

Depression, eating disorders, and carbohydrate craving are frequently seen in
alcoholics or recovering alcoholics. Accordingly, these disorders may share some
mediating pathways. It is now well-established that there is a genetic predisposition to alcoholism. Through genetic means, our laboratory has developed an
animal model of alcoholism. Free-fed Wistar rats were selectively bred for the
traits of alcohol-preference (the P line) and non-preference (the NP line). After
more than 20 generations of selection, the lines show a stable difference of more

than six-fold in voluntary ethanol consumption. We have now shown that the P line satisfies all the perceived requirements of an animal model of alcoholism. One major discovered difference between the P and the NP line is the lowered content of serotonin in certain brain regions of the P rats. Interestingly, fluoxetine curbs the alcohol-seeking behavior of the P rats; variation in the carbohydrate content of the diet, however, does not modify voluntary ethanol intake. The P rats are similar in body weight to the NP rats, but are more active in a novel environment than the NP rats.

REFERENCES

1. LI, T.-K. 1963. The absorption, distribution and metabolism of ethanol and its effects on nutrition and hepatic function. *In* Medical and Social Aspects of Alcohol Abuse. B. Tabakoff, P. B. Sutker & C. L. Randall, Eds.: 47–77. Plenum Press. New York.
2. VON KNORRING A.-L., C. R. CLONINGER, M. BOHMAN & S. SIGVARDSSON. 1983. An adoption study of depressive disorders and substance abuse. Arch. Gen. Psychiatry **40:** 943–950.
3. JONES, D. A., N. CHESHIRE & H. MOORHOUSE. 1985. Anorexia nervosa, bulimia and alcoholism: association of eating disorder and alcohol. J. Psychiatr. Res. **19:** 377–380.
4. YUNG, L., E. GORDIS & J. HOLT. 1983. Dietary choices and likelihood and abstinence among alcoholic patients in an outpatient clinic. Drug Alcohol Depend. **12:** 355–362.
5. CLONINGER, C. R., M. BOHMAN & S. SIGVARDSSON. 1981. Inheritance of alcohol abuse: cross-fostering analysis of adopted men. Arch. Gen. Psychiatry **38:** 861–868.
6. BOHMAN, M., S. SIGVARDSSON & C. R. CLONINGER. 1981. Maternal inheritance of alcohol abuse: cross-fostering analysis of adopted women. Arch. Gen. Psychiatry **38:** 965–969.
7. EDWARDS, G. & M. M. GROSS. 1976. Alcohol dependence: provisional description of a clinical syndrome. Br. Med. J. **1:** 1058–1061.
8. EDWARDS, G., A. ARIF & R. HODGSON. 1981. Nomenclature and classification of drug and alcohol related problems. Bull. W.H.O. **59:** 225–242.
9. CICERO, T. J. 1979. A critique of animal analogues of alcoholism. *In* Biochemistry and Pharmacology of Ethanol. E. Majchrowicz & E. P. Noble, Eds.: **2:** 533–560. Plenum Press. New York.
10. DEITRICH, R. A. & C. L. MELCHIOR. 1985. A critical assessment of animal models for testing new drugs for altering ethanol intake. *In* Research Advances in New Psychopharmacological Treatments for Alcoholism. C. A. Naranjo & E. M. Sellers, Eds.: 23–43. Excerpta Medica. Amsterdam, Netherlands.
11. MCCLEARN, G. E. & D. A. RODGERS. 1959. Differences in alcohol preference among inbred strains of mice. J. Stud. Alcohol **20:** 691–695.
12. MARDONES, J. 1960. Experimentally induced changes in the free selection of ethanol. Int. Rev. Neurobiol. **2:** 41–76.
13. ERIKSSON, K. 1968. Genetic selection for voluntary alcohol consumption in the albino rat. Science **159:** 739–741.
14. LI, T.-K., L. LUMENG, W. J. MCBRIDE & M. B. WALLER. 1979. Progress toward a voluntary oral consumption model of alcoholism. Drug Alcohol Depend. **4:** 45–60.
15. LI, T.-K., L. LUMENG, W. J. MCBRIDE & M. B. WALLER. 1981. Indiana selection studies on alcohol-related behavior. *In* Development of Animal Models as Pharmacogenetic Tools. G. E. McClearn, R. A. Deitrich & V. G. Erwin, Eds.: National Institute on Alcohol Abuse and Alcoholism Research Monograth 6. DHEW Publ. No. (ADM) 79–847. Washington, D.C.: Supt. of Docs., U.S. Govt. Print. Off., 171–191.
16. LUMENG, L., T. HAWKINS & T.-K. LI. 1977. New strains of rats with alcohol preference and nonpreference. *In* Alcohol and Aldehyde Metabolizing Systems. R. G. Thurman, J. R. Williamson, H. R. Drott & B. Chance, Eds.: vol. III, 537–544. Academic Press. New York.

17. WALLER, M. B., W. J. MCBRIDE, L. LUMENG & T.-K. LI. 1982. Induction of dependence on ethanol by free-choice drinking in alcohol-preferring rats. Pharmacol. Biochem. Behav. **16:** 501–507.
18. LUMENG, L. & T.-K. LI. 1986. The development of metabolic tolerance in the alcohol-preferring P rats: comparison of forced and free-choice drinking of ethanol. Pharmacol. Biochem. Behav. **25:** 1013–1020.
19. MURPHY, J. M., G. J. GATTO, M. B. WALLER, W. J. MCBRIDE, L. LUMENG & T.-K. LI. 1986. Effects of scheduled access on ethanol intake by the alcohol-preferring P line of rats. Alcohol **3:** 331–336.
20. WALLER, M. B., W. J. MCBRIDE, L. LUMENG & T.-K. LI. 1982. Effects of intravenous ethanol and of 4-methylpyrazole on alcohol drinking of alcohol-preferring rats. Pharmacol. Biochem. Behav. **17:** 763–768.
21. TULLIS, K. V., W. Q. SARGENT, J. R. SIMPSON & J. D. BEARD. 1977. An animal model for the measurement of acute tolerance to ethanol. Life Sci. **20:** 875–882.
22. GATTO, G. J., J. M. MURPHY, W. J. MCBRIDE, L. LUMENG & T.-K. LI. 1986. Acquisition of tolerance to ethanol through free-choice drinking in alcohol-preferring P rats. Alcoholism Clin. Exp. Res. **10:** 111 (Abstract).
23. PENN, P. E., W. J. MCBRIDE, L. LUMENG, T. M. GAFF & T.-K. LI. 1978. Neurochemical and operant behavioral studies of a strain of alcohol-preferring rats. Pharmacol. Biochem. Behav. **8:** 475–481.
24. MEISCH, R. A. 1977. Ethanol self-administration: Infrahuman studies. *In* Advances in Behavioral Pharmacology. T. Thompson & P. B. Dews, Eds.: **1:** 35–82. Academic Press. New York.
25. DEUTSCH, J. A. & W. T. HARDY. 1976. Ethanol tolerance in the rat measured by the untasted intake of alcohol. Behav. Biol. **17:** 379–389.
26. DEUTSCH, J. A. & N. Y. WALTON. 1977. A rat alcoholism model in a free-choice situation. Behav. Biol. **19:** 349–360.
27. WALLER, M. B., W. J. MCBRIDE, G. J. GATTO, L. LUMENG & T.-K. LI. 1984. Intragastric ethanol self-administration by ethanol-preferring and -nonpreferring lines of rats. Science. **225:** 78–80.
28. DEUTSCH, J. A. & A. EISNER. 1977. Ethanol self-administration in the rat induced by forced drinking of ethanol. Behav. Biol. **20:** 81–90.
29. FROEHLICH, J. C., J. HARTS, L. LUMENG & T.-K. LI. 1986. Differences in ethanol-induced conditioned taste aversion between P and NP rats. Alcoholism Clin. Exp. Res. **10:** 110 (Abstract).
30. PEKKANEN, L., K. ERIKSSON & M. SIHVONEN. 1978. Dietary-induced changes in voluntary ethanol consumption and ethanol metabolism in the rat. Br. J. Nutr. **40:** 103–113.
31. WILLIAMS, R. J., R. B. PELTON & L. L. ROGERS. 1955. Dietary deficiencies in animals in relation to voluntary alcohol and sugar consumption. Q. J. Stud. Alcohol **16:** 234–244.
32. BROWN, R. V. & D. P. HUTCHINSON. 1973. Nutrition and alcohol consumption in the Sinclair miniature pig. W. J. Stud. Alcohol **34:** 758–763.
33. DOLE, V. P., A. HO & R. T. GENTRY. 1985. Toward an analogue of alcoholism in mice: criteria for recognition of pharmacologically motivated drinking. Proc. Natl. Acad. Sci. USA **82:** 3469–3471.
34. WALLER, M. B., J. M. MURPHY, W. J. MCBRIDE, L. LUMENG & T.-K. LI. 1986. Effect of low dose ethanol on spontaneous motor activity in the alcohol-preferring (P) and -nonpreferring (NP) lines of rats. Pharmacol. Biochem. Behav. **24:** 617–623.
35. LUMENG, L., M. B. WALLER, W. J. MCBRIDE & T.-K. LI. 1982. Different sensitivities to ethanol in alcohol-preferring and -nonpreferring rats. Pharmacol. Biochem. Behav. **16:** 501–507.
36. WALLER, M. B., W. J. MCBRIDE, L. LUMENG & T.-K. LI. 1983. Initial sensitivity and acute tolerance to ethanol in the P and NP lines of rats. Pharmacol. Biochem. Behav. **19:** 683–686.
37. GATTO, G. J., J. M. MURPHY, W. J. MCBRIDE, L. LUMENG & T.-K. LI. 1986. Persistence of acute ethanol tolerance in alcohol-preferring (P) rats. Alcoholism Clin. Exp. Res. **10:** 111 (Abstract).

38. TABAKOFF, B. & R. F. RITZMAN. 1979. Acute tolerance in inbred and selected lines of mice. Drug Alcohol Depend. **4:** 87–90.

39. TABAKOFF, B., R. F. RITZMAN, T. S. RAJU & R. A. DEITRICH. 1980. Characterization of acute and chronic tolerance in mice selected for inherent differences in sensitivity to ethanol. Alcoholism Clin. Exp. Res. **4:** 70–73.

40. ERWIN, V. G., G. E. MCCLEARN & A. R. KUSE. 1980. Interrelationships of alcohol consumption actions of alcohol and biochemical traits. Pharmacol. Biochem. Behav. **13:** Suppl. 1, 297–302.

41. NIKANDER, P. & L. PEKKANEN. 1977. An inborn alcohol tolerance in alcohol-preferring rats. The lack of relationship between tolerance to ethanol and brain microsomal Na^+, K^+-ATPase activity. Psychopharmacology (Berlin) **51:** 219–233.

42. MURPHY, J. M., W. J. MCBRIDE, L. LUMENG & T.-K. LI. 1982. Regional brain levels of monoamines in alcohol-preferring and -nonpreferring lines of rats. Pharmacol. Biochem. Behav. **16:** 145–149.

43. MURPHY, J. M., W. J. MCBRIDE, L. LUMENG & T.-K. LI. 1986. Alcohol preference and regional brain monoamine contents of N/Nih heterogeneous stock rats. Alcohol Drug Res. **7:** 33–39.

44. AMIT, S., E. A. SUTHERLAND, K. GILL & S. O. OGREN. 1984. A review of its effects on ethanol consumption. Neurosci. Biobehav. Rev. **8:** 35–54.

45. MURPHY, J. M., M. B. WALLER, G. J. GATTO, W. J. MCBRIDE, L. LUMENG & T.-K. LI. 1985. Monoamine uptake inhibitors attenuate ethanol intake in alcohol-preferring (P) rats. Alcohol **2:** 349–352.

46. WALLER, M. B., J. M. MURPHY, W. J. MCBRIDE, L. LUMENG & T.-K. LI. 1985. Studies on the reinforcing properties of ethanol in alcohol-preferring P rats. Alcoholism Clin. Exp. Res. **9:** 207 (Abstract).

Dietary Treatments of Obesity

WILLIAM BENNETT

Harvard Medical School Health Letter
Department of Continuing Education
Harvard Medical School
Boston, Massachusetts 02115

DIETARY TREATMENTS OF OBESITY

It is generally taken to be self-evident that overeating is the cause of obesity. Thus, most treatments for obesity consist of efforts to reduce the client's caloric intake. Although the modalities currently in use may appear quite disparate, they are virtually all based on one guiding principle: an acceptable level of body fat not only can, but must be achieved through dietary restriction.

Most of the conceivable strategies seem to have been employed. The least subtle are surgical operations designed to interfere with ingestion: jaw-wiring and gastric limitation procedures. These operations are an attempt to put caloric intake outside the patient's control. Analogous to surgery in this respect are rigid reducing diets. Such regimens span the gamut from specially formulated liquid rations to the type of plan that is based on a set of fixed menus or some kind of conversion chart. These approaches, which have been the focus of much investigative effort in the past decade, are united by the philosophy that the overweight person cannot be trusted, at least for a time, to choose types and quantities of food appropriately. They attempt to take the locus of control away from the treated subject. Surgical intervention and extreme diets, of which the protein-sparing modified fast is currently the most used, are not ordinarily first-line treatments. They tend to be reserved for people who are extremely obese and have failed in earlier efforts to achieve weight control.

Unlike the drastic modalities that attempt to remove control from the patient, primary therapy for obesity has often been based on the assumption that people are capable of controlling their weight through will power but get fat by making innocent errors of judgment. It is this latter class of interventions that I shall discuss.

Until about 25 years ago, such treatment usually consisted of efforts to educate clients about the caloric content of familiar foods and give some kind of instruction in dietary limit-setting. By the beginning of the 1960s, the failure of this strategy was apparent.[1]

The time was ripe for a motivational theory that would explain why people who should know better, and who do not like being fat, still allow themselves to overeat. Elaborated in a paper, "The Control of Eating" by Ferster, Nurnberger, and Levitt, this theory became the foundation of behavior modification as a treatment for obesity.[2] A few years later, Stuart's 1967 report of success, using behavioral control of overeating to produce weight loss in eight women, appeared.[3] There followed an outpouring of research on behavior modification. By now it is generally accepted as the first-line treatment for people who are mildly obese.[4] Strictly speaking, behavior modification is a set of generic techniques that can be used to alter habitual behaviors, but as applied to obesity, it is in practice a dietary therapy; most behavior-modification programs identify overeating as the principal target behavior for modification.

Thus, despite some rather obvious differences, the methods I have listed so far all belong to the same school of thought, sharing a common model of the mechanism by which fat stores are maintained or can be altered. This is the "balance-sheet" model. Its major tenets are that food withheld is fat lost, daily caloric imbalances summate in a fairly simple fashion to produce gain or loss of fat, energy storage is not subject to any appreciable degree of regulation by the body, and eating behavior is quantitatively the most important variable contributing to fat accumulation.

Although balance-sheet treatments are now regarded as standard, there is an older dietary concept that has persisted in popular culture while almost vanishing from the mainstream of medical science. This is the notion that altering the composition of diet—usually the proportion of macronutrients—is a more efficient way to alter body fat stores than straightforward restriction of calories.

For about a century, marked at the beginning by William Banting's 1863 bestseller, *Letter on Corpulence*,[5] and at the end by Alfred Pennington's 1953 paper "Reorientation on Obesity" in the *New England Journal of Medicine*,[6] one particular form of this theory enjoyed a fairly high level of credibility. This was the belief that carbohydrates are the guilty nutrient, whereas fat and protein if anything, are protective. The most extreme statement of this view appeared in Herman Taller's popular book *Calories Don't Count* (1961).[7] Werner's paper challenging Pennington,[8] and Kinsell's response to Pennington and Taller,[9] discredited this version of the dietary-composition theory, and probably diverted attention from alternative formulations of it.

Nevertheless, the bias in favor of low-carbohydrate diets persisted in popular works, such as *The Scarsdale Diet*,[10] in some professional articles,[11,12] and in one group of workers committed to the protein-sparing modified fast, which, it is claimed, induces less hunger when carbohydrate content is low.[13] This claim has also been challenged,[14,15] and a recent report indicates that restricting carbohydrate intake may be one of the features of a weight-loss regimen that lowers resting metabolic rate.[16]

Within the past decade, attempts to bring about weight loss by adjusting composition of diet have regained a modicum of respectability. Currently in vogue are recommendations that fat intake be reduced to very low levels and that carbohydrate intake be high rather than low.[17] Sugar, despite its impeccable status as a carbohydrate, still tends be disallowed by most diet therapists, though the empirical basis for this practice is difficult to ascertain.

There remains an undercurrent of hope at the fringes of obesity research that manipulating one or several micronutrients will provide the clue to successful weight control. In the past five years or so, speculation about the effects of chromium, carnitine, lipoic acid, glycerol, and gamma-linolenic acid has appeared in the literature,[18] as have unsubstantiated claims for the effectiveness of a variety of amino-acid supplements.[19] Tryptophan has been put to a more rigorous, albeit short-term test, with equivocal results.[20] And a hardy perennial, nonnutritive fiber in the diet, has blossomed again in several recent studies, indicating that short-term weight loss is favored by high fiber intake.[21-23]

As a primary therapeutic approach to obesity, dietary therapy has been under active study for a little more than 50 years. In retrospect, the clinical research (and by extension, treatment programs) can be criticized on two grounds: theory and results.

THEORY OR TAUTOLOGY?

A recent, and useful, editorial on the complications of very-low-calorie diets begins with the statement, "Once we attain our adult size, usually by age 18 to 20, chronic overeating with a positive caloric balance results in obesity."[24] Sentences of this type permeate the literature on obesity. They have, unfortunately, one serious flaw. They do not mean anything. No plausible definition of the term *overeating* is independent of the observation that the person or animal in question is overweight. If eating behavior did not produce deposits of body fat, we could not call it overeating. Thus, to say that people get fat because they overeat is no different from saying that the sun comes up because it is morning. The assertion is, in its way, true, and it relates to a physical reality, but it is empty of content because it simply restates the definition of terms.

The first law of thermodynamics, by the way, is irrelevant to this discussion, although it is often brought in. The law constrains the equations that can be written to describe energy flow, but it does not explain how or why a body allocates its available energy to useful work, metabolic heat, or storage as fat. Indeed, the second law, which is sometimes cited by people who confuse it with the first, is probably more germane. The second law points out that real systems have rather wide latitude in the efficiency with which they convert incoming energy to mechanical work or heat. The efficiency of a system, or the way it allocates available energy, cannot be predicted a priori, but as a matter of observation it is always less than 100 percent.

These points are not logic-chopping. Such sentences as the one I just quoted can be decomposed into two propositions: positive caloric balance is equivalent to obesity (a tautology) and animals are heterotrophic, which is a meaningful, but not terribly specific or helpful point to make. To leap from the true and self-evident, but vacant, identification of overeating with obesity to the conclusion that control of food intake is the sole or most important modality for reversing the condition is as unwarranted as inferring that we could make the sun rise by taking suitable measures to make it be morning. Yet this is precisely the intellectual maneuver that launches the two fundamental papers on behavior modification as a treatment for obesity.

Ferster began his theoretical case for behavior therapy with the proposition, "excessive eating results in increased body fat and this is aversive to the individual. The problem is therefore to gain control of the factors which determine how often and how much one eats."[2] Keeping this tack, Stuart opened his seminal report of a treatment success with the following statement (citing the U.S. Public Health Service as its source): "Only two common characteristics have been observed in obese persons: a tendency to overeat and a tendency to underexercise."[3] Of course. The conclusion is foregone in the prefixes; if there is fat on a body, ipso facto it has overeaten, underexercised, or undermetabolized. Indeed, all three are automatically true, and the choice between them is arbitrary. It thus becomes highly unclear what kind of observation could have been made that would incriminate any one or two of these factors and not the third. Field studies on energy intake and expenditure of obese people have yielded, at best, equivocal results from attempts to measure differences between the caloric intake of fat and lean people,[25-27] though output studies suggest that obese adults, but perhaps not children, expend less energy than do their lean counterparts.[27,28]

To a considerable degree, even those laudable efforts to obtain firm data on the input/output characteristics of fat people are beside the point, because a positive finding with respect to any one of them begs the crucial question: Why is energy balance achieved at a particular level of fat storage and not some other? If one person is shown to exercise less than the other, and to be fatter, lack of exercise does not directly explain the obesity, because intake could have been adjusted to compensate for reduced output. Why wasn't it?

The common response to this dilemma is to ignore it. Overeating is accepted as the cause of overweight, and overeating is explained by characterizing food as an attractive nuisance that induces people to consume calories that they do not, in some mystical sense, really want. This was the essence of Ferster's argument, and it is uttered all the time by people who are in the busines of treating obesity. But inasmuch as the consequence (obesity) is used as its own explanation, this line of reasoning leads nowhere. I harp on this point for three reasons. The kind of thinking I am describing has been scientifically unproductive; it has yielded little discernible progress in the treatment of obesity; and it forms the basis for instruction that is given to patients in behavioral weight-loss programs. There is, thus, not only an intellectual, but an ethical problem pervading dietary treatments of obesity.

RATS, FOOD, AND FAT

Nothing I have said is intended to deny what is irrefutable: that manipulating an organism's food intake can lead to changes of body weight and body fat stores. Clearly it can. But 40 years ago there was unequivocal evidence from animal experiments that caloric intake could be uncoupled from weight gain, and since then the observation has often been repeated under other conditions.

Rats subjected to ventromedial hypothalamic (VMH) lesions can massively increase their fat stores without increasing their total caloric intake, as Brooks and Lambert showed in 1946.[29] Rats made to lose weight on amphetamine or fenfluramine regain their weight after the drugs are withdrawn without eating more than they did under treatment.[30] When refed, fasted rats regain their lost weight without full dietary replacement of the caloric deficit.[31] When given granulated sugar or fat along with chow, rats of some strains will gain weight without measurably increasing their total caloric intake (unlike rats given sugar water, which do both).[32,33] Genetically obese strains of mice and rats become obese even when restricted by pair-feeding to the intake of litter-mate controls. Such animals, when fasted to normal weight, retain a higher content of body fat than their equal-weight controls.[34–37]

There is, in other words, ample reason from animal experimentation to question the notion that altering food intake is an efficient, or even an effective, way of regulating body fat content. Short-term deprivation regularly and consistently lowers body fat content. But this finding may be simply irrelevant to the long-term concerns of free-living people or, for that matter, rodents. Too many steps intervene between food choice and fat storage for it even to be likely that manipulating caloric intake has the therapeutic value ascribed to it.

A principal reason that caloric restriction is likely to be ineffective as a long-term method of weight control is that it represents a highly unstable strategy for maintaining a given level of body fat. Human beings, without the most rigid instructions and controls, are not cognitively equipped to monitor caloric intake with anything like the precision required to prevent major changes in body fat stores.[38] On the basis of current experience with eating disorders, it would appear that at least some dieters pass an emotional point of no return, after which either habitual self-starvation or a cycle of binge-purge eating becomes established and, in either case, becomes exceedingly difficult to reverse. Thus, there is at least room to question whether most human beings are endowed with the cognitive and emotional equipment needed to permit conscious, intentional regulation of caloric intake, that is, regulation tight enough to permit stable weight maintenance over long periods of time.

SLENDER EVIDENCE

Reports of research on dietary treatment of obesity began to appear in the medical literature in the nineteenth century, but the first report giving sufficient data to permit some evaluation of outcome appeared in 1931.[39] In 1959, Stunkard and McLaren-Hume searched for and reviewed the available outcome studies. They found only eight papers meeting quite minimal standards for the reporting of data. In summarizing thier pioneering efforts at metastatistical analysis, these authors wrote, "the ambiguity of reported results has obscured the relative ineffectiveness" of outpatient treatment for obesity.[1] They found that the modal weight loss of the 1368 patients whose experience had been recorded in their eight studies was less than 10 pounds.

Twenty years later, Wing and Jeffery published a second metastatistical analysis of weight loss and maintenance.[40] They included in their analysis any study published between 1966 and 1977 "presenting enough information to compute the average number of pounds lost in treatment for a minimum of five overweight, healthy adult outpatients." Of the studies reviewed by Wing and Jeffery, 57, reporting data on 3,864 subjects, were primarily dietary in orientation, either straightforward reducing regimens or programs of behavior modification. Wing and Jeffery found that the average subject in these studies weighed 185 pounds at intake. The average weight loss of the people in the behavior-modification and reducing-diet groups, during a treatment typically lasting 11 weeks, was 16.5 pounds, or 8.9% of the entry weight.

Does this represent progress in the effectiveness of treatments developed in the interval between Stunkard and McLaren-Hume's survey? It is impossible to know whether the modest gain represented a real change in effectiveness of therapy, simply reflected a higher average weight of the clients entering the later group of studies, or resulted from a process of self-censorship in the research community, such that studies with poor results were not published.

In any case, weight loss logged during a 2- to 3-month period of research is hardly crucial information. What one wants to know is the results at follow-up, preferably after several years. Wing and Jeffery were able to find 34 reports that included follow-up statistics. The 308 clients treated with behavior modification, at a follow-up interval of about 6 months, had increased their weight loss by about half a pound. The 158 subjects in the diet studies had regained nearly 4 pounds at an average follow-up of 32 weeks.

In 1981, Foreyt, Goodrick, and Gotto analyzed the results of 16 studies reporting a one-year follow-up of behavior modification.[41] Data on 592 of the 858 subjects who entered these studies were available. This subset had lost a mean of 13.2 pounds during treatment periods averaging 12 weeks; at one year they had only maintained this weight loss, not increased it. If we make the rigorous assumption that the 266 people lost to follow-up had remained at or returned to their starting weight, this figure 13.2 pounds at one year diminishes to 4.1 pounds. Thus, at one year, the subjects had achieved, at best, a 7% reduction of their mean intake weight of 198 pounds or, at worst, a 2.2% reduction.

Among the reports analyzed by Foreyt, Goodrick, and Gotto, was a paper by Stalonas, Johnson, and Christ, which was right in the middle of the pack, with a mean weight loss of 11 pounds at the end of treatment and a total weight loss of 13.6 at one year.[42] Based on this study, two of the investigators published a popular book with the following statement about their behavioral program: "it has been subjected to stringent scientific tests—and it works! Not only do those who follow it lose weight but, more important, they maintain the weight loss after a one-year follow-up period, and many keep losing. This is accomplished in only ten weeks of formal exposure to the program." They promised their readers that "new eating and exercise habits . . . will be second nature to you."[43] When the authors returned to their subjects at the end of 5 years, however, they found that the average weight change of the subjects was no longer a loss but a gain of 1.49 pounds over intake weight.[44]

SINCE 1976

Through a MEDLINE search and from cross-checking citations from one study to another, I have located 26 papers published in the years 1977–1985 that meet the following criteria: there were more than five people in the study as a whole, a mean entry weight was given, the number of participants in the study was specified (though how many were present at each phase was sometimes unclear), and mean weight loss was reported at one or more times during or after the period of intervention.[44-69] I doubt whether this sample is exhaustive, but it seems quite representative of what there is to be found in the medical literature of the last decade.

Many of these studies included more than one treatment group. I coded each separately and included only those that had been the object of some intervention (thus excluding wait-list or attentional controls). I included only interventions that appeared to be primarily aimed at lowering caloric intake. In some studies, an exercise prescription was also employed, and this is potentially an important confounding factor. In all, there were 66 subgroups with a total of 1861 subjects. Mean weight at entry for the 1861 subjects was 207 pounds. The following variables were used for analysis: year of publication of the study, number of subjects, weight at entry, maximum percentage of intake weight lost (virtually always recorded at some point during the initial phase of intensive treatment or at the end of it), percentage of intake weight lost at last follow-up, and length of time to last follow-up.

Maximum Loss

The mean of the maximum losses reported in these studies was 8.5% of intake weight; the median was 6.8 percent. This is no different from the mean reported by Wing and Jeffery a decade ago: 8.9% of entry weight. This comparison must not, I should note, be overinterpreted as describing some kind of reality in the world of weight-loss efforts. It merely describes a trend recorded in the literature on this subject, and suggests that no material progress is being registered by interventions regarded as worthy of reporting.

Nevertheless, within the period from 1977 to 1985 a distinct time trend does appear. The maximum percentage weight loss does increase over this period, from about 6 percent to about 12 percent. Intake weight, however, also increases.

Stepwise regression analysis suggests that the higher intake weight of subjects in the later studies is the single most important factor accounting for the greater percentage of body weight they report being lost. (Fatter people evidently lose not only more pounds, but a higher percentage of their intake weight.) Intake weight accounts for about 27% of the variance in maximum reported weight loss. When both intake weight and year of publication are used in the model, however, 40% of the variance is accounted for, suggesting that some feature of these studies besides their tendency to report on progressively heavier patients was positively affecting outcome.

Loss at Follow-Up

Half of the 66 subgroups were followed for 52 weeks or less from the time of entry into the study. The remainder had follow-up times ranging from 52 to 520 weeks, and there was a slight, salutary tendency for longer follow-ups in the later studies. Interpreting the overall trends in the entire group of studies is made difficult by the fact that most of them produced a slight effect and measured it for a brief time. The ultimate weight loss reported in most of these studies was 6% or less of intake weight, an essentially trivial result given that the median intake weight was 195 pounds (mean was 201). And most of them report follow-ups well under two years. This large cluster of subgroups recording a weight loss that is negligible, with a follow-up time that is immaterial given the duration of most weight problems, tends to obscure any time trend in the data and to limit the opportunities for statistical analysis.

Simple correlations do not reflect any relationship between percentage weight loss at last follow-up and time to follow-up, although it is apparent from FIGURE 1 that the subgroups reporting larger losses tend to lie on a declining slope. If the results from the total sample are weighted by the number of participants in the study, a negative correlation with duration of follow-up does appear (Pearson product-moment correlation = 0.33, probability <0.0001). Stepwise regression analysis of weight loss at follow-up indicates that intake weight itself is the single independent variable accounting for the largest share of the variance, but only 11% of it. Adding length of follow-up, which is negatively correlated, brings the level to 15 percent.

From a glance at FIGURE 1, it is can be seen that an appreciably higher percentage of weight loss for any given time was reported by 4 of the 66 subgroups. These were the studies of Palgi,[69] Wadden,[57] Andersen,[53] and Björvell.[67] There is also a second echelon of subgroups, parallel to the first but with a smaller effect at any given time. The trend in this second tier is fairly easily described: weight loss at follow-up is less than 15% of starting weight and decays to zero by five years. The 4 outliers, however, lie on a line that seems to go from a 20% loss at six months to zero at 10 years. These four exceptionally effective subgroups may well differ from the majority of studies mainly because of their selection criteria. Two of them[53,69] were all male, whereas the majority of subjects in the studies reviewed were female. In all four, the subjects were very obese: the average weight at entry of the two all-male groups was 264 pounds[69] and 303 pounds.[67] In Wadden's all-female group, the average weight of the 17 subjects was 238 pounds,[57] and in Andersen's group of 26 women and 4 men the median weight at entry was 253 pounds.[53] Treatment may also have differed, however, in that three of the interventions[57,67,69] stressed a program of intensive exercise and presented themselves as multidisciplinary. The program reported by Andersen was evidently confined to a very-low-calorie regimen with frequent follow-up visits to support maintenance of weight loss.

I would urge the reader not to take the numbers I have given as representing any very precise version of reality. Papers reporting on research studies are undoubtedly a biased sample of the universe of efforts at weight control. The quality of the data in this literature also leaves something to be desired. Although the reporting in the studies I included was more complete than in many that I did not include, it often was too partial and idiosyncratic to support firm conclusions about the progress made either by the study subjects themselves or by the field of weight management as a whole. For example, it is the norm in these studies to omit height from the subject variables reported. Frequently, data for males and

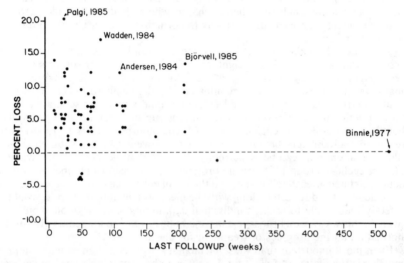

FIGURE 1. Dietary treatment of obesity, 1977–1985. The percent change of initial body weight at last reported follow-up is shown for 66 groups of patients in 26 reports on dietary treatment of obesity published between 1977 and 1984.[44-69] A total of 1861 subjects are included. There is a set of four outliers, Palgi,[69] Wadden,[57] Andersen,[53] and Björvell.[67] Of the remainder, the following generalization appears to hold: a 15% average weight loss is the maximum that a treatment group achieves, in a matter of weeks, and this loss decays toward zero at about five years. The exceptions are discussed in the text.

females are pooled in these studies, although there is reason to think that men and women react differently to weight loss regimens (and in any case, their average lean body mass is bound to be different).

METHODS AND ETHICS

There is an important distinction to be maintained between reporting and analyzing data. It is not unusual for a paper on treatment of obesity to give statistical interpretation of its results without also giving the data; this is particu-

larly seen in studies of behavior modification reported in the psychological literature. Nor is it uncommon to see excess weight given as a variable, with no clear
indication of the standard that is being applied and no effort to report actual
weight and height of the subjects. Excess weight is usually, but not always,
calculated by reference to the tables of desirable weight published by the Metropolitan Life Insurance Company. There are several reasons for not using these
tables. In the first place, the derivation of these tables is shrouded in some degree
of mystery; second, there are now two sets of tables, which are not identical;
third, the tables give a range of weights, 20–40 pounds for most heights, and it is
often unclear what point in this range was taken as the value to be subtracted from
the subject's entry weight in calculating percentage excess. Likewise, Feinstein's
reduction index,[70] which is based on difference between actual body weight and
the Metropolitan Life standard, should not be used in place of the actual data, but
only as an aid for analyzing them. On the whole, body-mass index (weight/
height^2) probably serves as the best way to normalize data for people of different
weight and height.

Any study that takes weight loss as one of its end points should include the
following information: weight, height, and body-mass index for subjects at entry,
then weight and body-mass index at each follow-up time. When expressed as
means, these values should be accompanied by the standard deviation, not the
standard error. Data for males and females should always be separated. If the
study contains more than one experimental group or a control group, the data
should be presented for each of them. (A common practice is to report entry
weights for all subjects but not the mean entry weight of the subgroups. It is
unlikely that entrants can be so perfectly allocated that the mean for the whole is
valid for each subgroup.) If there are drop-outs, the remaining number of subjects
should be stated at each follow-up, and the mean entry weight of this group should
be recalculated and reported along with the mean weight at follow-up. It would be
perfectly reasonable to present individual data in any study with 50 subjects or
fewer. In this way a weight-loss registry might be developed that could give usable
information on the progress of treatment for obesity.

Even more important than these elementary aspects of honest and complete
reporting is the matter of follow-up. It proves to be exceedingly easy to generate
statistically significant results by recruiting a population of people who are eager
to lose weight and engaging them in a behavioral/dietary treatment program.
Even acutely, however, these results hardly meet any other standard of significance. In addition, the longer the follow-up, the more trivial they become. I can
see no justification for planning or publishing a study that includes a follow-up of
less than three years, and even then, there are many studies that ought not to be
undertaken.

Data on the dietary treatment of obesity have been accumulating since 1931.
Nothing in the chronicle suggests that worthwhile progress has been made by
pursuing efforts to teach people more effective ways to restrict their food intake.
There is now enough information to permit the prediction that results will be
mediocre in the short run and after several years will be less than acceptable. The
burden should now be on the investigator to establish a strong reason for undertaking yet another study of intake restriction, including studies employing behavior modification aimed primarily at altering eating behaviors.

Committees reviewing the use of human subjects in these experiments should
not assume that they are ethically uncomplicated. The low probability that information of therapeutic value will result from such a study should weigh heavily in
any deliberation on whether to authorize it.

Relatively little is known about the experience, other than weight change, of participants in treatment studies. If there were significant adverse effects during or after the studies, it is highly unlikely that surveillance in most of research programs would detect them. Although some data indicate that people cheer up during behavior-modification programs,[58] the real question is how they feel weeks to months later, as they either fail to maintain their loss, or fail to reach the promised goal. To whom is the failure attributed, self or the investigator? Given the way behavioral interventions are presented to the subjects, it seems most probable that subjects blame themselves and not the therapists for failure they experience.

An important element of behavior modification is giving the client a model of his or her problem, one that focuses on eating behavior as the target for correction. An essential component of this model is the claim that it will be effective if the client believes it and acts accordingly. The model that appears to form the heart of most such programs, however, is at the very least seriously incomplete; there is good reason, as I have already pointed out, to assume it is simply wrong. In any case, the model has not produced results that would support claims of effectiveness—claims implying that failure must be the subject's fault. Is there any justification for engaging clients in a behavior-modification program that provides them with deceptive information?

The ethical questions that can be raised about research efforts also must be asked about the dietary programs for weight control that are carried on outside a research setting—commercial, hospital- or clinic-based, or self-help. Many such programs proffer treatment as though it were established as effective and safe. Nothing in the results published by research programs authorizes anyone to make such claims. It is incumbent upon any practitioner or enterprise claiming better results than those I have cited to provide the data to a disinterested scientific public. Until better results appear in the literature, the only honest way to characterize this type of intervention is to call it speculative, reserving the word *experimental* for those programs that are actually collecting data for publication.

Are there adverse physiological effects of weight loss and regain? There is some indication that participation in prior weight-loss efforts worsens the prognosis for subsequent weight loss.[71] If this is so, is it a result of various programs selecting hard cases, or is it, in effect, the treatment?

I can see little reason for intake restriction to receive continued support, either as a subject of research or as an accepted therapy for obesity. Bloodletting as a therapy for pneumonia was abandoned about a century before pencillin was discovered. It required a modicum of courage and good sense on the part of the practitioners who turned away from the practice, but there is no reason to believe their patients suffered from this lack of therapy.

DIRECTIONS

Abandoning intake control as the focus of efforts to treat obesity would not leave us without alternatives. Altering composition of the diet may be an effective tool after all. There are studies showing that fat or sugar intake can alter the body composition of laboratory rats without affecting their caloric intake.[32,33] Jeffrey Peck's elegant studies of this phenomenon suggest that nutrients may act directly on mechanisms that work to maintain body weight.[72,73] These findings need not fall into a tautological trap; they do not depend on a concept of overeating to explain the findings.

Mayer's fundamental observations of the relationship between physical activity and weight regulation[74,75] have not been refuted by recent studies showing that exercise produces weight loss without affecting caloric intake.[76,77] These and many other observations suggest that exercise is capable of reducing the level of body fat, quite apart from any effect on food consumption.

Exploration of micronutrient effects may also be worthwhile, if only because they have the potential to produce more interesting information at this point than studies of intake restriction. I think it plausible that micronutrients might have a drug-like effect on fat storage. If the goal is to treat obesity, however, such substances should be studied for their effect on body weight, not food intake.

The need at the moment, however, is for more and better basic research. I can see little justification for clinical efforts that continue to bark up the same old tautological tree.

SUMMARY

Dietary treatment of obesity is based on one or another of two premises: that the obese eat too much or that they eat the wrong things. The first is a tautology lacking explanatory power. The second is a meaningful and promising hypothesis but has yet to be effectively applied. At present, virtually all outpatient treatments of obesity, including behavior modification, are based on the first premise and consist of strategies for reducing the subject's caloric intake. Most such interventions produce short-term weight loss. Regain after the end of treatment remains the usual outcome.

A survey of studies published in the period 1977–1986 and reporting on dietary or behavioral treatment of obesity reveals that the maximum percentage of body weight lost is, on average, 8.5 percent—no different from the value, 8.9%, in similar studies from 1966–1976, as reviewed by Wing and Jeffery. The principal determinant of success in such programs appears to be the intake weight of the subjects: the higher the intake weight, the more successful the intervention will appear to be.

The goals and research methods of studies on dietary treatments for obesity are overdue for ethical as well as scientific reevaluation. The same may be said for the numerous programs providing such treatment outside the context of research.

REFERENCES

1. STUNKARD, A. & M. McLAREN-HUME. 1959. The results of treatment for obesity. Arch. Intern. Med. **103**: 79–85.
2. FERSTER, C. B., J. I. NURNBERGER & E. B. LEVITT. 1962. The control of eating. J. Mathetics **1**: 87–109.
3. STUART, R. B. 1967. Behavioral control of overeating. Behav. Res. Ther. **5**: 357–365.
4. STUNKARD, A. J. 1984. The current status of treatment for obesity in adults. In Eating and Its Disorders. A. J. Stunkard & E. Stellar, Eds.: 157–173. Raven Press. New York.
5. BANTING, W. 1864. Letter on Corpulence, Addressed to the Public. 3rd edit. Harrison. London.
6. PENNINGTON, A. W. 1953. A reorientation on obesity. N. Engl. J. Med. **248**: 959–964.
7. TALLER, H. 1961. Calories Don't Count. Simon and Schuster. New York.
8. WERNER, S. C. 1955. Comparison between weight reduction on a high-calorie, high-fat diet and on an isocaloric regimen high in carbohydrate. N. Engl. J. Med. **252**: 661–665.

9. KINSELL, L. W., B. GUNNING, G. D. MICHAELS, J. RICHARDSON, S. E. COX & C. LEMON. 1964. Calories do count. Metab. Clin. Exp. **13:** 195–204.
10. TARNOWER, H. & S. SINCLAIR-BAKER. 1978. The Complete Scarsdale Medical Diet. Rawson, Wade, New York.
11. YUDKIN, J. 1974. The low-carbohydrate diet. *In* Obesity Symposium: Proceedings of a Servier Research Institute Symposium held in December 1973. W. L. Burland, P. D. Samuel & J. Yudkin, Eds.: 271–280. Churchill Livingstone. Edinburgh.
12. GEISELMAN, P. J. & D. NOVIN. 1982. The role of carbohydrates in appetite, hunger and obesity. Appetite **3:** 203–223.
13. BISTRIAN, B. R., G. L. BLACKBURN, J. P. FLATT, J. SIZER, N. S. SCRIMSHAW & M. SHRMAN. 1976. Nitrogen metabolism and insulin requirements in obese diabetic adults on a protein-sparing modified fast. Diabetes **25:** 494–504.
14. BOGARDUS, C., B. M. LAGRANGE, E. S. HORTON & E. A. H. SIMS. 1981. Comparison of carbohydrate-containing and carbohydrate-restricted hypocaloric diets in the treatment of obesity. J. Clin. Invest. **68:** 399–404.
15. ROSEN, J. C., D. A. HUNT, E. A. H. SIMS & C. BOGARDUS. 1982. Comparson of carbohydrate-containing and carbohydrate-restricted hypocaloric diet in the treatment of obesity: effects on appetite and mood. Am. J. Clin. Nutr. **36:** 463–469.
16. HENDLER, R. G., M. WALESKY & R. S. SHERWIN. 1986. Sucrose substitution in prevention and reversal of the fall in metabolic rate accompanying hypocaloric diets. Am. J. Med. **81:** 280–284.
17. WURTMAN, J. J. 1983. The Carbohydrate Craver's Diet. Houghton Mifflin. Boston, MA.
18. MCCARTY, M. F. 1982. Orthomolecular aids for dieting. Med. Hypotheses **8:** 269–274.
19. GHADIMI, H. 1984. Amino acids and obesity. Pediatr. Ann. **13:** 557–563.
20. HERAIEF, E., P. BURCKHARDT, J. J. WURTMAN & R. J. WURTMAN. 1985. Tryptophan administration may enhance weight loss by some moderately obese patients on a protein-sparing modified fast (PSMF) diet. Int. J. Eating Disorders **4:** 281–292.
21. MICKELSEN, O., D. D. MAKDANI, R. H. COTTON, S. T. TITCOMB, J. C. COLMEY & R. GATTY. 1979. Effects of a high fiber bread diet on weight loss in college-age males. Am. J. Clin. Nutr. **32:** 1703–1709.
22. TUOMILEHTO, J., E. VOUTILAINEN, J. HUTTUNEN, S. VINNI & K. HOMAN. 1980. Effect of guar gum on body weight and serum lipids in hypercholesterolemic females. Acta Med. Scand. **208:** 45–48.
23. HYLANDER, B. & S. ROSSNER. 1983. Effects of dietary fiber intake before meals on weight loss and hunger in a weight-reducing club. Acta Med. Scand. **213:** 217–220.
24. MOSS, A. J. 1985. Caution: Very-low-calorie diets can be deadly [editorial]. Ann. Int. Med. **102:** 121–123.
25. COLL, M., A. MEYER & A. J. STUNKARD. 1979. Obesity and food choices in public places. Arch. Gen. Psychiatry **36:** 795–797.
26. WOOLEY, S., O. W. WOOLEY & S. DYRENFORTH. 1979. Theoretical, practical, and social issues in behavioral treatments of obesity. J. Appl. Behav. Anal. **12:** 3–25.
27. GARROW, J. S. 1974. Energy Balance and Obesity in Man. North-Holland, Amsterdam, and London.
28. THOMPSON, J. K., G. J. JARVIE, B. B. LAHEY & K. J. CURETON. 1982. Exercise and Obesity: Etiology, Physiology, and Intervention. Psychol. Bull. **91:** 55–79.
29. BROOKS, C. M. & E. F. LAMBERT. 1946. A study of the effect of limitation of food intake and the method of feeding on the rate of weight gain during hypothalamic obesity in the albino rat. Am. J. Physiol. **147:** 695–707.
30. LEVITSKY, D. A., B. J. STRUPP & J. LUPOLI. 1981. Tolerance to anorectic drugs: Pharmacological or artifactual? Pharmacol. Biochem. Behav. **14:** 661–667.
31. LEVITSKY, D. A., I. FAUST & M. GLASSMAN. 1976. The ingestion of food and the recovery of body weight following fasting in the naive rat. Physiol. Behav. **17:** 575–580.
32. KANAREK, R. B. & N. ORTHEN-GAMBILL. 1982. Differential effects of sucrose, fructose and glucose on carbohydrate-induced obesity in rats. J. Nutr. **112:** 1546–1554.
33. OSCAI, L. B., M. M. BROWN & W. C. MILLER. 1984. Effect of dietary fat on food intake, growth and body composition in rats. Growth **48:** 415–424.

34. Cox, J. E. & T. L. Powley. 1977. Development of obesity in diabetic mice pair-fed with lean siblings. J. Comp. Physiol. Psychol. **91:** 347–358.

35. Bray, G. A., D. A. York & R. S. Swerloff. 1973. Genetic obesity in rats. 1. The effects of food restriction on body composition and hypothalamic function. Metab. Clin. Exp. **22:** 435–442.

36. Deb, S. & R. J. Martin. 1975. Effects of exercise and of food restriction on the development of spontaneous obesity in rat. J. Nutr. **105:** 543–549.

37. Stolz, D. J. & R. J. Martin. 1982. Role of insulin in food intake, weight gain and lipid deposition in the Zucker obese rat. J. Nutr. **112:** 997–1002.

38. Wing, R. R. & L. H. Epstein. 1981. Prescribed level of caloric restriction in behavioral weight loss programs. Addict. Behav. **6:** 139–144.

39. Fellows, H. H. 1931. Studies of relatively normal obese individuals during and after dietary restrictions. Am. J. Clin. Med. **181:** 301–312.

40. Wing, R. R. & R. W. Jeffery. 1979. Outpatient treatments of obesity: a comparison of methodology and clinical results. Int. J. Obesity **3:** 261–279.

41. Foreyt, J. P., G. K. Goodrick & A. M. Gotto. 1981. Limitations of behavioral treatment of obesity: Review and analysis. J. Behav. Med. **4:** 159–174.

42. Stalonas, P. M., W. G. Johnson & M. Christ. 1978. Behavior modification for obesity: The evaluation of exercise, contingency management and program abstinence. J. Consult. Clin. Psychol. **46:** 463–469.

43. Johnson, W. G. & P. M. Stalonas. Weight No Longer. 1981. Pelican. Gretna, LA.

44. Stalonas, P. M., M. G. Perri & A. B. Kerzner. 1984. Do behavioral treatments of obesity last? A five-year follow-up investigation. Addict. Behav. **9:** 175–183.

45. Binnie, G. A. C. 1977. Ten-year follow-up of obesity. J. Royal Coll. Gen. Pract. **27:** 492–495.

46. Iselin, H. U. & P. Burckhardt. 1982. Balanced hypocaloric diet versus protein-sparing modified fast in the treatment of obesity: a comparative study. Int. J. Obesity **6:** 175–181.

47. Armstrong, S., C. Shahbaz & G. Singer. 1981. Inclusion of meal-reversal in a behaviour modification program for obesity. Appetite **2:** 1–5.

48. Wing, R. R., L. H. Epstein & B. Shapira. 1982. The effect of increasing initial weight loss with the Scarsdale diet on subsequent weight loss in a behavioral treatment program. J. Consult. Clin. Psychol. **50:** 446–447.

49. Bolocofsky, D. N., D. Spinler & L. Coulthard-Morris. 1985. Effectiveness of hypnosis as an adjunct to behavioral weight management. J. Clin. Psychol. **41:** 35–41.

50. Long, C. G., C. M. Simpson & E. A. Allott. 1983. Psychological and dietetic counseling combined in the treatment of obesity: A comparative study in a hospital outpatient clinic. Hum. Nutr. Appl. Nutr. **37A:** 94–102.

51. Holm, R. P., M. T. Taussig & E. Carlton. 1983. Behavioral modification in a weight-reduction program. J. Am. Diet. Assoc. **83:** 170–174.

52. O'Brien, M. H., K. W. Samonds, V. A. Beal, D. W. Hosmer & J. O'Donnell. 1982. Incorporating transactional analysis into a weight loss program. J. Am. Diet. Assoc. **81:** 450–453.

53. Andersen, T., O. G. Backer, K. H. Stokholm & F. Quaade. 1984. Randomized trial of diet and gastroplasty compared with diet alone in morbid obesity. N. Engl. J. Med. **310:** 352–356.

54. DeWolfe, J. A. & E. Jack. 1984. Weight control in adolescent girls: A comparison of the effectiveness of three approaches to follow-up. J. Student Health **54:** 347–349.

55. Perri, M. G., R. M. Shapiro, W. W. Ludwig, C. T. Twentyman & W. G. McAdoo. 1984. Maintenance strategies for the treatment of obesity: An evaluation of relapse prevention training and posttreatment contact by mail and telephone. J. Consult. Clin. Psychol. **52:** 404–413.

56. Donahoe, C. P., D. H. Lin, D. S. Kirschenbaum & R. E. Keesey. 1984. Metabolic consequences of dieting and exercise in the treatment of obesity. J. Consult. Clin. Psychol. **52:** 827–836.

57. Wadden, T. A., A. J. Stunkard, K. D. Brownell & S. C. Day. 1984. Treatment of

obesity by behavior therapy and very low calorie diet: A pilot investigation. J. Consult. Clin. Psychol. **52:** 692–694.
58. JEFFERY, R. W., W. M. BJORNSON-BENSON, B. S. ROSENTHAL, R. A. LINDQUIST & S. L. JOHNSON. 1984. Behavioral treatment of obesity with monetary contracting: two-year follow-up [brief report]. Addict. Behav. **9:** 311–313.
59. AJA, J. H. 1977. Brief group treatment of obesity through ancillary self-hypnosis. Am. J. Clin. Hypn. **19:** 231–234.
60. BLACK, D. R. & C. E. LANTZ. 1984. Spouse involvement and a possible long-term follow-up trap in weight loss. Behav. Res. Ther. **22:** 557–562.
61. VAN SETERS, A. P., M. L. BOUWHUIS-HOOGERWERF, B. M. GOSLINGS, L. VAN NIEUWKOOP, H. VAN SLOOTEN & T. STRUIJK-WIELINGA. 1982. Langdurige behandleing van patiënten met vetzucht door middel van mazindol en een vermageringsdieet [Protracted treatment of obese patients with mazindol and a low-energy diet]. Ned. Tijdschr. Geneeskd. **12:** 990–994.
62. O'NEIL, P. M., H. S. CURREY, A. A. HIRSCH, F. E. RIDDLE, C. I. TAYLOR, R. J. MALCOLM & J. D. SEXAUER. 1979. Effects of sex of subject and spouse involvement on weight loss in a behavioral treatment program: A retrospective investigation. Addict. Behav. **4:** 167–177.
63. LORO, A. D., E. B. FISHER & J. C. LEVENKRON. 1979. Comparison of established and innovative weight-reduction treatment procedures. J. Appl. Behav. Anal. **12:** 141–155.
64. HALL, S. M., A. BASS & J. MONROE. 1978. Continued contact and monitoring as follow-up strategies: A long-term study of obesity treatment. Addict. Behav. **3:** 139–147.
65. BROWNELL, K. D., J. H. KELMAN & A. J. STUNKARD. 1983. Treatment of obese children with and without their mothers: Changes in weight and blood pressure. Pediatrics **71:** 515–523.
66. GÖTESTAM, K. G. 1979. A three year follow-up of a behavioral treatment for obesity. Addict. Behav. **4:** 179–183.
67. BJÖRVELL, H. & S. RÖSSNER. 1985. Long term treatment of severe obesity: four year follow up of results of combined behavioural modification programme. Br. Med. J. **291:** 379–382.
68. MACMAHON, S. W., G. J. MACDONALD, L. BERNSTEIN, G. ANDREWS & R. B. BLACKET. 1985. A randomized controlled trial of weight reduction and metoprolol in the treatment of hypertension in young overweight patients. Clin. Exp. Pharmacol. Physiol. **12:** 267–271.
69. PALGI, A., J. L. READ, I. GREENBERG, M. A. HOEFER, B. R. BISTRIAN & G. L. BLACKBURN. 1985. Multidisciplinary treatment of obesity with a protein-sparing modified fast: Results in 668 outpatients. Am. J. Public Health **75:** 1190–1194.
70. FEINSTEIN, A. R. 1959. The measurement of success in weight reduction: An analysis of methods and a new index. J. Chron. Dis. **10:** 439–457.
71. ADAMS, S. O., K. E. GRADY, C. H. WOLK & C. MUKAIDA. 1986. Weight loss: A comparison of group and individual interventions. J. Am. Diet. Assoc. **86:** 485–490.
72. PECK, J. W. 1978. Rats defend different body weights depending on palatability and accessibility of their food. J. Comp. Physiol. Psychol. **92:** 555–570.
73. PECK, J. W. 1979. Active regulation to be lean by rats with ventromedial hypothalamic lesions. J. Comp. Physiol. Psychol. **93:** 695–707.
74. MAYER, J., N. B. MARSHALL, J. J. VITALE, J. H. CHRISTENSEN, M. B. MASHAYEKHI & F. J. STARE. 1954. Exercise, food intake, and body weight in normal rats and genetically obese adult mice. Am. J. Physiol. **177:** 544–548.
75. MAYER, J., P. ROY & K. P. MITRA. 1956. Relation between caloric intake, body weight, and physical work: Studies in an industrial male population in West Bengal. Am. J. Clin. Nutr. **4:** 169–175.
76. WOO, R., J. S. GARROW & F. X. PI-SUNYER. 1982. Effect of exercise on spontaneous calorie intake in obesity. Am. J. Clin. Nutr. **36:** 470–477.
77. WOO, R., J. S. GARROW & F. X. PI-SUNYER. 1982. Voluntary food intake during prolonged exercise in obese women. Am. J. Clin. Nutr. **36:** 478–484.

Mood and Food

A Psychopharmacological Enquiry

TREVOR SILVERSTONE

Academic Unit of Human Psychopharmacology
St. Bartholomew's Hospital
London, England

Major depressive episodes, as defined in DSM III are frequently accompanied by marked changes in appetite. These changes can take a number of forms. In mild to moderate depression, appetite may either increase or decrease. In one survey, 14% of the patients had noted their appetite to have increased when depressed, with 66% noting a decrease.[1] In another series, the proportion noting an increase in appetite was 27%, wheres 54% experienced a decrease in appetite.[2] In both series the degree of appetite change, whether up or down, was related to the severity of the depressive illness.

A more selective alteration in appetite occurs in seasonal affective disorder where there is typically a heightened desire for carbohydrates.[3] Almost 80% describe what the authors call carbohydrate craving, some preferring sweets and chocolates, others starches. There is frequently a concomitant increase in weight.

In the most severe form of depressive illness, referred to in DSM as a major depressive episode with melancholia, a profound reduction in appetite is the rule. In his classic description of melancholia, Sir Aubrey Lewis states: "Depressive states are almost invariably characterized during the greater part of their course by disinclination for food".[4] More recent clinical surveys of this condition have similarly found that the majority of patients so diagnosed lose their appetite, with many consequently having an appreciable weight loss. Nelson and his colleagues[5] reported that 32 (74%) of their 43 melancholic patients had a decreased appetite, with six of them having lost weight. Comparing depressed patients who were classified as melancholic according to DSM III, with those who were not, Davidson and Turnbull[6] recently reported that 22 (81%) of the 27 melancholics had experienced a lowering of appetite with none noting an increase. Of the 65 patients in the nonmelancholic group, 39 (60%) had a lower appetite than usual, whereas 9 (14%) had a greater appetite. Corresponding weight changes occurred in similar proportions of patients in each group.

Although the exact pathogenesis of the various subtypes of depressive illness remains unresolved, there is a general consensus that alteration in one or more neurotransmitter pathways is involved in some way, either primarily or secondarily.[7] Many of the insights that have been gained into the pathogenetic mechanisms have been obtained through studying the actions of centrally acting drugs on the symptomatology of these illnesses. Among the drugs that can be used in this manner are antidepressants, which not only affect the underlying mood state but that also have a direct effect on appetite itself. Two such antidepressant drugs are amitriptyline, which increases appetite, particularly the desire for sweet foods,[8] and fluoxetine, which has an appetite suppressant effect.[9] The observation that these two drugs have opposite effects on appetite can perhaps best be explained by the fact that they also have opposing effects on serotoninergic (5-HT) neurotransmission. Amitriptyline reduces 5-HT neurotransmission by blocking 5-HT receptors,[10] whereas fluoxetine enhances it by slowing the removal of 5-HT from the synaptic cleft through inhibition of reuptake into the presynaptic neurone.[11]

Other drugs that block 5-HT receptors also increase appetite and food intake in a similar manner to amitriptyline. Included in this group are cyproheptadine[12] and metergoline.[13] Drugs that enhance 5-HT neurotransmission include tryptophan, a 5-HT precursor, and d-fenfluramine, which releases 5-HT from the presynaptic neurone (see Garattini, this volume). Both suppress appetite and food intake in human subjects.[13]

In order to explore in more detail the role of 5-HT in human feeding, we have examined the interaction of the 5-HT receptor blocker metergoline with that of the 5-HT releaser fenfluramine. One of our aims was to shed some light on the distortion of appetite that occurs in seasonal affective disorders.

In this work we have used subjective measures of hunger and objective measures of food intake to evaluate the changes in appetite and food intake occurring in response to metergoline and fenfluramine.

Visual analog scales (VAS) were used for the rating of subjective changes of hunger and mood; for the objective measurement of food intake we employed the automated solid food dispenser developed in our laboratory.[14]

When given to 14 healthy male volunteer subjects, metergoline (which in animals is a relatively selective 5-HT receptor blocker) significantly increased their intake of sweet foods as compared to placebo; the intake of nonsweet foods was unaffected (Goodall and Silverstone, this volume). Thirty mg d-fenfluramine countered this effect. Thus, in metergoline we have a 5-HT receptor blocking drug, which enhances particularly the desire for sweet foods, and a 5-HT–enhancing drug, fenfluramine, which counters this effect. Could it be that the craving for sweet food seen in seasonal affective disorder is also due to a relative reduction in central 5-HT neurotransmission? If so, 5-HT–enhancing drugs such as d-fenfluramine and fluoxetine should be particularly effective in its treatment.

Let us now turn to melancholia, that form of depressive disorder in which appetite and food intake are profoundly suppressed. What light can the psychopharmacology of appetite-suppressant drugs throw on the underlying neurochemical disturbances? To this end we have carried out a series of experiments on the clinical psychopharmacology of amphetamine.

Amphetamine is a drug with potent anorectic, stimulant, and euphoriant properties in human subjects.[15] In laboratory animals, amphetamine has been shown to act in the brain largely by releasing preformed dopamine (DA) and noradrenaline (NA) from presynaptic neurones.[16] Given this dual pattern of neurochemical actions, it could be that the anorectic effect of amphetamine was mediated through one neurotransmitter, whereas its stimulant and euphoriant activity was related to an action on the other.

We have attempted to resolve this point by examining the interaction of amphetamine with a number of relatively specific receptor-blocking compounds and observing the resulting psychological changes. We began by studying the role of central DA pathways by using the selective DA receptor-blocking drug pimozide (PMZ), to determine the effect of DA receptor blockade on amphetamine's stimulant and euphoriant activity.[17]

We administered a single oral dose of 2 mg PMZ, or matching placebo, two hours before giving a single oral dose of 10 mg dextroamphetamine (d-Amp) or a second matching placebo to eight healthy female subjects. The subjects completed VAS ratings for arousal, mood, and hunger before receiving the first tablet and at hourly intervals thereafter for the next six hours. We observed a significant increase in subjective arousal after d-Amp, which was attenuated by pretreatment with 2 mg PMZ. This finding strongly suggests that the stimulant action of d-Amp is mediated through central DA pathways.

Hunger ratings, which were markedly reduced by d-Amp remained unaffected by PMZ, indicating that d-Amp–induced anorexia, in contrast to its stimulant effect, is not mediated primarily through DA pathways.

To study the role of NA pathways, we used the alpha-1 receptor-blocking drug thymoxamine (TMX), which is considered to have a relatively specific action on these receptors.[18] It has been shown to be active centrally. In our first experiments with TMX, we administered 80 and 160 mg TMX, or matching placebo one hour before giving a single oral dose of 20 mg d-Amp to 12 healthy male volunteers. As far as subjective mood ratings were concerned, TMX, if anything, increased d-Amp–induced euphoria and irritability. A similar pattern was seen in the VAS arousal ratings, with TMX enhancing the effect of d-Amp. In contrast to what was observed with d-Amp–induced arousal, d-Amp–induced anorexia was partially attenuated by the higher dose of TMX. This finding suggests that d-Amp anorexia may well be NA-mediated, a view consistent with some of the animal data.[19] In a second study, however, involving healthy female subjects in which we measured food intake directly in addition to assessing subjective hunger, we failed to replicate our previous finding that TMX attenuates d-Amp anorexia. But in this second study, food intake was measured two hours after the drug had been given, whereas the most marked effect of TMX in the first study had not occurred until some three to four hours after it had been given. Thus, the lack of agreement in the two studies may well be more of a reflection of the methodological differences between them than a true pharmacological inconsistency.

We found propranolol (PPL), a centrally active beta-NA receptor-blocking drug,[20] to be completely without effect on either d-Amp–induced arousal or anorexia in normal female volunteers. Nor did it influence the reduction of food intake brought about by d-Amp. Such a complete lack of interaction between d-Amp and PPL argues strongly against a primary involvement of beta-NA receptors in d-Amp–induced arousal or anorexia.

From our human volunteer studies, we can be reasonably confident that the stimulant and euphoriant actions of d-Amp are mediated through central DA pathways. The situation with regard to the mediation of d-Amp anorexia is less clear-cut than that of arousal; certainly neither DA or beta-NA receptors appear to be primarily involved. Whether alpha-NA receptors are, remains unresolved; in one study there did appear to be a definite interrelationship between the alpha-NA receptor-blocking drug TMX and d-Amp anorexia.

If it is confirmed that d-Amp anorexia is mediated through central NA pathways, then the possibility arises that other anorectic states, which occur in depressive illness, may be a consequence of an abnormality in central NA neurotransmission. In order to test this possibility, we examined the effect of a single intravenous injection of 15 mg methylamphetamine (m-Amp) as compared to sterile water under strict double blind conditions in 21 depressed subjects.[21] The question we were asking was, If methylamphetamine improved the mood of any of our depressed patients, was there an associated improvement in appetite, as normally occurs during recovery from a depressive illness, or was any such improvement in appetite suppressed by the direct anorectic action of the drug? Two intriguing findings emerged. First, as was expected from previous uncontrolled studies,[22] only a third of our twenty-one patients responded to m-Amp (but not to placebo) with an unequivocal improvement in mood. The majority showed no such response. This lack of response may reflect an underlying lowering of responsiveness in central DA pathways in these severely depressed patients. A differential response of this kind to a standardized pharmacological challenge raises the real possibility of delineating different categories of depressive illness on pharmacological grounds, a psychopharmacological nosology as it were. The other intriguing finding that emerged from our m-Amp study in depressed patients was that of the seven who responded to m-Amp with a marked improvement in mood, six experienced a concomitant increase in hunger. If d-Amp anorexia is in fact NA-mediated, then the absence of m-Amp–induced anorexia in these patients could reflect a reduction in central NA neurotransmission. There is already good neuroendocrinological evidence that central NA neurotransmission is reduced in depressive illness.[23]

Thus, the study of appetite in healthy human subjects, and the way in which centrally acting drugs affect it, can throw light on neurochemical abnormalities that may form the basis of a number of depressive states. In particular, our results are consistent with the view that seasonal affective disorder may be related to a reduction in central 5-HT neurotransmission. Melancholia on the other hand appears to be associated with a reduction in central DA neurotransmission in the majority of cases; there is, however, a sizable minority of about one-third of patients with melancholia who appear DA-responsive but NA nonresponsive.

I think we can safely conclude that mood and food are indeed inextricably linked, although the linkages involved are complex and varied.

REFERENCES

1. PAYKEL, E. S. 1977. Depression and appetite. J. Psychosom. Res. **21:** 401–407.
2. HARRIS, B., J. YOUNG & B. HUGHES. 1984. Appetite and weight change in patients presenting with depressive illness. J. Affective Dis. **6:** 331–339.
3. ROSENTHAL, N. E., D. A. SACK, J. C. GILLIN, A. J. LEWY, F. K. GOODWIN, Y. DAVENPORT, P. S. MUELLER, D. A. NEWSOME & T. A. WEHR. 1984. Seasonal affective disorder. Arch. Gen. Psychiatry **41:** 72–80.
4. LEWIS, A. J. 1934. Melancholia: a clinical survey of depressive states. J. Ment. Sci. **80:** 277–378.
5. NELSON, J. C., C. MAZURE, D. M. QUINLAN & P. I. HARLOW. 1984. Drug responsive symptoms in melancholia. Arch. Gen. Psychiatry **41:** 663–668.
6. DAVIDSON, J. & C. D. TURNBULL. 1986. Diagnostic significance of vegetative symptoms in depression. Br. J. Psychiatry **148:** 442–446.
7. ZIS, A. P. & F. K. GOODWIN. 1982. The amine hypothesis. In Handbook of Affective Disorders. E. S. Paykel, Ed.: 175–190. Churchill Livingstone. Edinburgh.
8. PAYKEL, E. S., P. S. MULLER & O. O. DE LA VERGNE. 1973. Amitriptyline, weight gain and carbohydrate craving: a side effect. Br. J. Psychiatry **123:** 501–507.
9. FERGUSON, J. M. 1986. Fluoxetine induced weight loss in humans. In Disorders of Eating Behaviour: A Psycho-neuroendocrine approach. E. Ferrari, Ed. Pergamon Press. Oxford.
10. MAI, J., A. LEWANDOWSKA & A. RAWLOW. 1979. Central antiserotonin action of amitriptyline. Pharmacopsychiat. **12:** 281–285.
11. WONG, D. T., F. P. BYMASTER, J. HORNING & B. B. MOLLOY. 1975. A new selective inhibitor for uptake of serotonin into synaptasomes of rat brain. J. Pharmacol. Exp. Ther. **193:** 804–811.
12. SILVERSTONE, T. & D. SCHUYLER. 1975. The effect of cyproheptadine on hunger, calorie intake and body weight in man. Psychopharmacologia **40:** 335–340.
13. SILVERSTONE, T. & E. GOODALL. 1984. The clinical pharmacology of appetite suppressant drugs. Int. J. Obesity **8** (Suppl. 1): 23–33.
14. SILVERSTONE, T., J. FINCHAM & J. BRYDON. 1980. A new technique for the continuous measurement of food intake in man. Am. J. Clin. Nutr. **3:** 1852–1855.

15. SILVERSTONE, T. & B. WELLS. 1980. Clinical psychopharmacology of amphetamine and related compounds. *In* Amphetamines and Related Stimulants. J. Caldwell, Ed.: 147–159. CRCV Press. Boca Raton, Fla.

16. CARLSSON, A. 1970. Amphetamine and brain catecholamines. *In* Amphetamine and Related Compounds. E. Costa & S. Garattini, Eds.: 289–300. Raven Press. New York.

17. ANDEN, N. E., S. G. BUTCHER, H. CORRODI, F. FUXE & U. UNGERSTEDT. 1979. Receptor activity and turnover of dopamine noradrenaline after neuroleptics. Eur. J. Pharmacol. **11:** 303–314.

18. BESSER, G. M., P. BUTLER, J. G. RATCLIFFE, L. REES & P. YOUNG. 1968. Release by amphetamine in man of growth hormone and corticosteroids: the effects of thymoxamine and propranolol. Br. J. Pharmacol. **39:** 196–197.

19. AHLSKOG, J. E., 1974. Food intake and amphetamine anorexia after selective forebrain norepinephrine loss. Brain Res. **82:** 211–240.

20. PATEL, L. & P. TURNER. 1981. Central actions of beta-adrenoreceptor blocking drugs in man. Res. Rev. **1:** 387–410.

21. COOKSON, J. & T. SILVERSTONE. 1986. The effects of methylamphetamine on mood and appetite in depressed patients; a placebo controlled study. Int. Clin. Psychopharmac. **1:** 127–133.

22. CHECKLEY, S. A. 1978. A new distinction between the euphoric and the antidepressant effect of methylamphetamine. Br. J. Psychiatry **133:** 416–423.

23. CHECKLEY, S. A., I. B. GLASS, C. THOMPSON, T. CORN & R. ROBINSON. 1984. The GH response to clonidine in endogenous as compared to reactive depression. Psychol. Med. **14:** 773–777.

New Developments in Pharmacological Treatments for Obesity

ANN C. SULLIVAN, SUSAN HOGAN,
AND JOSEPH TRISCARI

Research Division
Hoffmann-La Roche Inc.
Nutley, New Jersey 07110

THERAPEUTIC GOALS

Obesity is a major health problem, which is caused by a chronic imbalance between energy intake and energy expenditure. The treatment of obesity is largely ineffective in the majority of patients, particularly when long-term results are considered. Clearly, greater effectiveness is required than can be achieved with diet restriction (with or without the use of anorectics), behavior modification, and exercise.

From our perspective, drug treatment of obesity is still in its infancy, and significant opportunities exist for future therapeutics to treat this important disease. The currently available appetite suppressants, which act by central mechanisms have several major disadvantages, including limited effectiveness, side effects on the central nervous system, development of tolerance, and abuse potential.

There is a significant need for safe and efficacious drugs as an adjunct to diet restriction and exercise programs to increase the loss of body fat and to prevent weight regain once weight loss has been achieved. Pharmacological treatment of obesity, depending on severity, may necessitate intervention at one or more sites simultaneously to circumvent the multiple compensatory systems, which are working to maintain an elevated body fat level in the obese patient. For severe forms of obesity, the simultaneous use of several drugs with different mechanisms of action may be required to achieve optimal loss of body fat. Certain subtypes of obese patients may be more responsive to one type of mechanistic approach. These important issues cannot be resolved until clinical evaluations of drugs with unique and different mechanisms of action are conducted.

There are many sites where intervention can create a reduction in body fat. Three broad approaches can be taken: reduce energy intake, decrease energy storage, and enhance energy expenditure. FIGURE 1 outlines schematically a number of potential targets for pharmacological intervention that could result in decreased body fat in obese subjects. This paper will focus on one example of each of these broad approaches: chlorocitric acid (Ro 21-7716), a peripherally acting appetite suppressant to reduce energy intake; Ro 22-0654, an inhibitor of lipid synthesis that accelerates the oxidation of fat to decrease energy storage, and Ro 16-8714, a beta-agonist to enhance energy expenditure.

It is too early to know whether these experimental approaches will provide the safe and efficacious drugs that are required to promote weight loss and to prevent weight regain once desirable body weight has been achieved. The need for such drugs, however, is tremendous, and the commitment in research and development for such agents must be sustained.

269

ENERGY   ENERGY   ENERGY
INTAKE   STORAGE   EXPENDITURE

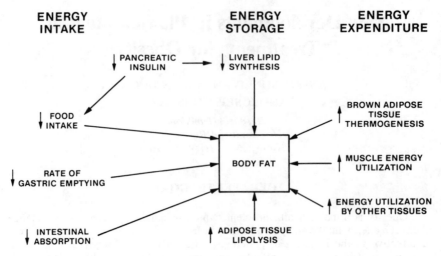

FIGURE 1. Sites of pharmacological intervention in obesity.

SUPPRESSION OF ENERGY INTAKE

Regulation of food intake is a complex process consisting of both central and peripheral elements and involving integration by the brain of a variety of signals from peripheral organs transmitted by neurotransmitters, peptides, hormones, and metabolites.[1] The traditional pharmacological approach to treating obesity consists of an appetite suppressant as an adjunct to dietary restriction. Drugs affecting appetite can be categorized as primarily acting directly on either the brain or a peripheral site(s). Anorectic drugs available today all have direct central nervous system (CNS) sites of action and appear to lower food intake by potentiating central dopaminergic, adrenergic, or serotonergic mechanisms.

The limited effectiveness and CNS side effects of the centrally acting anorectics have encouraged the search for appetite suppressants that function at peripheral sites. The upper gastrointestinal tract is thought to be the site of action of the anorectic agent, chlorocitric acid (Ro 21-7716). This compound reduced food intake dose-dependently in normal and obese rats and dogs.[2] When chronically administered to rats, chlorocitric acid reduced body weight through a selective reduction in body lipid levels.[3] No CNS side effects were observed in these studies, and there was no development of tolerance to the anorectic effect. In rats, chlorocitric acid delayed gastric emptying and changed circulating levels of certain hormones such as gastric inhibitory polypeptide, pancreatic polypeptide, and insulin.[4] A synergistic effect on appetite suppression was observed when cholecystokinin and cholorocitric acid were given simultaneously to rats,[5] further implicating the upper gastrointestinal tract as a key site of anorectic action. The precise mechanism of action of chlorocitric acid is still unclear, however.

The effect of chlorocitric acid on human eating behavior and body weight was examined recently in an inpatient double-blind study.[6] After 7 days of chlorocitric acid (approximately 8 mg/kg/day) treatment, obese men lost more weight or gained less by an average of 3.5 lb (1.6 kg) compared to a 7-day placebo period (p < 0.02; FIGURE 2). During drug treatment, cumulative food intake was reduced 1644 kcal; the average daily food intake for all conditions was 4510 kcal. There were no reliable differences in hunger ratings or gastric emptying. No clinically significant adverse effects were observed. Additional clinical studies of longer duration are needed to confirm the antiobesity effect of chlorocitric acid and to further define whether the anorectic effects observed reliably in rats and dogs can be reproduced in obese subjects.

REDUCTION OF ENERGY STORAGE

One of the metabolic changes observed in genetically obese rodents is increased fatty acid synthesis.[7] Enhanced fatty acid synthesis contributes significantly to lipid accumulation in adipose tissue of rodents fed high carbohydrate diets.[8] Although increased lipogenesis is sometimes associated with obesity in humans, its significance as a contributing factor toward adiposity remains unclear.[7] Inhibition of lipid synthesis as a strategy for reducing body lipid levels has not been evaluated in human obesity, although several experimental compounds have shown antiobesity effects in rodents.[7]

Ro 22-0654 is particularly interesting because it suppresses the biosynthesis and enhances the oxidation of fatty acids. This dual action has been demonstrated in rats *in vitro* in hepatocytes and perfused liver, and *in vivo*.[9–11] Chronic administration of Ro 22-0654 to lean and genetically obese Zucker rats reduced body weight gain and body fat levels selectively; body protein levels were unchanged.[9,10] These antiobesity effects were more pronounced in the genetically obese compared to lean rats. The efficiency of energy utilization was lowered by Ro 22-0654, because the amount of weight gained per gram of food eaten was reduced significantly.

The effects of Ro 22-0654 on diet-induced obese rats are reported here, and FIGURE 3 illustrates the marked reduction in the rate of body weight gained,

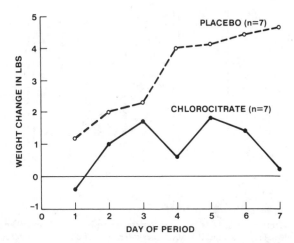

FIGURE 2. Mean daily body weight change of obese subjects given chlorocitrate (300 mg t.i.d.) or placebo one to two hours before meals for 7 days in a double-blind study.[6]

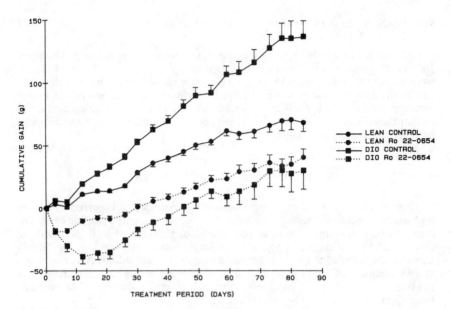

FIGURE 3. Effect of Ro 22-0654 given as a dietary admixture to lean (103 mg/kg/day) and diet-induced obese (105 mg/kg/day) rats on cumulative body weight gain for 84 days.

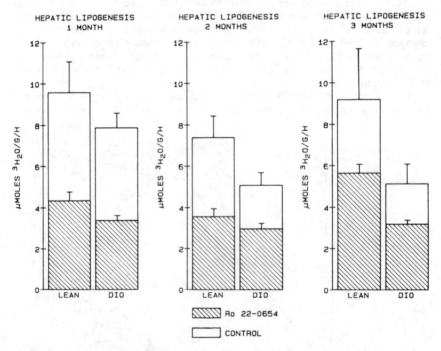

FIGURE 4. Effect of Ro 22-0654 given as a dietary admixture to lean (103 mg/kg/day) and diet-induced obese (105 mg/kg/day) rats on *in vivo* rates of hepatic lipogenesis (μmoles ^3H_2O incorporated into fatty acids per g liver per hr; for method see reference 8) determined after 1, 2, and 3 months of treatment.

272

particularly in the treated diet-induced obese rats. Once dietary obesity was produced in rats, as described previously,[12] Ro 22-0654 (105 mg/kg/day) was administered as a dietary admixture for 86–94 days. The observed reductions in weight gain were caused by decreased body fat levels and not by changes in body protein content (data not shown). Energy utilization was reduced significantly by Ro 22-0654 treatment, since the amount of weight gained per gram of food eaten was decreased (data not shown). This reduced energy utilization could be due to decreased hepatic lipogenesis[9–11] and increased fatty acid oxidation.[10] FIGURE 4

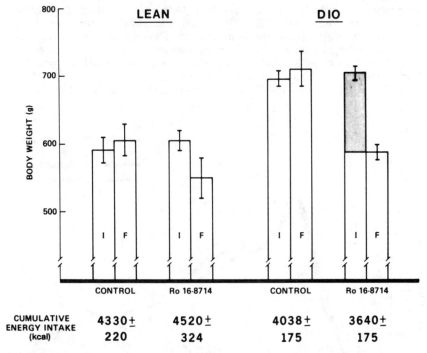

| CUMULATIVE ENERGY INTAKE (kcal) | 4330± 220 | 4520± 324 | 4038± 175 | 3640± 175 |

FIGURE 5. Effect of Ro 16-8714 (13 mg/kg/day), given orally by intubation for 6 weeks to lean and diet-induced obese (DIO) rats, on body weight and cumulative energy intake. I = initial body weight, F = final body weight.

shows that Ro 22-0654 caused a sustained inhibition of hepatic lipogenesis *in vivo* in both lean and diet-induced obese rats, inasmuch as reduced rates were observed in rats after 1, 2, and 3 months of 22-0654 treatment.

ENHANCEMENT OF ENERGY EXPENDITURE

Impaired thermogenesis is an important contributor to excessive lipid deposition in genetic and diet-induced obese rodents.[13] The extent of impaired thermogenic responsiveness in human obesity is less clear. A reduced metabolic rate, however, after even mild weight loss has been shown in many clinical studies. This reduction in metabolic rate makes continual weight loss more difficult to achieve. Thus, the pharmacological stimulation of thermogenesis appears to be a rational target for antiobesity action.

Three new thermogenic agents have been described recently. BRL 26830A, Ro 16-8714, and LY 104119 appear to enhance lipolysis and energy expenditure by a direction stimulation of β-adrenoreceptors.[14-16] Chronic administration of these drugs reduced body weight gain and body fat in genetically obese rodents, and to a lesser extent in their lean littermates.

Potent antiobesity effects were also observed when diet-induced obese rats were treated with Ro 16-8714 (13 mg/kg/day) for 6 weeks (FIGURE 5). Body lipid levels were reduced by more than 50% in both lean and obese treated rats (data not shown). Energy expenditure, as indicated by increased oxygen consumption, was enhanced significantly in both lean and diet-induced obese rats treated with Ro 16-8714 (FIGURE 6). Ro 16-8714 stimulated thermogenesis persisted for at least 6 hours following oral administration of 4.3 mg/kg.

BRL 26830A and Ro 16-8714 are currently undergoing clinical evaluation.

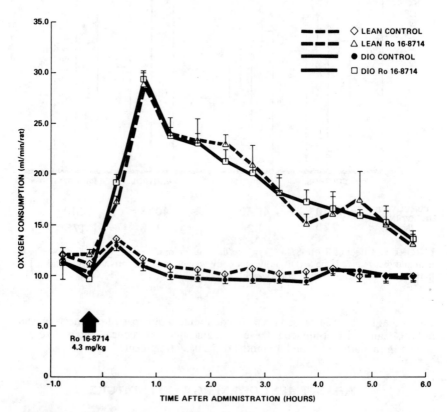

FIGURE 6. Effect of Ro 16-8714 (4.3 mg/kg) on oxygen consumption in lean and diet-induced obese (DIO) rats after 34–37 days of treatment.

Preliminary results reported in abstract form confirm the thermogenic effect of BRL 26830A[17] in obese subjects and Ro 16-8714 in normal weight males.[18] Heart rate, however, was elevated at doses of Ro 16-8714 that increased energy expenditure significantly.[18] Weight loss was reported in one study with BRL 26830A[17] but was not seen in a second trial with refractory obese women.[19]

One important issue with all β-agonists is their selectivity regarding β-adrenoreceptors in cardiac tissue versus tissues responsible for lipolysis (adipose tissue) and thermogenesis. Stimulation of thermogenesis without tachycardia is a major hurdle these drugs must overcome to be used safely. If a safe calorigenic agent able to correct inherent defects in thermogenesis and/or overcome the inevitable lowering of metabolic rate that occurs during caloric restriction could be identified, such a compound could have significant potential for use as an antiobesity agent.

REFERENCES

1. SULLIVAN, A. C. & R. GRUEN. 1985. Mechanisms of appetite modulation by drugs. Fed. Proc. Fed. Am. Soc. Exp. Biol. 44: 139–144.
2. SULLIVAN, A. C., W. DAIRMAN & J. TRISCARI. 1981. (—)-Threochlorocitric acid: A novel anorectic agent. Pharmacol. Biochem. Behav. 15: 303–310.
3. TRISCARI, J. & A. C. SULLIVAN. 1981. Studies on the mechanism of action of a novel anorectic agent, (—)-threo-chlorocitric acid. Pharmacol. Biochem. Behav. 15: 311–318.
4. TRISCARI, J., S. R. BLOOM, T. GAGINELLA, T. O'DORISIO & A. C. SULLIVAN. 1985. Effects of an anorectic agent (Ro 21-7716) on meal stimulated hormone levels. Int. J. Obesity 9: A101.
5. TRISCARI, J., S. HOGAN, D. NELSON, W. DANHO & A. C. SULLIVAN. 1985. Synergistic effect of CCK-8 and Ro 21-7716 on food intake. Fed. Proc. Fed. Am. Soc. Exp. Biol. 44: 1162.
6. HESHKA, S., C. NAUSS-KAROL, A. NYMAN, K. REISEN, H. R. KISSILEFF, K. P. PORIKOS & J. G. KRAL. 1985. Effects of chlorocitrate on body weight in obese men on a metabolic ward. Nutr. Behav. 2: 233–239.
7. SULLIVAN, A. C., J. G. HAMILTON & J. TRISCARI. 1983. Metabolic inhibitors of lipid biosynthesis as anti-obesity agents. In Biochemical Pharmacology of Obesity. P. B. Curtis-Prior, Ed.: 311–337. Elsevier Science Publishers.
8. PEARCE, J. 1983. Fatty acid synthesis in liver and adipose tissue. Proc. Nutr. Soc. 42: 263–271.
9. TRISCARI, J. & A. C. SULLIVAN. 1984. Antiobesity effects of a novel lipid synthesis inhibitor (Ro 22-0654). Life Sci. 34: 2433–2442.
10. TRISCARI, J. & A. C. SULLIVAN. 1984. Anti-obesity activity of a novel lipid synthesis inhibitor. Int. J. Obesity 8(Suppl. 1): 227–239.
11. YAMAMOTO, M., N. FUKUDA, J. TRISCARI, A. C. SULLIVAN & J. A. ONTKO. 1985. Decreased hepatic production of very low density lipoproteins following activation of fatty acid oxidation by Ro 22-0654. J. Lipid Res. 26: 1196–1204.
12. LEVIN, B. E., J. TRISCARI & A. C. SULLIVAN. 1983. Altered sympathetic activity during development of diet-induced obesity in rat. Am. J. Physiol. 244: R347–R355.
13. LEVIN, B. E. 1986. Neurological regulation of body weight. CRC Crit. Rev. Clin. Neurobiol. 2: 1–60.
14. ARCH, J. R. S., A. T. AINSWORTH, R. D. M. ELLIS, V. PIERCY, V. E. THODY, P. L. THURLBY, C. WILSON, S. WILSON & P. YOUNG. 1984. Treatment of obesity with thermogenic β-adrenoceptor agonists: studies on BRL 26830A in rodents. Int. J. Obesity 8(Suppl. 1): 1–11.
15. MEIER, M. K., L. ALIG, M. E. BÜRGI-SAVILLE & M. MÜLLER. 1984. Phenethanolamine derivatives with calorigenic and antidiabetic qualities. Int. J. Obesity 8(Suppl. 1): 215–225.

16. YEN, T. T., M. M. MCKEE & N. B. STAMM. 1984. Thermogenesis and weight control. Int. J. Obesity 8(Suppl. 1): 65–78.
17. ZED, C. A., G. S. HARRIS, P. J. HARRISON & G. H. ROBB. 1985. Antiobesity activity of a novel β-adrenoreceptor agonist (BRL 26830A) in diet-restricted obese subjects. Int. J. Obesity 9: 231.
18. HENNY, C., Y. SCHUTZ, A. BUCKERT, M. MEYLAN, E. JEQUIER & J. P. FELBER. 1986. Thermogenic effect of the new β-adrenoreceptor agonist Ro 16-8714 in healthy male volunteers. Fifth International Congress on Obesity. Jerusalem, Israel.
19. CHAPMAN, B. J., D. FARQUHAR, S. GALLOWAY, G. K. SIMPSON & J. F. MUNRO. 1985. The effects of BRL 26830A, a new β-adrenoceptor agonist in refractory obesity. Int. J. Obesity 9: 230.

Pharmacological Treatments That Affect CNS Activity: Serotonin

C. NATHAN AND Y. ROLLAND

Institut de Recherches Internationales Servier
92202 Neuilly, France

It is only within the last 10 years that the potential contribution of serotonin (5-HT) to the control of food intake and body weight has even been considered. This notion was put forward only after the accumulation of a great deal of evidence pointing to the influence of catecholamines on energy regulation. Research on 5-HT is currently being undertaken within a framework in which the extreme complexity of food intake control and body weight regulation is being increasingly recognized. This, in turn, has contributed to the abandonment of the somewhat simplistic view that obesity is a solitary homogeneous disease for which only a defect of total food intake has to be considered. Today the concept of obesity as a single clinical entity is being replaced by the concept of several forms of obesity, corresponding to different pathological syndromes and involving complex etiologies and mechanisms. Accordingly, when studying energy input, we must consider not only total intake but also the qualitative patterns that could lead to hyperphagia: patterns of eating behavior (binging, snacking, the sizes and distribution of meals); food choice, particularly the consumption of carbohydrates, fats, and protein; environmental events, including stressors and other emotional stimuli; the hedonic value of food (its perceived pleasantness and satisfaction); and eating sensations and the perception of hunger and fullness.

In conjunction with energy input, it is also necessary to consider energy utilization, peripheral metabolism, and their possible modifications in different types of obesity. Such considerations have led to the recognition that body weight regulation is the result of the complex interaction of both central and peripheral mechanisms. These mechanisms involve a variety of neurochemical systems, including catecholamines, serotonin, probably GABA, and a number of neuropeptides (particularly beta-endorphin, a kappa opiate system, CRF, and neuropeptide Y). These may be active in both the central nervous system and peripheral tissues. The treatment of obesity (and of eating disorders) should therefore be considered qualitatively, and should involve a search for selective therapeutic approaches.

Within this framework, the analysis of serotonin systems should lead to a clearer definition of the role of 5-HT, not only in the control of food intake, but also on general metabolism and, ultimately, on body weight regulation. This, in turn, will lead to both a better understanding of the physiology and pathophysiology of energy regulation, and will also bring considerable therapeutic benefit through the search for advanced forms of serotoninergic treatment and the understanding of their mode of action.

277

SEROTONINERGIC COMPOUNDS AND WEIGHT EVOLUTION

The contribution of serotonin to weight regulation is now fully recognized: stimulation or manipulation that enhances serotonin tone can lead to weight loss. On the other hand, destruction or inhibition of serotoninergic pathways in animals leads to obesity (for review, see references 1, 2). Nevertheless, the serotoninergic hypothesis applied to certain forms of human obesity has hardly begun to be explored.

The class of serotoninergic drugs involves various serotonin agonists, which differ markedly in their neurochemical mode of action. They can enhance serotonin release from nerve terminals, and/or inhibit its reuptake, and/or act at the postsynaptic levels by activating different serotoninergic receptors, as shown, for instance, in TABLE 1. This can result in various prominent pharmacological effects, and lead to different clinical applications. Until recently, the majority of serotoninergic drugs were developed mostly for their antidepressant effect, and little attention was directed towards effects on body weight. Among those, the fenfluramines emerge as being the only drugs developed for their dominant effect on body weight. These compounds, first dl-fenfluramine (Ponderal), and more recently dexfenfluramine (Isomeride), act mainly by releasing serotonin (5-HT) from nerve terminals and inhibiting its reuptake.[3] Dexfenfluramine is more active and more specific in its action than the racemic compound because it is devoid of any direct antidopaminergic activity at pharmacological dosage. Its main metabolite, d-norfenfluramine, is also active, though through a slightly different serotoninergic mechanism.[4] On the other hand, l-fenfluramine is not active.

It is well-known that the racemic compound, dl-fenfluramine, decreases weight in animals (for review, see reference 5). The dextroisomer, dexfenfluramine, has been studied more recently.[6–9] In normal weight or obese (cafeteria) rats, chronic administration of the drug (from 12 up to 76 days) decreases weight. Weight loss is dose-dependant, continues throughout the entire treatment period with no tolerance, and is much more marked in obese than in normalweight animals; in long-term studies with obese or old fat animals,[7] weight increases after withdrawal of the drug, but does not seem to regain the level of control groups.

In human obesity, the weight-lowering effect of dl-fenfluramine has long been recognized (for review, see references 5, 10, 11). The usual dosage is between 60 to 120 mg/day. The clinical efficacy of dexfenfluramine in reducing body weight in obese patients has been reported more recently. The product was administered twice daily (15 mg × 2) in four double-blind placebo-controlled studies.[12,13] After three months of treatment, mean weight loss was significantly greater in the dexfenfluramine group (−24.9 ± 2.1% of initial overweight) as compared to the

TABLE 1. Selection Criteria and Weight Loss after Treatment for Three Months with Dexfenfluramine in Four Double-Blind Placebo-Controlled Studies[12]

	Selection Criteria	Weight Loss (kg)
Unselected obesity	no run-in	10.2 ± 0.8
Refractory obesity	no run-in	5.3 ± 0.8
Unselected obesity	one month run-in diet alone	4.9 ± 0.5
Refractory obesity	one month run-in diet alone	2.8 ± 0.6

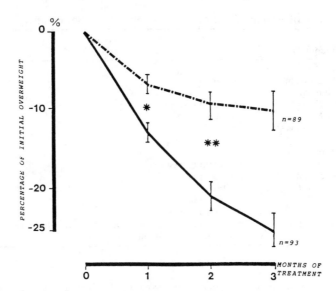

FIGURE 1. Weight loss expressed as percentage of initial overweight:

$$\frac{\text{initial weight} - \text{final weight}}{\text{initial weight} - \text{ideal weight}}$$

Obese patients are treated for three months with dexfenfluramine (solid line) or placebo (dotted line). ** $p < 0.01$; * $p < 0.05$ between the two groups.[12]

placebo group ($-10.8 \pm 2.6\%$) (FIG. 1). Significant weight loss occurred after one month. Interestingly, the rate of weight loss was also significant after two and three months. It is to be noted that the difference in weight loss between placebo and drug-treated patients was similar in each of the four studies, which confirms the efficiency of the drug; on the other hand, the absolute weight loss of the dexfenfluramine-treated groups varied (from 10.2 ± 0.8 kg to 2.8 ± 0.6 kg) and depended on the selection criteria (unselected or refractory obesity, with or without a run-in period on diet alone) (TABLE 2).

The persistent effect of the drug was confirmed in another study,[14] where dexfenfluramine was administered for six months to obese patients; mean weight loss increased over the entire study. The rate of weight loss decreased during the last three months, but mean weight was significantly lower after six months, compared with the weight at the end of the first three-month treatment period (FIG. 2). In these studies, the drug was well-tolerated. Acceptability was better than that usually observed with *dl*-fenfluramine, presumably due to the absence of the specific antidopaminergic activity of *l*-fenfluramine.[15]

These results indicate clearly that at least some serotoninergic compounds can be useful for treating obesity. Fenfluramines are representative of this category of drugs, and experiments with these compounds can be used to exemplify the properties of the class. Not all serotoninergic compounds, however, may produce identical effects, and the degree to which they induce weight loss may vary from one product to another in clinical use. A tendency to lose weight has been ob-

TABLE 2. Mode of Action of Various Compounds on the Serotoninergic System

Compounds	Serotoninergic Activity
tryptophan 5-hydroxytryptophan	precursor
fluoxetine, fluvoxamine, citalopram, ORG 6582, RU 25591, LM 5008, cianopramine, femoxetine, zimelidine	serotonin uptake inhibitor
dl-fenfluramine, dexfenfluramine	serotonin releaser
l-fenfluramine, CM 57373, PK 5078, PK 7059	serotonin uptake inhibitor
MCPP, CM 57493	postsynaptic 5-HT receptor agonist
quipazine MK 212	postsynaptic 5-HT; receptor agonist; serotonin releaser and serotonin-uptake inhibitor

served in depressed patients treated with fluoxetine,[16,17] femoxetine,[18] and fluvoxamine,[19] which contrasts with the weight gain observed with the nonserotoninergic antidepressants. The weight-lowering effect of these antidepressants has been considered. In obese patients, significant weight loss was described with zymeldine,[20] although further development of the drug was stopped, due to toxicological effects. Significant weight loss was also described with fluoxetine in obese and nonobese animals (10 mg/kg, i.p. 10 days),[21,22] and in obese humans. In a recent eight-week study conducted on obese patients randomly allocated to

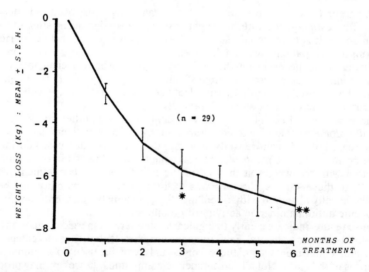

FIGURE 2. Weight loss expressed in kilograms after six months of treatment with dexfenfluramine. * < between 0 and 3 months; ** < between 3 and 6 months.[14]

placebo, benzphetamine, and fluoxetine,[23] a mean dose of 65 mg/day of fluoxetine significantly reduced weight, the effect being comparable to that of benzphetamine.

The mediation of the weight-reducing effect of serotoninergic compounds by way of an enhancement of the serotoninergic tone has been further demonstrated by observations made in drugs and in serotonin antagonists. Serotonin antagonists, which decrease serotonin tone, can lead to an increase in body weight. Chronic administration of methylsergide and cyproheptadine, two serotonin receptor antagonists, has been shown to be capable of inducing weight gain in animals and patients (for review, see references 24–27).

From the results obtained with dexfenfluramine in obesity, it appears evident that not all patients lose weight equally. A basic problem that yet remains to be solved is that of determining the characteristics of those patients who respond to the drug. A first step is to analyze the effect of serotoninergic drugs on the abnormal parameters in obesity liable to be serotonin-dependent.

SEROTONINERGIC COMPOUNDS AND TOTAL CALORIC INTAKE

The serotoninergic system affects to varying degrees a variety of processes involved in weight regulation. The most striking effect is the reduction of total caloric intake when the serotoninergic system is activated. This has been clearly demonstrated by manipulations that enhance the serotoninergic tone. Lesions and depletion of the brain serotoninergic system may also lead to an increase in food intake.[24,28–30]

In animals, a decrease in caloric intake has been shown to occur after a single administration of a large number of serotoninergic compounds. The most extensive works to date concern *dl*-fenfluramine (for review, see references 5, 24, 29, 31–36) and, more recently, dexfenfluramine:[3,6–9,32,37] the dose-inhibiting food intake by 50% in deprived animals ranges from 1 to 3 mg/kg. Many serotoninergic products share the same activity, the effectiveness depending on the compound (TABLE 3), although not all serotoninergic compounds are active in decreasing food intake: LM 5008, for example, is without effect.[35] For clinical purposes, the effect of such a drug must be considered from various aspects: the first is obviously the action on caloric intake in humans, but the second is the existence, at doses that effectively reduce food intake, of other effects that may not be therapeutically beneficial in obesity.

Numerous serotonin-dependent effects may be observed to various degrees with each serotoninergic drug, but the intensity of any effect in particular and the dose at which it appears are usually specific to each compound. Differences in the neurochemical mechanism of action and/or the kinetic characteristics of the drug determine its suitability for different clinical applications. Thus, a therapeutic index ensuring efficiency and safety is especially important for drugs used in obesity or feeding disorders, because until now, they have been considered comfort drugs.

A good illustration of this problem is the serotoninergic compound CM 57 227, which stimulates serotonin release and inhibits its reuptake, and exerts a powerful influence on food intake in animals.[39,44] In humans, at doses of 20 and 40 mg, its effect on caloric intake is clear, but its adverse effects, that is, persistent nausea and vomiting, render it unsuitable for therapeutic application in obesity.[44]

It is well-established that *dl*-fenfluramine decreases caloric intake at meal times in humans.[10,25,38–40] This action is dose-dependent,[41] and the usual dosage administered ranges from 60 to 120 mg/day. The main reported side effects are drowsiness, nausea, diarrhea, dry-mouth, and pollakiuria. Dexfenfluramine is more potent and better tolerated, and this was clearly demonstrated by T. Silverstone in a dose-range study comparing different doses of dl-fenfluramine, d-fenfluramine, and placebo[42] (FIGURES 3 and 4). These results were confirmed by J. Duchier in another study, comparing only the usual daily dosage (60 mg) of dl-fenfluramine with half this dosage of dexfenfluramine (30 mg), and placebo[43] (FIGURES 5 and 6).

Up to now, very few studies have been published on the effects of other serotoninergic drugs on food intake in humans. The serotonin precursor, l-tryptophan (TRP), however, has recently been studied.[25,45] Two or three grams of TRP decrease food intake at meal times by 18–20% compared to placebo, though with decreased mental alertness, dizziness, and drowsiness.[45] The serotoninergic mediation of fenfluramine activity on food intake is further illustrated by its inhibi-

TABLE 3. Mean Active Dose of Various Serotoninergic Compounds on Food Intake in Animals

Compounds	Mean Dose Active on Food Intake (mg/kg)	Reference
tryptophan	50	24, 30
5-HTP	37–50	34, 116
5-HT	125	
fluoxetine	10–15	21, 122
ORG 6582	20	29
RU 25591	20–40	115
LM 5008	no effect	35
dl-fenfluramine	2.5–5	32
dexfenfluramine	1–3	32, 117, 118
l-fenfluramine	>10	32, 117
CM 57373	7.5	44
MCPP	2.5	35
CM 57493	10	44
quipazine	5	35, 36, 117
MK 212	1.5–3	119, 120, 121

tion by serotonin antagonists, methergoline or methylsergide, or by brain serotonin depletion (for review, see reference 15).

Proof of the inverse effect, namely an increase of food intake by serotoninergic antagonists, is less conclusive. One possible explanation is that they are not purely serotonin antagonists, but possess other aminergic properties that could interfere with serotonin-linked action on food intake. Nevertheless, cyproheptadine and pizotifen have been reported to increase appetite and food intake in humans.[24,25,27,30,46] Methylsergide, a 5-HT antagonist used in the prophylaxis of migraine, increases food intake in animals[24,47,48] and has on rare occasions been found to stimulate appetite in humans.[24,30] Methergoline has also been reported to increase food intake in humans, whereas hunger was not affected.[25]

The persistence of a decreased effect on food intake after chronic administration of serotoninergic drugs in obese humans remains to be determined. From animal studies, it appears that fenfluramine and dexfenfluramine have no persis-

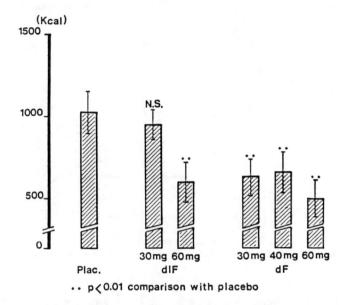

FIGURE 3. Total caloric intake at meal time after a single administration of different doses of *dl*-fenfluramine (dlF) and dexfenfluramine (dF) compared to placebo. Double-blind crossover study in latin-square design.[42]

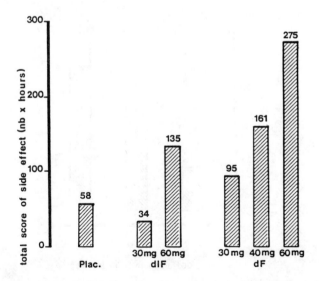

FIGURE 4. Total score of side effects (number × duration) after a single administration of different doses of *dl*-fenfluramine (dlF) and dexfenfluramine (dF) compared to placebo. Double-blind crossover study in latin-square design.[42]

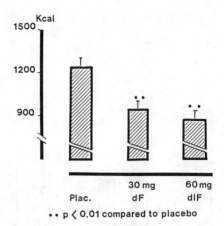

FIGURE 5. Total caloric intake at meal time after two-day administration of 30 mg of dexfenfluramine (dF), 60 mg of dl-fenfluramine (dlF) and placebo. Double-blind crossover study.[43]

tent effect on food intake after chronic administration in normal animals,[4–8] whereas weight loss clearly persists. This tolerance is less obvious for obese cafeteria-treated animals,[8] which suggests that the effect of fenfluramine compounds on food intake could be dependent upon the basal status of weight and feeding patterns, which could in turn reflect different states of equilibrium regarding monoamine and neuropeptide tone. Tolerance to the anorectic effect of the

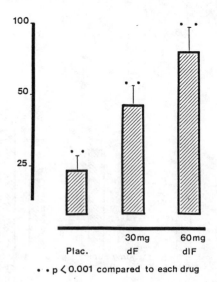

FIGURE 6. Total score of side effect (number × duration × intensity) after two-day administration of 30 mg of dexfenfluramine (dF), 60 mg of dl-fenfluramine (dlF) and placebo. Double-blind crossover study.[43]

fenfluramines has been widely discussed and depends upon the feeding regime employed and the mode of administration of the drug. This has led to the search for other activities that could explain the effect on weight evolution.

SEROTONINERGIC COMPOUNDS AND EATING BEHAVIOR

The activation of the serotoninergic pathway is not the only way of inhibiting food intake, and the effects of modulation of the catecholaminergic system have been recognized for a number of years. Interestingly, the way in which these two systems affect the behavioral aspect of global food intake seems to be different: the serotoninergic system is involved in satiation, and its stimulation decreases meal size and duration (the opposite effect is observed after an alpha-adrenergic stimulation); conversely, activation of the dopaminergic system decreases meal frequency.[24,29,30,33,49,50]

The behavioral aspect of feeding inhibition with serotoninergic drugs thus differs almost entirely from that obtained with catecholaminergic compounds. Studies conducted with fenfluramine on the structure of feeding behavior indicate that the drug does not lead to a general inhibition of eating, nor does it introduce abnormal patterns of behavior capable of interfering with the natural expression of eating. The drug appears to produce a significant readjustment in eating pattern by diminishing meal size, slowing down the rate of eating, and producing a negligible effect on meal initiation.[30] A similar effect on the pattern of eating has been observed with tryptophan, fluoxetine, and Org 6582.[29]

These findings are commonly referred to as the satieting effect of these drugs and may correlate to the concept of an integrative hypothalamic satiety structure in the ventromedial hypothalamus (VMH), more specifically, the paraventricular and medial hypothalamus. This structure stops the feeding process, unlike the lateral area, which initiates feeding. This concept has recently been reviewed by Grossman.[51] The neurotransmitters involved in this VMH structure are serotonin, which induces satiety, and the alpha-adrenergic system, which is an inhibitor.[52] Of particular interest is the fact that this area seems to integrate hedonic sensory inputs, inasmuch as VMH-lesioned rats are hyperreactive to hedonic factors.[53–56]) This seems to indicate that hedonic as well as nutritive considerations need to be taken into account with reference to satiety. This hypothesis correlates well with the observed more pronounced effect of dexfenfluramine on food intake in rats fed with palatable food (cafeteria) as opposed to chow diet.[8]

The fact that the reduction of food intake with serotoninergic agents implies an enhancement of the satiety mechanism (reduced meal size, slower rate of eating), through increased resistance to hedonic cues, may have clinical implications because the inability of some obese patients to resist the temptation of palatable food is well recognized. In humans, such a satiating effect, associated with decreased hedonic pressure, has been demonstrated for *dl*-dexfenfluramine and dexfenfluramine. Blundell has shown that *dl*-fenfluramine reduces meal size and slows down the rate of eating in normal volunteers.[57] Wooley[58,59] has shown that the product reduces appetite for palatable food after a caloric load. In these two experiments, the effect of amphetamine was different.

More recently, Blundell[60] analyzed the effect of dexfenfluramine, using a sophisticated paradigm. Human volunteers were asked to select highly preferred foods, carbohydrate (CHO) or protein, from a check list. They were given a standard meal and received dexfenfluramine or placebo in random order. Absorption of the standard meal reduced the hedonic perception of preferred food, and

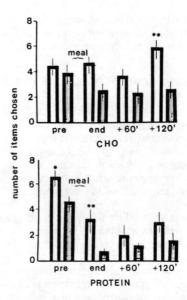

FIGURE 7. Effect of dexfenfluramine (shaded columns) and placebo (solid columns) on the selection of highly preferred food items from a checklist before and after a standard meal. Comparison between the two treatments, * $p < 0.05$; ** $p < 0.001$.[60]

dexfenfluramine administration induced a further reduction of the preference for both CHO and protein, its effect being particularly pronounced after the meal. In the same study, the number and the size of eating episodes, that is, meals and snacks, were recorded during four days, and dexfenfluramine administration was shown to decrease the number of midsize eating episodes, that is, snacks (FIG-

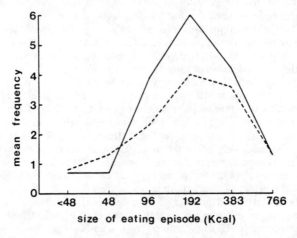

FIGURE 8. Effect of dexfenfluramine (broken line) and placebo (solid line) on the number of eating episodes of different size during three days of administration.[60]

URES 7 and 8). From these data, it clearly appears that dexfenfluramine can decrease caloric intake by increasing satiety, decrease the hedonic pressure for food, and thereby decrease the caloric content of the meal and the amount of interprandial eating episodes.

SEROTONINERGIC COMPOUNDS AND MACRONUTRIENT SELECTION

Recent works on the regulation of food intake have provided data demonstrating that, in addition to total energy regulation, the intake of macronutrients is independently regulated. Musten et al.[61] showed that rats regulate their protein intake independently of total energy consumption, and Wurtman et al.[62] showed that CHO intake is also controlled independently. As demonstrated elsewhere by Wurtman in another chapter, serotonin plays a large part in this regulation, by way of insulin secretion, which enhances the plasma ratio of tryptophan to neutral amino acids and allows tryptophan to enter the brain and increase serotonin synthesis. Enhancement of serotonin activity reduces subsequent CHO intake, while preserving normal protein intake.[63] This is true not only for meal to meal regulation, but also for long-term regulation, as demonstrated by the chronic increase of CHO intake and suppression of protein intake that occurs when serotoninergic transmission is impaired, for example, after depletion of brain 5-HT.[64] This regulating effect of 5-HT on CHO is independent of the sweetness of food, as demonstrated by Wurtman and Wurtman.[65]

Some recent works have focused on the possibility in humans of such a selective abnormality in food choice with enhancement of carbohydrate intake. This was achieved by using food containing specific macronutrients and simultaneously analyzing the total energy intake together with the ratio and total amounts of CHO, protein, and fat intake, respectively. Such patients were described by Wurtman and Wurtman[66] as carbohydrate cravers. In the main, such patients are obese.[67] Interestingly, their craving for carbohydrates concerns principally snacks and appears at particular times of the day. Yet they do not manifest totally uncontrolled carbohydrate consumption, as in binges, and they differ from bulimic patients. These behavioral disturbances suggest a deficiency in central serotoninergic transmission, this deficiency possibly originating from a central and/or a peripheral defect in the regulatory loop. For instance, insulin deficiency and insulin resistance, which are often increased by a commonly used low CHO diet, may decrease the $\frac{TRP}{Neutral\ AA}$ plasma ratio. A particularly low ratio has, in fact, been observed in certain obese diabetic and nondiabetic patients.[62,68] This specific increase of CHO intake has also been observed in women with premenstrual syndrome,[69-71] in anxiety,[72] and in stress situations.[73] More recently, Rosenthal has described an atypical type of depression, called the seasonal affective disorder, which occurs in autumn and winter;[74] two-thirds of these patients complain of carbohydrate craving as one of the earliest symptoms,[75] usually accompanied by weight increase. Wurtman[76] has shown that dl-fenfluramine, tryptophan, and fluoxetine selectively reduce high carbohydrate diet intake in rats. The effect was most marked with dexfenfluramine, which was found to be twice as potent as the racemic compound, whereas l-fenfluramine produced no effect.[77,78] Quipazine[50] and MK 212[78] would also seem to share the same effect. On the other hand, and as further evidence for the serotoninergic CHO preference hypothesis, Leibowitz has found that antiserotoninergic drugs such as cyproheptadine enhance carbohydrate and fat intake.[50] Other neurochemical systems are obviously involved in the control of macronutrient selection and/or preference: it has been shown, for example, that norepinephrine selectively increases CHO consumption.[50] Whereas amphetamines selectively decrease protein and/or fat consumption,[34,79] lithium and chlorimipramine increase CHO consumption.[79]

Studies were undertaken in humans to determine if dexfenfluramine might selectively affect the disturbance in eating behavior manifested by carbohydrate-craving obese patients.[80] Twenty such patients, whose craving for carbohydrates in the form of snacks was established at the beginning of the study, were randomly allocated to dexfenfluramine (15 mg p.o. twice daily) or placebo, for two eight-day

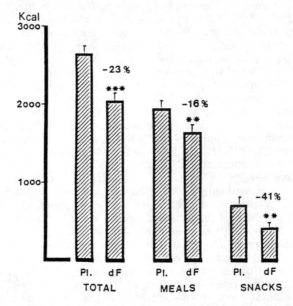

FIGURE 9. Effect of dexfenfluramine (dF) compared with placebo (Pl) on daily caloric intake in obese carbohydrate cravers. Comparison between the two treatments, *** p < 0.0001; ** p < 0.001.[80]

periods, in a double-blind, cross-over design. They were given self-selected meals and had free access to a vending machine for snacks. The caloric and macronutrient content of foods were previously assessed in a way that made possible the analysis of total food intake, macronutrient selection, and feeding pattern. The results revealed that, after eight days of treatment, dexfenfluramine selectively decreases the abnormal pattern characterized by high CHO snacks, with no significant effect on protein consumption. The resultant drug effect was twice as great on the calories absorbed as snacks, as compared to the calories absorbed at meal times (FIGURES 9–11).

Interestingly, this effect was observed after subchronic treatment. In a more recent study,[81] where medium-term (three months) treatment with d-fenfluramine was pursued and the results compared to those for placebo, the effect was con-

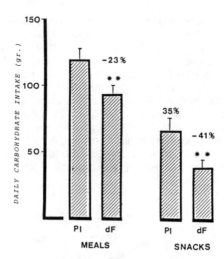

FIGURE 10. Effect of dexfenfluramine (dF) compared to placebo (Pl) on daily carbohydrate intake in obese carbohydrate cravers. Comparison between the two treatments, ** p < 0.001.[80]

firmed, and a significant weight loss was achieved in those carbohydrate-craving obese patients, although patients had been told not to modify their usual diet.

SEROTONINERGIC COMPOUNDS AND STRESS-INDUCED AND COMPULSIVE EATING

The important role of emotional factors in overeating has long been recognized, and stress associated with traumatic emotional events has been held re-

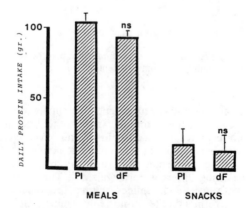

FIGURE 11. Effect of dexfenfluramine (dF) compared to placebo (Pl) on daily protein intake in obese carbohydrate cravers. Comparison between the two treatments; ns, not significant.[80]

sponsible for certain cases of obesity.[82–84] Overeating is generally recognized as alleviating the distress, dysphoric state, anxiety, or depressive reaction caused by these events. Overeating and weight gain may appear after dramatic events (*e.g.*, death of a parent) but also occur as a result of everyday frustrating experiences. The eating pattern of such subjects is often characterized by compulsive eating. Stress and emotional disturbance have been responsible for such well-known eating disorders as the night-eating syndrome[85] and bulimia.[86] From these data, the potential impact of serotoninergic compounds for treating stress-induced obesity or eating disorders in humans must be considered.

In animals, stress-induced eating has also been well described. An experimental model, based on the tail-pinch technique was developed by Antelman and coworkers,[87] in order to mimic stress-induced eating. With this technique, consid-

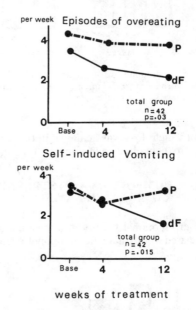

FIGURE 12. Effect of dexfenfluramine (dF) compared to placebo (Pl) on episodes of overeating and self-induced vomiting in bulimic patients.[98]

erable weight gain can be observed after repeated stimulation over a long period of time. It is now recognized that serotonin, among other brain neurotransmitters, is important in inhibiting stress-induced eating.[88] Tail-pinch overeating is reduced by manipulations that enhance brain serotoninergic activity.[89]

The effect of various serotoninergic drugs on stress-induced eating in animals was analyzed using different paradigms.[90–93] The most extensive studies were performed with the fenfluramines, either the racemic compound (*dl*-fenfluramine), its active metabolite (*dl*-norfenfluramine), and more recently the dextroisomer, dexfenfluramine. It was demonstrated that these compounds were able to abolish or markedly decrease stress-induced overeating, triggered by tail pinching.[92] By contrast, nonserotoninergic drugs such as amphetamine, methyl-

phenidate, and mazindol at equianorectic doses were unable to inhibit this hyperphagia.[91] The degree of inhibition depended on the severity of the stress, and was
more marked in tail-pinching than in 2-deoxyglucose- (2 DG) induced hyperphagia: 2 DG is considered to be a very strong metabolic stressor[94] and is, inciden-
tally, less representative of mild environmental stress as experienced in everyday
life. Other serotoninergic compounds were also tested: quipazine, fluoxetine, and
MK 212[37,90,94] were able to reduce stress-induced overeating but differed in the
intensity of their effect.

The clinical implication of these results as regards such drugs as dexfenfluramine is obvious, and it would seem that this compound must necessarily be
more effective than other nonserotoninergic anorectic drugs in those cases of
human overeating and obesity where stress and emotional factors play a major
part. Observations from Wurtman and Wurtman suggest that CHO cravers must
also, to some extent, belong to this category.[80] The relationship between stress,
compulsive eating behavior, and food preference remains to be investigated more
fully.

In bulimia, a possible abnormality of the serotoninergic system, that is, decreased serotonin turnover, has been suggested.[95] In two separate double-blind
placebo-controlled studies, Russell[96] and Blonin[97] have shown the effectiveness of
dl-fenfluramine in alleviating bulimic symptoms. In a recent placebo-controlled
study using dexfenfluramine at a daily dose of 30 mg, Russell demonstrated that
the product reduces the episodes of overeating and vomiting[98] (FIG. 12). The same
tendency was reported by Freeman with fluoxetine in an open trial.[99]

SEROTONINERGIC COMPOUNDS AND METABOLIC ACTIVITY

That these drugs affect food intake does not rule out the possibility of their
acting on other components of weight regulation. In body-weight regulation, eating behavior and peripheral metabolism are closely interrelated. In most cases of
obesity, abnormal glucose tolerance and insulin sensitivity, as well as abnormal
lipid metabolism, are frequent and suggest impaired fuel-utilization, which could
lead to impaired energy expenditure. This notion of impairment of basal energy
expenditure, however, in obese patients is not generally accepted. This is perhaps
due to the difficulty of setting up precisely defined, valid, and reliable basic
parameters and a precise classification of obese patients (e.g., gynoid and android; hypertrophic and hyperplastic) who possibly present different metabolic
abnormalities. Impairment of diet-induced thermogenesis, especially glucose-induced thermogenesis, appears to exist in some obese patients,[100] and an attempt
to define a subgroup of obesity with abnormal glucose-induced thermogenesis has
been made.[101] A relationship has recently been suggested between impaired insulin sensitivity and abnormal glucose-induced thermogenesis.[101] In this context, it
is interesting to consider the metabolic activities observed with the fenfluramines.
Improvements in insulin sensitivity and glucose tolerance in obese diabetics after
chronic treatment with dl-fenfluramine have been reported, even in the absence of
any weight loss.[102–104] Improvement in insulin sensitivity as well as hypolipidemic
actions have also been shown in various in vivo and in vitro animal experiments
with dl-fenfluramine.[104–110] More recently, Levitsky described an enhancement of
the thermogenic effect of a gastric glucose load in fenfluramine-treated rats. No
such effect was observed after fat intake or in fasted animals.[110] This effect of
fenfluramine in potentiating diet-induced thermogenesis was dose-dependent and

significantly greater in diabetic animals when compared with controls.[111] With regard to thermogenesis, G. Bray's group has recently described an increased binding of guanosine diphosphate to brown adipose tissue mitochondria in fenfluramine-treated rats.[112] This same effect on diet-induced thermogenesis has recently been confirmed by Even for dexfenfluramine, and a connection has been suggested between this and the effect on food intake.[113] The same group also described increased thermogenesis in rats during physical activity after treatment with dexfenfluramine.[114] These effects could be partly responsible for the weight-lowering effect of the drugs.

An interesting hypothesis concerning the mechanism underlying these metabolic activities involves the attenuated effect of stress hormones. In a recent publication, Brindley[6] has shown that chronic treatment with dexfenfluramine reduces the stress reaction after an acute load of fructose, as measured by a plasmatic corticosterone level; simultaneously, the concentration of fatty acids and of glycerol also decreased. In another experiment, chronic treatment with dexfenfluramine also decreased the stress response to urethane injection, as measured by the blood adrenaline concentration. This effect contrasts with the results obtained after d-amphetamine treatment.[6]

These findings should be examined in the light of 1) several reports on the links between corticosteroids and obesity, implying a relationship between corticosteroids and clinical diseases and the causative role of corticosteroids in experimental, genetic, or cafeteria-induced animal obesities (for review, see reference 115); and 2) the action of serotoninergic compounds on stress-induced feeding behavior and obesity, already discussed in this paper.

DISCUSSION AND CONCLUSION

From the different serotoninergic drugs available for clinical use, the fenfluramines emerge as the only ones that have been widely studied for their activity in obesity. The good clinical acceptability of dexfenfluramine has made possible an extensive series of investigations that highlight its specific activity as a serotoninergic drug. The weight-lowering effect of this compound has been shown to be associated with a reduction in caloric intake at meal times, together with specific modifications of eating behavior and eating pattern. These involve a greater satiating effect of food, a reduced hedonic perception of highly preferred nutrients, a decreased intake in the number of abnormally high carbohydrate-rich snacks, and a diminution in emotional or stress-induced eating. The changes evoked in fuel utilization include possible modifications of insulin secretion and activity, stress-hormone secretion, and diet-induced thermogenesis.

The particular interest represented in studying the selective action of dexfenfluramine with regard to the various aspects of weight regulation is the possibility it holds forth of determining a specific clinical profile of activity, which will, we hope, lead to a high level of clinical efficacy in the case of selected obese patients possessing the appropriate characteristics. From the results obtained with dexfenfluramine, it may be advanced that such patients display an overresponsiveness to iterative stimuli (hedonic and emotional cues), and it is tempting to suggest that in the presence of a state of imbalance, dexfenfluramine acts mainly as a modulator of these hyperstimulated states. It is obvious that further studies are needed in order to verify such a hypothesis and, equally, to spotlight other important questions that have not been discussed in this paper, such as 1) the extent of the effect of dexfenfluramine on the gastrointestinal system and the role of the latter in the mechanism of its action; 2) the confirmation of the metabolic activity of dexfenfluramine in human obesity and the interest it represents in obesity associated with metabolic disorders such as diabetes; 3) the general concept of the existence of an effect that will "in fine" lower a body weight set point; and 4) the prospect of long-term drug therapy in certain types of obesity.

In conclusion, the action of serotoninergic drugs in treating obesity underlines the importance of the as yet unresolved problem, consisting of the classification of the different subtypes of obesity on the basis of various parameters, such as eating behavior, macronutrient selection, emotional state, metabolic and hormonal equilibrium, and fat cell distribution.

ACKNOWLEDGMENTS

We would like to express our sincere thanks to Professors B. Guy-Grand, J. Blundell, and S. Nicolaidis for their respective contributions over the years to the elaboration of these concepts, and to the first two of the above-mentioned authorities for their invaluable help in preparing this paper.

REFERENCES

1. STUNKARD, A. J., Ed. 1980. Obesity. W. B. Saunders Company. Philadelphia.
2. NICOLAIDIS, S. Ed. Appetite 1986. Academic Press. London.
3. GARATTINI, S., S. CACCIA, T. MENNINI, R. SAMANIN, S. CONSOLO & H. LADUNSKI. 1979. Curr. Med. Res. Opin. 6(1): 15–27.
4. GARATTINI, S. & R. SAMANIN. 1981. S. Garattini & R. Samanin, Eds. Raven Press. New York.
5. ROWLAND, N. 1986. Prog. Neurobiol. In press.
6. BRINDLEY, D. N., J. SAXTON, H. SHAHIDULLAH, M. ARMSTRONG & E. H. MANGIAPANE. 1985. In Metabolic Complications of Human Obesities. J. Vague, P. Bjorntorp, B. Guy-Grand, M. Rebuffe-Scribe & P. Vague, Eds.: 207–217. Excerpta Medica. Amsterdam.
7. FANTINO, M. & F. FAION. 1985. In Metabolic Complications of Human Obesities. J. Vague, P. Bjorntorp, B. Guy-Grand, M. Rebuffe-Scribe & P. Vague, Eds.: 185–198. Excerpta Medica. Amsterdam.
8. BLUNDELL, J. E. & A. J. HILL. 1985. In Metabolic Complications of Human Obesities. J. Vague, P. Bjorntorp, B. Guy-Grand, M. Rebuffe-Scribe & P. Vague, Eds.: 199–206. Excerpta Medica. Amsterdam.
9. FANTINO, M., F. FAION & Y. ROLLAND. 1986. Appetite 7: 115–126.
10. SILVERSTONE, T., Ed. 1982. Drugs and Appetite. T. Silverstone, Ed.: 81–92. Academic Press. London.
11. NOBLE, R. E. 1979. Curr. Med. Res. Opin. 6(1): 169–179.
12. NATHAN, C. 1985. In Metabolic Complications of Human Obesities. J. Vague, P. Bjorntorp, B. Guy-Grand, M. Rebuffe-Scribe & P. Vague, Eds.: 229–234. Excerpta Medica. Amsterdam.
13. FINER, N., D. CRADDOCK, R. LAVIELLE & N. KEEN. 1985. Curr. Ther. Res. Clin. Exp. 38(6): 847–854.
14. FINER, N., D. CRADDOCK, R. LAVIELLE & H. KEEN. 1986. Submitted to Int. J. Obesity.
15. GARRATINI S., T. MENNINI, C. BENDOTTI, R. INVERNIZZI & R. SAMANIN. 1986. Appetite 7: 15–38.
16. FEIGHNER, J. P. 1985. J. Clin. Psychiatry 46: 369–372.
17. BREMNER, J. D. 1984. J. Clin. Psychiatry 45: 414–419.

18. SHEDEGAARD, J., P. CHRISTIANSEN & B. SKRUMSAGER. 1981. Int. J. Obesity **5:** 377.
19. GUY, W., W. H. WILSON, T. A. BAN, D. L. KING, G. MANOV & O. K. FJETLAND. 1984. Psychopharmacol. Bull. **20**(1): 73–78.
20. SIMPSON, R. J., D. J. LAWTON, M. H. WATT & B. TIPDLAY. 1981. Br. J. Clin. Pharmacol. **11:** 96–98.
21. WONG, D. T. & T. T. YEN. 1985. Fed. Proc. Fed. Am. Soc. Exp. Biol. **44:** 1162.
22. REID, L. R., P. G. THRELKELD & D. T. WONG. 1984. Pharmacologist **26:** 184.
23. FERGUSON, J. M. 1986. *In* Disorders in Eating Behaviour. Advances in the Biosciences. Pergamon Press. Oxford. In press.
24. BLUNDELL, J. E. 1977. Int. J. Obesity **1**(1): 15–42.
25. SILVERSTONE, T. & E. GOODALL. 1986. Appetite **7:** 85–97.
26. SILVERSTONE, T. & E. GOODALL. 1986. *In* Pharmacology of Eating Disorders. Carruba M. O. & J. E. Blundell, Eds.: 141–150. Raven Press. New York.
27. SILVERSTONE, T. & D. SCHUYLER. 1975. Psychopharmacologia **40:** 335–340.
28. HOEBEL, B. G. 1976. *In* Brain—stimulated reward. A. Wauquier, Ed.: 335–372. Elsevier. Amsterdam.
29. BLUNDELL, J. E. & J. C. LATHAM. 1978. *In* Central Mechanisms of Anorectic Drugs. S. Garattini & R. Samanin, Eds.: 83–109. Raven-Press. New York.
30. BLUNDELL, J. E. 1984. Neuropharmacology **23**(12 B): 1537–1551.
31. PINDER, R. M., R. N. BROGDEN, P. R. SAWYER, T. M. SPEIGHT & G. S. AVERY. 1975. Drugs **10:** 241–323.
32. LE DOUAREC, J. C., H. SCHMITT & M. LAUBIE. 1966. Arch. Int. Pharmacoclin. **161**(1): 206–232.
33. BLUNDELL, J. E. & M. B. LESHEM. 1975. *In* Recent Advances in Obesity Research. A. Howard, Ed.: 368–371. Newman. London.
34. BLUNDELL, J. E. & R. A. MCARTHUR. 1979. Br. J. Pharmacol. **67:** 436–438.
35. SAMANIN, R., T. MENNINI & S. GARRATINI. 1980. Prog. Neuro-psychopharmacol. Biol. Psychiat. **4:** 363–369.
36. GARATTINI, S. & R. SAMANIN, Eds. 1978. Central Mechanism of Anorectic Drugs. Raven Press. New York.
37. ROWLAND, N. E. & J. CARLTON. 1986. *In* Disorders in Eating Behaviour, Advances in the Biosciences. Pergamon Press. Oxford. In press.
38. SILVERSTONE, T. 1981. Int. J. Obesity **5**(1): 88.
39. BLUNDELL, J. E. 1980. *In* Obesity. A. J. Stunkard, Ed.: 182–207. W. B. Saunders Company. Philadelphia.
40. SILVERSTONE, T. 1981. *In* Anorectic Agents. S. Garratini & R. Samanin, Eds.: 211–222. Raven Press. New York.
41. KIRIAKIDES, M. & T. SILVERSTONE. 1979. Curr. Med. Res. Opin. **6**(1): 180–187.
42. SILVERSTONE, T. 1986. *In* Body Weight Control. A. E. Bender & L. J. Brooks, Eds. Churchill Livingstone. London. In press.
43. DUCHIER, J. Personal communication.
44. RONCUCCI, R., G. F. MIRANDA & M. VERRY. 1985. *In* Novel Approaches and Drugs for Obesity. A. C. Sullivan & S. Garattini, Eds.: 103–118. J. Libbey and Cie., New York.
45. HROBOTICKY, N., L. A. LEITER & G. H. ANDERSON. 1985. Nutr. Res. **5:** 595–607.
46. BERGEN, S. S. 1964. Am. J. Dis. Child. **108:** 270–273.
47. BAXTER, M. G., A. A. MILLER & F. E. SOROKO. 1970. Br. J. Pharmacol. **39:** 229–230.
48. BLUNDELL, J. E. & M. B. LESHEM. 1975. J. Pharm. Pharmacol. **27**(1): 31–37.
49. HOEBEL, B. G. 1971. Ann. Rev. Physiol. **33:** 533–568.
50. LEIBOWITZ, S. & G. SHOR-POSNER. 1986. Appetite **7:** 1–14.
51. GROSSMAN, S. P. 1984. *In* Eating and its Disorders. A. J. Stunkard & E. Stellar, Eds.: 5–13. Raven Press. New York.
52. HOEBEL, B. G. 1984. Eating and its Disorders. A. J. Stunkard & E. Stellar, Eds.: 220–224. Raven Press. New York.
53. GROSSMAN, S. P. 1975. Psychol Rev. **82:** 200–224.
54. GROSSMAN, S. P. 1979. Ann. Rev. Psychol. **30:** 209–242.
55. KING, B. M. 1980. Neurosci. Biobehav. Rev. **4**(2): 151–160.
56. SCLAFANI, A. 1978. Neurosci. Biobehav. Rev. **2:** 339–355.

57. BLUNDELL, J. E., C. LATHAM. E. MONIZ, R. MCARTHUR & P. ROGERS. 1979. Curr. Med. Res. Opin. 6(1): 34–54.
58. WOOLEY, O. W., S. C. WOOLEY, B. S. WILLIAMS & C. NURRE. 1977. Int. J. Obesity 1(3): 293–300.
59. WOOLEY, O. W., S. C. WOOLEY & J. C. LEE. 1979. Curr. Med. Res. Opin. 6(1): 83–90.
60. HILL, A. J. & J. BLUNDELL. 1986. In Disorders in Eating Behaviour. Advances in the Biosciences. Pergamon Press. Oxford. In press.
61. MUSTEN, B., D. PEACE & G. H. ANDERSON. 1974. J. Nutr. 194: 563–572.
62. WURTMAN, R. J. & J. J. WURTMAN. 1984. Eating and its Disorders. A. J. Stunkard & E. Stellar, Eds.: 77–86. Raven Press. New York.
63. ANDERSON, G. H., E. T. S. LI & N. T. GLANVILLE. 1984. Brain Res. Bull. 12: 167–173.
64. ASHLEY, D. V. M., D. U. COSCINA & G. H. ANDERSON. 1979. Life Sci. 24: 973–984.
65. WURTMAN, J. J. & R. J. WURTMAN. 1979. Curr. Med. Res. Opin. 6(Suppl. 1): 28–33.
66. WURTMAN, J. J., R. J. WURTMAN, J. H. GROWDON, P. HENRY, A. LIPSCOMB & S. H. ZEISEL. 1981. Int. J. Eating Disorders 1: 2–15.
67. WURTMAN, J. J. & R. J. WURTMAN. 1982/83. J. Psychiatr. Res. 17(2): 213–221.
68. ASHLEY, D. V. M., M. O. FLEURY, A. GOLAY, E. MAEDER & P. D. LEATHWOOD. 1985. Am. J. Clin. Nutr. 42: 1240–1245.
69. SMITH, S. & C. SAUNDERS. 1969. Psychosom. Med. 31: 281–287.
70. DALVIT & M. C. PHILLIPS. 1983. Physiol. Behav. 31: 209–212.
71. HROBOTICKY, N., L. A. LEITER & G. H. ANDERSON. 1985. Int. J. Obesity 9: 145.
72. CRADDOCK, D. 1973. In Obesity and its Management. A. E. Bender & L. J. Brookes, Eds.: 2nd edition. 16–52. Churchill Livingstone. Edinburgh.
73. LEWIS, B. E. 1980. A multiple predictor approach to body weight regulation. Ph.D. Thesis, Clark University. Worcester, MA.
74. ROSENTHAL, N. H. & M. H. HEFFERNAN. 1985. In Nutrition and the Brain. R. J. Wurtman & J. J. Wurtman, Eds.: 7: 139–166. Raven Press. New York.
75. ROSENTHAL, N. E., D. A. SACK, S. P. JAMES, B. L. PARRY, W. B. MENDELSON, L. TAMARKIN & T. A. WEHR. 1984. Presented at the New York Academy of Sciences, November 1984.
76. WURTMAN, J. J. & R. J. WURTMAN. 1979b. Life Sci. 24: 895–904.
77. HIRSCH, J. A., S. GOLDBERG & R. J. WURTMAN. 1982. J. Pharm. Pharmacol. 34(1): 18–21.
78. MOSES, P. L. & R. J. WURTMAN. 1984. Life Sci. 35: 1297–1300.
79. KANAREK, R. B., L. HO & R. G. MEADE. 1981. Pharmacol. Biochem. Behav. 14: 539–542.
80. WURTMAN, J. J., R. J. WURTMAN, S. MARK, R. TSAY, W. GILBERT & J. GROWDON. 1985. Int. J. Eating Disorders 4(1): 89–99.
81. WURTMAN, S. 1986. In Body Weight Control. A. E. Bender & L. J. Brookes, Eds. Churchill Livingstone, London. In press.
82. BRUCH, E. 1973. In Eating Disorders. Basic Books. New York.
83. HAMBURGER, W. W. 1951. Med. Clin. North Am. 35: 483.
84. STUNKARD, A. J., W. I. GRACE & H. G. WOLFF. 1955. Am. J. Med. 19: 78–86.
85. STUNKARD, A. J. 1967. In Comprehensive Text Book of Psychiatry. 2nd edition. M. Freedman, L. Kaplan & J. Sadock, Eds.: 2: 1648–1655. Williams & Wilkins. Baltimore.
86. PYLE, R. L., J. E. MITCHELL & E. D. ECKERT. 1981. J. Clin. Psychiatry 42: 60–64.
87. ANTELMAN, S. M., H. SZECHTMAN, P. CHIN & A. E. FISHER. 1975. Brain Res. 99: 319.
88. MORLEY, J. E., A. S. LEVINE & N. E. ROWLAND. 1983. Life Sci. 32: 2169–2182.
89. ANTELMAN, S. M. & A. R. CAGGIULA. 1977. In Animal Models in Psychiatry and Neurology. p. 227. Pergamon Press. New York.
90. ANTELMAN, S. M., N. ROWLAND & D. KOCAN. 1981. Anorectic Agents: Mechanisms of Action and Tolerance. S. Garattini & R. Samanin, Eds.: 45–63. Raven Press. New York.
91. ANTELMAN, S. M., A. R. CAGGIULA, A. J. EICHLER & R. R. LUCIK. 1979. Curr. Med. Res. Opin. 6: 73–82.

92. ROWLAND, N., S. M. ANTELMAN & D. KOCAN. 1982. Eur. J. Pharmacol. 81: 57–77.
93. CARRUBA, M. O., S. RICCIARDI, P. SPANO & P. MANTEGAZZA. 1985. Life Sci. 36: 1739–1749.
94. ANTELMAN, N. E., S. M. ROWLAND & T. J. BARTNESS. 1985. Life Sci. 36: 2295–2300.
95. KAYE, W. E., M. H. EBERT, H. E. GWIRTSMAN & S. WEISS. 1984. Am. J. Psychiatry 141(12): 1598–1601.
96. ROBINSON, P. H., S. A. CHELKLEY & G. M. F. RUSSELL. 1985. Br. J. Psychiatry 146: 169–176.
97. BLOUIN, A., E. PEREZ, J. BLOUIN, T. BUSHNIK, E. MULDER & C. ZURO. 1986. Second International Conference on Eating Disorders. 19–20 April, 1986. New York.
98. RUSSELL, G. M. F. 1986. Second International Conference on Eating Disorders. 19–20 April, 1986. New York.
99. FREEMAN, C. P. 1986. Second International Conference on Eating Disorders. 19–20 April, 1986. New York.
100. SCHUTZ, V., T. BESSARD & E. JECQUIER. 1984. Am. J. Clin. Nutr. 40: 542–552.
101. FELIG, P. 1984. Clin. Physiol. 4: 267–273.
102. VERDY, M. L., L. CHARBONNEAU, I. VERDY, R. BELANGER, E. BOLTE & J. L. CHIASSON. 1983. Int. J. Obesity 7(4): 289–297.
103. VERDY, M. L., J. L. CHIASSON, P. HAMMET & I. VERDY. 1983. Union Med. Can. 112(10): 1–3.
104. DANNENBURG, W. N. 1983. In Biochemical Pharmacology of Obesity. Curtis Prior Pb Ed. 263–283. Elsevier. Amsterdam.
105. BRINDLEY, D. N. 1983. In Biochemical Pharmacology of Obesity. Curtis Prior Pb Ed. 285–308. Elsevier. Amsterdam.
106. TURNER, P. 1978. Int. J. Obesity 2(3): 343–348.
107. TURNER, P. 1979. Curr. Med. Res. Opin. 6(1): 101–105.
108. TURNER, P., L. A. BICHI, H. SLUSARCZYK & C. S. FRANKLIN. 1982. Int. J. Obesity 6(4): 411–415.
109. GEELEN, M. J. H. 1983. Biochem. Pharmacol. 32(22): 3321–3324.
110. SHUSTER, J. A. & D. A. LEVITSKY. 1982. Fed. Proc. Fed. Am. Soc. Exp. Biol. 41(4): 3926.
111. STALLONE, D. D. & D. A. LEVITSKY. 1984. Fed. Proc. Fed. Am. Soc. Exp. Biol. 43(4): 1062.
112. LUPIEN, J. R. & G. A. BRAY. 1985. Pharmacol. Biochem. Behav. 23: 509–513.
113. EVEN, P. 1986. Ninth International Conference on the Physiology of Food and Fluid Intake. 7–11 July, 1986. Seattle.
114. NICOLAÏDIS, S. & P. EVEN. 1986. Pharmacology of Eating Disorders. M. O. Carruba & J. Blundell, Eds.: 117–133. Raven Press. New York.
115. BRAY, G. A. 1985. In Metabolic Complications of Human Obesities. J. Vague, P. Bjorntorp, B. Guy-Grand, M. Rebuffe-Scribe & P. Vague, Eds.: 97–103. Excerpta Medica. Amsterdam.
116. DUMONT, C., J. LAURENT, A. GRANDADAM & J. R. BOISSIER. 1981. Life Sci. 28: 1939–1945.
117. ROWLAND, N. E. & J. CARLTON. 1986. Appetite 7: 71–83.
118. SAMANIN R., C. BENDOTTI, G. CANDELARESI & S. GARRATINI. 1977. Life Sci. 21: 1259–1266.
119. CLINESCHMIDT, B. V., J. C. McGUFFIN & A. B. PFLUEGER. 1977. Eur. J. Pharmacol. 44: 65–74.
120. CLINESCHMIDT, B. V., J. C. McGUFFIN, A. B. PFLUEGER & J. A. TORATO. 1978. Br. J. Pharmacol. 62: 579–589.
121. CLINESCHMIDT, B. V., H. M. HANSON, A. B. PFLUEGER & J. C. McGUFFIN. 1977. Psychopharmacology 55: 27–33.
122. GOODIE, A. J., E. V. THORNTON, T. J. WHEELER. 1976. J. Pharm. Pharmacol. 28: 318–320.

Centrally Active Peptides

Are They Useful Agents in the Treatment of Obesity?[a]

A. S. LEVINE

Neuroendocrine Research Laboratory
Veterans Administration Medical Center
Minneapolis, Minnesota 55417
and
Department of Food Science and Nutrition
University of Minnesota
St. Paul, Minnesota 55108

Over the past decade we have become aware of the important role that amino acids and peptides play as neurotransmitters. Along with the catecholamines these neurotransmitters are involved in the regulation of food intake, and to some extent these substances may effect energy expenditure.[1-3] The sites of action of the various neuropeptides that are involved in the control of food intake are not clear. For example, cholecystokinin appears to act as a satiating factor at a peripheral level in rats,[4] whereas in sheep it appears to act centrally.[5] What is clear, however, is that the eventual effect of the peptide on food intake involves the entire nervous system. It is the origin of neurotransmission that often is unknown. Those gut peptides that were originally identified in the gastrointestinal tract often are also present in the brain and spinal cord.[6] To further complicate the situation, these peptides can act as paracrine, autocrine, endocrine, and neurocrine substances.

Various animal studies indicate that peptides can affect food intake by direct or indirect effects. Neuropeptides may alter the ability of an animal to eat by decreasing food-seeking behavior, by sedating the animal, by making the animal ill, or by causing hypotension and various other indirect effects.[6] They may also alter the transit time of food through the gastrointestinal tract, make an animal extremely thirsty, alter taste perception, and alter the half-time that food remains in the stomach. Presently, it is not understood why some peptides decrease food intake and why others increase food intake.

The focus of this brief review is on the use of peptides, which seem to act at the central nervous system level as pharmacologic agents that may be useful in the treatment of obesity (and other eating disorders). This is a difficult task because only a few neuropeptides have been given to humans, and it is questionable whether they act in the periphery or in the central nervous system. The majority of the studies have involved antagonists of the endogenous opioids.

Portoghese had reported in 1966 that only the (−) enatiomers of opiates were active, indicating that opiates acted stereospecifically.[7] Avram Goldstein, in 1971, found that opiates bound to homogenates of mouse brain in a stereospecific fashion.[8] This result was questioned because the binding was minimal. By 1973,

[a] The preparation of this manuscript was supported, in part, by Veterans Administration Research Funds.

297

however, several groups had reported that opiates bound avidly to homogenates of mammalian nervous system tissue.[9-11] Furthermore, this binding was correlated to the bioactivity of the opioids. The fact that opiates bound to animal tissue hinted at the possibility that animals might, like plants, produce opiate-like compounds. Several laboratories found in the mid-1970s that extracts of rat brain inhibited the contraction of guinea pig ileum and mouse vas deferens, responses that are found in in vitro studies of these smooth muscles[12-15] following the addition of opiates. Such extracts were found to contain two pentapeptides, which were named enkephalins.[13] In 1976, beta-endorphin was isolated from pituitary by Li and his colleagues.[16] The most potent of all endogenous opioids, dynorphin, was identified by Goldstein and coworkers in 1979.[17] In the past five years, the endogenous opioid peptides have been classified into three families: the pro-opiomelanocortin, pro-enkephalin, and pro-dynorphin families.

Opioids are known to affect consummatory behaviors as well as a variety of other functions including smooth muscle contraction, gastric acid secretion, immune competence, memory, and pain.[18-21] In 1929, Babour et al. reported that water intake was enhanced in rats that were morphine-dependent.[22] The first report of morphine-induced feeding was published by Martin et al. in 1963.[23] Grandison and Guidotti reported in 1977 that hypothalamic administration of beta-endorphin resulted in an increase in food intake.[24] Other studies have indicated that blockade of the opioid receptor can result in a decrease in food intake. Naloxone has been reported to decrease food intake in a variety of species under a variety of conditions (see references 25 and 26).

Further evidence for an opioid involvement in energy balance has accumulated based on measurements of opioid levels in obese animals. Margules et al. showed that the concentrations of beta-endorphin is increased in the hypothalamus and pituitary of genetically obese rats and mice compared with their lean littermates.[27] Levels of beta-endorphin have also been measured in obese and lean humans. In 1980, Givens and colleagues demonstrated elevated levels of beta-endorphin in obese women who had oligoamenorrhea.[28] Other investigators have reported that both plasma and cerebrospinal fluid (CSF) beta-endorphin are increased in obese patients. Genazzani and colleagues[29] found that obese children and adolescents had fasting levels of beta-endorphin that were approximately twice the concentration of the nonobese controls. Two laboratories have found that when CSF is fractionated, beta-endorphin is elevated in only one of the fractions.[30,31] Further evidence that beta-endorphin levels may be linked to energy expenditure is the correlation between beta-endorphin and body weight.

Animal studies have indicated that a variety of opioid ligands can stimulate feeding. Opioid agonists of the mu, kappa, and delta receptors have been shown to reliably stimulate food intake following intraventricular injection. One of the most potent opioid stimulators of feeding is the mixed agonist/antagonist butorphanol tartrate.[25,26] This substance is a kappa/sigma agonist and a mu antagonist. In a preliminary trial,[32] we administered this substance in two doses to nonobese subjects following an overnight fast. The subjects were then allowed to choose between three different sandwiches for six hours following injection of the drug. At the high dose, 20 μg/kg, total caloric intake decreased from 666 ± 83 to 377 ± 54 kcal. Naloxone (6 μg/kg) partially reversed this effect (470 ± 30 kcal). In a second study,[33] we found that at a dose of 1 μg/kg, butorphanol increased food intake. The ten individuals ingested 510 kcal during the six-hour period when given saline; after butorphanol tartrate administration, however, they ate 845 kcal during this time period. When butorphanol and naloxone were injected together, the butorphanol effect was eliminated.

In a group of methadone addicts in our medical center we found that food ingestion was greatly enhanced in some of the subjects.[34] One subject, for example, injested about 13,500 kcal/day and was normal weight for height. The major source of calories for this subject was cola drinks. This could be due to a craving for sweet substances or a desire for fluid ingestion. Studies from the early part of this century indicated that opiates stimulate fluid ingestion. In contrast to our finding in these methadone patients, animals appear to favor high fat diets rather than high carbohydrate diets following opioid administration.[35,36] These studies, however, did not directly address the ingestion of sweet substances. The decreased energy efficiency noted in the methadone addicts suggests that opioids may be involved in energy balance. Early studies by Barbour[37] indicated that morphine may alter metabolic rate.

It is well-known from the animal literature that blockade of opioid receptors results in the decrease of food intake. Therefore, it seemed reasonable to test the effects of the opioid antagonists, naloxone and naltrexone, on energy intake in humans. The first reports were anecdotal in nature. Schwartz, in 1980,[38] attempted to convince a group of colleagues that naloxone might suppress appetite. As he stated, "the suggestion was met with that eloquent silence which juniors reserve for elders who cannot be defied openly." He therefore decided to conduct a trial on himself in which he would not need any permission from the authorities nor the cooperation of others. On and off for a 48-day period he ingested various doses of naloxone. He found, when the bathroom scale functioned, that he was losing weight during the period of naloxone administration. He stated that naloxone "strengthens the resolve, a decision already made, not to eat." It did not result in a psychic wiring of jaws. In the same year Kyriakides et al.[39] reported that naloxone (1.6 mg) decreased food intake in two male patients with Prader-Willi syndrome. A third female patient was unaffected by naloxone. In two female twins given 0.4 mg of naloxone twice a day, food intake and body weight was reported to be decreased. A reduction in appetite and body weight has been noted in opiate addicts receiving naloxone as a treatment method. Atkinson reported in 1982[40] that naloxone decreased food intake in a group of obese humans. Wherein 2 mg of intravenously administered naloxone had no effect on a meal given 30 minutes later, 15 mg of naloxone (5 mg IV bolus followed by an infusion at 5 mg/hour) decreased food intake by 29% in the obese subjects compared with saline infusion. Atkinson did not observe this effect in lean subjects. Wolkowitz et al.[41] reported that obese subjects decreased ingestion of food about three and eight hours after infusion of 0.5 mg/kg of naloxone. O'Brien and colleagues[42] studied the effect of naloxone on subjective indices of appetite in massively obese subjects. With cumulative doses as high as 40 mg of naloxone given intravenously, no alterations in subjective measures of appetite, hunger, mood, or opiate withdrawal-like symptoms were noted. Also, no changes in heart rate, skin temperature, respiratory rate, or change in pupil size were noted.

Other investigators have reported that naloxone decreases food intake in non-obese subjects. Trenchard and Silverstone conducted a dose-response study of the effects of naloxone on food intake, using an automated food dispenser.[43] A dose of 0.8 mg of naloxone failed to decrease food intake statistically, whereas 1.6 mg of naloxone decreased food intake by about 25 percent. This effect reached significance 2 hours after food was made available and was maximal at 2½ hours. Cohen et al.[44] found that 2 mg/kg of naloxone decreased eating 2¾ and 7¾ hours after drug administration in normal weight individuals. It should be noted that in neither of the above studies were subjective ratings of hunger altered. This is in agreement with the study of O'Brien et al.[42] as discussed above. Thompson and colleagues found that 2-deoxy-D-glucose–induced food intake was inhibited by naloxone administration.[45]

Since these studies were conducted, several investigators have evaluated the effects of the long-acting opiate antagonist, naltrexone. In addition to being longer acting, naltrexone can be given orally because a large percentage of the drug is not taken up by the liver on the initial passage. Doses of up to 150 mg/day of naltrexone decreased food intake as reported by diary in 6 out of 10 normal subjects.[46] Unfortunately body weight and food intake were not measured in this study. In four former addicts, Sternbach et al.[47] noted that 150 mg/day naltrexone decreased body weight (2–5 kg) after two to six weeks. These data led several investigators to conduct carefully controlled double-blind studies testing the efficacy of naltrexone on long-term body weight loss. The results have been less than encouraging. Atkinson gave 60 obese subjects placebo or naltrexone (50 and 100 mg) for eight weeks and found no significant weight loss.[48] The female subjects, however, lost 1.7 kg during the study. Diary keeping demonstrated no differences in food intake at any time during the study. Malcolm and colleagues studied the effect of 200 mg of naltrexone or placebo for eight weeks and found no effects.[49] A dose of 300 mg naltrexone given daily also had no effect in another study.[49a] Maggio et al. found that doses of 100, 200, and 300 mg of naltrexone for three days each (versus placebo), during a 28-day study period, had no effect on food intake or body weight.[50] In several of these studies, liver enzymes were elevated, and in fact in one study[49a] this resulted in cessation of the drug trial.

Sleep apnea is known to occur in obese humans in the form of Pickwickian syndrome. Atkinson and colleagues[51] studied the effect of naloxone infusion versus saline infusion on the frequency and severity of sleep apnea. A bolus of 5 mg of naloxone followed by a constant infusion of 5 mg/hour throughout the night decreased the average maximal oxyhemoglobin desaturation. These data suggest that naloxone infusion may be useful in reducing sleep apnea in obese humans, without a resultant weight loss.

Thus, opioid blockade is not an effective means of long-term weight management. This may be due to the well-known tolerance effects that occur after chronic opioid administration. Also, the antagonists used may not have potent effects on the specific opioid receptor most important to food intake. The development of more selective antagonists may prove to be useful in further evaluating the effect of opioid blockade on food intake and body-weight regulation.

Another family of peptides that can increase food intake in animals is the pancreatic polypeptide family. Clark et al.[52] were the first investigators to publish data demonstrating that human pancreatic polypeptide and neuropeptide Y (NPY) increased feeding in rats. Stanley and Leibowitz[53,54] found that doses as low as 78 pmoles stimulate food intake when injected into the paraventricular nucleus (PVN) of the hypothalamus. Our laboratory reported that NPY stimulated feeding in a very potent manner after central administration during the daytime, during the nighttime, and after food deprivation.[55] NPY also stimulated drinking behavior, but less so when food was not present. Peptide YY (PYY), another member of the pancreatic polypeptide family, also increases food intake in a potent manner.[56] Because NPY coexists with norepinephrine in some neurons, we thought that NPY might act in conjunction with norepinephrine (also known to stimulate food intake). We, and others,[54,55] did not find that the alpha antagonist phentolamine was capable of blocking the NPY effect. Several other lines of evidence also indicate that these peptides do not act directly together to stimulate food intake.

NPY is a more potent orexigenic agent than any of the opioid peptides. Naloxone, however, when given either periphally or centrally can block the NPY effect (reference 55 and unpublished data). We have also recently found that the opioid receptor alkylating agent, β-CNA, can block NPY-stimulated feeding. The same dose of β-CNA also blocked dynorphin-induced feeding (unpublished results). Such data suggest some type of association between opioid and NPY-induced feeding.

In light of the potent effects of NPY on feeding, it seems likely that human studies with this agent will follow. Antagonists of NPY need to be developed in order to investigate the possible role that NPY might play in obesity. Stanley and Leibowitz have, in fact, shown that repeated administration of NPY can result in an increase in food intake and in fat mass in rats.

A variety of peptides have been reported to decrease food intake. Gut peptides such as cholecystokinin (CCK) and bombesin have been demonstrated to decrease food intake in animals and humans. Inasmuch as it is believed that these peptides act peripherally, they have been discussed in a separate paper in this volume. It is important to note, however, that it is not entirely clear where CCK and bombesin act in humans and in animals. For example, Gibbs[57] argued that bombesin acts peripherally because nonspecific behaviors (excessive grooming) occur after central injection, but not following peripheral administration. Ladenkeim and Ritter[58] have reported, however, that small amounts of bombesin injected directly into the fourth ventricle suppress feeding without any accompanying nonspecific behaviors. Other anorectic peptides such as calcitonin appear to act more potently when administered centrally to experimental animals.[59,60] Calcitonin levels are increased following a meal, but the levels following a meal are not sufficient to decrease food intake.[61] Calcitonin has been reported to decrease food intake in humans, but not in a consistent manner. For example, Paget patients receive calcitonin chronically and do not all lose weight or decrease food intake. Some patients experience nausea associated with calcitonin.

Stress has been associated with alterations in food intake in animals and humans. Corticotropin-releasing factor (CRF), a peptide assumed to be released during stress, stimulates the pituitary secretion of ACTH and beta-lipotropin/ beta-endorphin. It increases heart rate, oxygen consumption, and causes an increase in arterial pressure after administration.[62] Several groups have demonstrated that CRF decreases food intake in rats and results in increased grooming behavior.[63,64] Hypophysectomy has no effect on the anorectic actions of CRF, suggesting that CRF affects these behaviors independently of the release of pro-opiomelanocortin.[64] These data suggest that CRF might be an important factor involved in the control of food intake in animals. CRF has been given to humans; its possible effects on food intake and energy expenditure, however, have not been examined.

From animal studies we know that a variety of neuropeptides either decrease or increase food intake. The few peptides that have been administered to humans to alter consummatory behaviors have not yielded results that indicate that any one peptide will control obesity. It is more likely that, to avoid tolerance, a regimen of peptides involving cyclic administration will be needed to regulate energy balance. As we have known for many decades, obesity is a disease the cause and treatment of which is elusive.

REFERENCES

1. MORLEY, J. E. & A. S. LEVINE. 1985. Pharmacology of eating behavior. Annu. Rev. Pharmacol. Toxicol. **25:** 127–145.
2. MORLEY, J. E. 1980. The neuroendocrine control of appetite: The role of the endogenous opiates, cholecystokinin, TRH, gamma-amino butyric acid and the diazepam receptor. Life Sci. **27:** 355–368.

3. LEIBOWITZ, S. F. 1980. Neurochemical systems of the hypothalamus: Control of feeding and drinking behavior and water electrolyte excretion. *In* Handbook of the Hypothalamus. P. J. Morgane & J. Panksepp, Eds.: **3:** 299–437. Raven Press. New York.

4. DELLA-FERA, M. A., C. A. BAILE, B. S. SCHNEIDER & J. A. GRINKER. 1981. Cholecystokinin-antibody injected in cerebral ventricles stimulates feeding in sheep. Science **212:** 687–689.

5. DELLA-FERA, M. A. & C. A. BAILE. 1979. Cholecystokinin octapeptide: Continuous picomole injections into the cerebral ventricles suppress feeding. Science **206:** 471–473.

6. KREIGER, D. T. & J. B. MARTIN. 1981. Brain peptides. N. Engl. J. Med. **304:** 876–885; 944–951.

7. PORTOGHESE, P. S. 1966. Stereochemical factors and receptor interactions associated with narcotic analgesics. J. Pharm. Sci. **55:** 865–887.

8. GOLDSTEIN, A., L. I. LOWNEY & B. K. PAL. 1971. Stereospecific and non-specific interactions of the morphine congener levorphanol in subcellular fractions of the mouse brain. Proc. Natl. Acad. Sci. USA **68:** 1742–1747.

9. PERT, C. B. & S. H. SNYDER. 1973. Opiate receptor: demonstration in nervous tissue. Science **179:** 1011–1014.

10. SIMON, E. J., J. M. HILLER & J. EDELMAN. 1973. Stereospecific binding of the potent analgesic ³H-etorphine to rat brain homogenate. Proc. Natl. Acad. Sci. USA **70:** 1947–1949.

11. TERENIUS, L. 1973. Characteristics of the "receptor" for narcotic analgesics in synaptic plasma membrane fractions from rat brain. Acta Pharmacol. Toxicol. **33:** 377–384.

12. HUGHES, J., T. SMITH, B. MORGAN & L. FOTHERGILL. 1975. Purification and properties of enkephalin: the possible endogenous ligand for the morphine receptor. Life Sci. **16:** 1753–1758.

13. HUGHES, J., T. W. SMITH, H. W. KOSTERLITZ, L. A. FOTHERGILL, B. A. MORGAN & H. R. MORRIS. 1975. Identification of two related pentapeptides from the brain with potent opiate agonist activity. Nature (London) **258:** 577–579.

14. PASTERNAK, G., R. GOODMAN & S. H. SNYDER. 1975. An endogenous morphine-like factor in mammalian brain. Life Sci. **16:** 1765–1769.

15. TERENIUS, L. & A. WAHLSTROM. 1975. Search for an endogenous ligand for the opiate receptor. Acta Physiol. Scand. **94:** 74–81.

16. LI, C. H. & D. CHUNG. 1976. Isolation and structure of a untriakontapeptide with opiate activity from camel pituitary glands. Proc. Natl. Acad. Sci. USA **73:** 1145–1148.

17. GOLDSTEIN, J. M., S. TACHIBANA, L. I. LOWNEY, M. HUNKAPILLER & L. HOOD. 1979. Dynorphin-(1-13), an extraordinarily potent opioid peptide. Proc. Natl. Acad. Sci. USA **76:** 6666–6670.

18. AKIL, H., S. J. WATSON, E. YOUNG, M. E. LEWIS, H. KHACHATURIAN & J. M. WALKER. 1984. Endogenous opioids: Biology and function. Annu. Rev. Neurosci. **7:** 223–255.

19. MARTIN, W. R. 1984. Pharmacology of opioids. Pharmacol. Rev. **35:** 283–323.

20. MORLEY, J. E. 1981. The endocrinology of opiates and opioid peptides. Metab. Clin. Exp. **30:** 195–209.

21. MORLEY, J. E. 1983. Neuroendocrine effects of endogenous opioid peptides in human subjects. A review. Psychoneuroendocrinology **8:** 361–379.

22. BARBOUR, H. G., L. G. HUNTER & C. H. RICHEY. 1929. Water metabolism and related changes in fat-fed and fat-free fed dogs under morphine addiction and acute withdrawal. J. Pharmacol. Exp. Ther. **36:** 251–277.

23. MARTIN, W. R., A. WIKLER, C. G. EADES & F. T. PESCOR. 1963. Tolerance to and physical dependence on morphine in rats. Psychopharmacology **4:** 247–260.

24. GRANDISON, L. & A. GUIDOTTI. 1977. Stimulation of food intake by muscimol and beta-endorphin. Neuropharmacology **16:** 533–536.

25. MORLEY, J. E., A. S. LEVINE, G. K. YIM & M. T. LOWY. 1983. Opioid modulation of appetite. Neurosci. Biobehav. Rev. **7:** 281–305.

26. LEVINE, A. S., J. E. MORLEY, B. A. GOSNELL, C. J. BILLINGTON & T. J. BARTNESS. 1985. Opioids and consummatory behavior. Brain Res. Bull. **14:** 663–672.
27. MARGULES, D. L., B. MOISSET, M. J. LEWIS, H. SHIBUYA & C. B. PERT. 1978. β-endorphin is associated with overeating in genetically obese mice (ob/ob) and rats (fa/fa). Science **202:** 988–991.
28. GIVENS, J. R., E. WIEDEMANN, R. N. ANDERSEN & A. E. KITABCHI. 1980. β-endorphin and β-lipotropin plasma levels in hirsute women: correlation with body weight. J. Clin. Endocrinol. Metab. **50:** 975–976.
29. GENAZZANI, A. R., F. FACCHINETTI, F. PETRAGLIA, C. PINTOR & R. CORDA. 1986. Hyperendorphinemia in obese children and adolescents. J. Clin. Endocrinol. Metab. **62:** 36–40.
30. FRAIOLI, F., A. FABBRI, C. MORETTI, C. SANTORO & A. ISIDORI. 1981. Endogenous opioid peptides and neuroendocrine correlations in a case of congenital indifference to pain. Endocrinology **108:** 238A.
31. KROTKIEWSKI, M., B. FABERBERG, P. BJORNTORP & L. TERENIUS. 1983. Endorphins in genetic human obesity. Int. J. Obesity **7:** 597–598.
32. MORLEY, J. E., A. S. LEVINE, B. A. GOSNELL & C. J. BILLINGTON. 1984. Which opioid receptor mechanism modulates feeding? Appetite **5:** 61–68.
33. MORLEY, J. E., S. PARKER & A. S. LEVINE. 1985. The effect of butorphanol tartrate on food and water consumption in humans. Am. J. Clin. Nutr. **42:** 1175–1178.
34. TALLMAN, J., M. WILLENBRING, G. CARLSON, M. BOOSALIS, D. KRAHN, A. S. LEVINE & J. E. MORLEY. 1984. Effect of chronic methadone use in humans on taste and dietary preference. Fed. Proc. Fed. Am. Soc. Exp. Biol. **43:** 1058A.
35. MARKS-KAUFMAN, R. & R. B. KANAREK. 1981. Modifications in nutrient selection induced by naloxone in rats. Psychopharmacology **74:** 321–324.
36. MARKS-KAUFMAN, R. & B. J. LIPELES. 1982. Patterns of nutrient selection in rats orally self-administering morphine. Nutr. Behav. **1:** 33–46.
37. BARBOUR, H. G., D. E. GREGG & L. G. HUNTER. 1930. The calorigenic action of morphine as revealed by addiction studies. J. Pharmacol. Exp. Ther. **40:** 433–465.
38. SCHWARTZ, T. B. 1980. Naloxone and weight reduction: an exercise in introspection. Trans. Am. Clin. Climatol. Assoc. **92:** 103–110.
39. KYRIAKIDES, M., T. SILVERSTONE, W. JEFFCOATE & B. LAURANCE. 1980. Effect of naloxone on hyperphagia in Prader-Willi syndrome. Lancet **i:** 876–877.
40. ATKINSON, R. L. 1982. Naloxone decreases food intake in obese humans. J. Clin. Endocrinol. Metab. **55:** 196–198.
41. WOLKOWITZ, O. M., A. R. DORAN, M. R. COHEN, R. M. COHEN, T. N. WISE & D. PICKAR. 1985. Effect of naloxone on food consumption in obesity. N. Engl. J. Med. **313:** 327.
42. O'BRIEN, C. P., A. J. STUNKARD & J. TERNES. 1982. Absence of naloxone sensitivity in obese humans. Psychosom. Med. **44:** 215–218.
43. TRENCHARD, E. & T. SILVERSTONE. 1983. Naloxone reduces the food intake of normal human volunteers. Appetite **4:** 43–50.
44. COHEN, M. R., R. M. COHEN, D. PICKAR & D. L. MURPHY. 1985. Naloxone reduces food intake in humans. Psychosom. Med. **47:** 132–138.
45. THOMPSON, D. A., S. L. WELLE, U. LILAVIVAT, L. PENICAUD & R. G. CAMPBELL. 1982. Opiate receptor blockade in man reduces 2-deoxy-D-glucose-induced food intake but not hunger, thirst, and hypothermia. Life Sci. **31:** 847–852.
46. HOLLISTER, L. E., K. JOHNSON, D. BOUKHABZA & H. K. GILLESPIE. 1981. Aversive effects of naltrexone in subjects not dependent on opiates. Drug Alcohol Depend. **3:** 37–41.
47. STERNBACH, H., W. ANNITTO, A. L. C. POTTASH & M. S. GOLD. 1982. Diurnal variation of erythrocyte sedimentation rate related to feeding. Lancet **i:** 388–389.
48. ATKINSON, R. L., L. K. BERKE, C. R. DRAKE, M. L. BIBBS, F. L. WILLIAMS & D. L. KAISER. 1985. Effects of long-term therapy with naltrexone on body weight in obesity. Clin. Pharmacol. Ther. **38:** 419–422.
49. MALCOLM, R., P. M. O'NEIL, J. D. SEXAUER, F. E. RIDDLE, H. S. CURREY & C. COUNTS. 1985. A controlled trial of naltrexone in obese humans. Int. J. Obesity **9:** 347–353.

49a. MITCHELL, J. E., J. E. MORLEY & D. HATSUKAMI. 1984. A double-blind, placebo controlled trial of naltrexone in obese males. The Neural and Metabolic Bases of Feeding. University of California, Davis. p. 69.

50. MAGGIO, C. A., E. PRESTA, E. P. BRACCO, J. R. VASSELLI, H. R. KISSILEFF & S. A. HASHIM. 1984. Naltrexone and human feeding behavior: a dose-ranging inpatient trial in moderately obese men. Neural and Metabolic Bases of Feeding. University of California, Davis. p. 68.

51. ATKINSON, R. L., P. M. SURATT, S. C. WILHOIT & L. RECANT. 1985. Naloxone improves sleep apnea in obese humans. Int. J. Obesity 9: 233–239.

52. CLARK, J. J., P. S. KALRA, W. R. CROWLEY & S. P. KALRA. 1984. Neuropeptide Y and human pancreatic polypeptide stimulate feeding behavior in rats. Endocrinology 115: 427–429.

53. STANLEY, B. G. & S. F. LEIBOWITZ. 1984. Neuropeptide Y: Stimulation of feeding and drinking by injection into the paraventricular nucleus. Life Sci. 35: 2635–2642.

54. STANLEY, B. G. & S. F. LEIBOWITZ. 1985. Neuropeptide Y injected in the paraventricular hypothalamus: A powerful stimulant of feeding behavior. Proc. Natl. Acad. Sci. USA 82: 3940–3943.

55. LEVINE, A. S. & J. E. MORLEY. 1984. Neuropeptide Y: A potent inducer of consummatory behavior in rats. Peptides 5: 1025–1029.

56. MORLEY, J. E., A. S. LEVINE, M. GRACE & J. KNEIP. 1985. Peptide YY (PYY)—A potent orexigenic agent. Brain Res. 341: 200–203.

57. GIBBS, J. 1985. Effect of bombesin on feeding behavior. Life Sci. 37: 147–153.

58. LADENKEIM, E. E. & R. C. RITTER. 1985. Suppression of food intake by low dose infusion of bombesin into the fourth ventricle. Soc. Neurosci. Abstr. 11(2): 343.

59. FREED, W. J., M. J. PERLOW & R. D. WYATT. 1979. Calcitonin: Inhibitory effect on eating in rats. Science 206: 850–852.

60. LEVINE, A. S. & J. E. MORLEY. 1981. Reduction of feeding in rats by calcitonin. Brain Res. 222: 187–191.

61. TALMAGE, R. V., S. H. POPPELT & C. W. COOPER. 1975. Relationship of blood concentration of calcium, phosphorus, gastrin, and calcitonin to the onset of feeding in the rat. Proc. Soc. Exp. Biol. Med. 149: 855–859.

62. BROWN, M. R., L. A. FISHER, J. RIVIER, J. SPIESS, C. RIVIER & W. VALE. 1982. Corticotropin-releasing factor: Effects on the sympathetic nervous system and oxygen consumption. Life Sci. 30: 207–210.

63. BRITTON, D., G. KOOB, J. RIVIER & W. VALE. 1982. Intraventricular corticotropin-releasing factor enhances behavioral effects of novelty. Life Sci. 31: 363–367.

64. MORLEY, J. E. & A. S. LEVINE. 1982. Corticotropin releasing factor, grooming and ingestive behaviors. Life Sci. 31: 1459–1464.

Mechanical Treatment for Obesity

J. F. MUNRO, I. C. STEWART, P. H. SEIDELIN,
H. S. MACKENZIE, AND N. G. DEWHURST

Eastern General Hospital
Edinburgh, Scotland

INTRODUCTION

The management of obesity involves not only the promotion of weight loss but also the treatment of coexistent complications or associated conditions, both medical and psychological. Indeed, in some circumstances, weight reduction itself may be of only secondary importance. Life-long modification of eating habits remains the cornerstone of effective weight reduction. A number of additional therapies, however, have been developed to assist the more morbidly obese with weight loss. These include various mechanical methods of promoting weight loss.

JEJUNOILEAL BYPASS SURGERY

Small bowel surgery for morbid obesity was developed in the late 1960s[1] and within a few years was being used extensively. The weight loss thus produced was substantial and often sustained, but in individual subjects its magnitude was unpredictable. It carried an immediate postoperative mortality and was associated with a large number of postoperative complications, including the risk of life-threatening liver failure.[2] Although still recommended in some countries,[3,4] there is increasing consensus that the overall hazards outweigh the potential advantages.[5,6] Indeed, many subjects, at first delighted by their progress, thereafter have become disillusioned, so that the successes of the 1970s have become the failures of the 1980s.

GASTRIC SURGERY

The use of gastric bypass operation for weight reduction was first described in 1967. Since then, a remarkable variety of gastric exclusion operations have been described. These include various gastric bypass procedures[7-12] and horizontal gastroplasty.[13-15] More recently, vertical banding gastroplasty has been introduced.[16-18] Others have evaluated a gastric banding procedure[19-21] or the use of a gastric clip gastroplasty.[22] Sometimes, these procedures have been combined with various degrees of wrapping of the stomach with polypropylene mesh. Gastric wrapping has also been used in combination with fundoplication.[19]

Initial weight loss is comparable to that obtained by jejunoileal bypass but usually stops after about eighteen months. The most severely obese expect to lose the most, but nonetheless are liable to a plateau while still substantially overweight.[9] Thenafter, it anything, there is a tendency towards weight regain. This is possibly associated with stomal dilatation, a problem that may be difficult to confirm except endoscopically and that seems particularly prone to develop following horizontal gastroplasty,[23] a procedure that is falling out of favor.

In a number of series, reporting 150 or more operations, the overall operative mortality was less then 1% with a morbidity of 10–15 percent.[9,13,14,24-30] Most of the complications that occur are those associated with the hazards of any intraabdominal surgery in the grossly obese, including a high incidence of postoperative hypoxemia.[31] Specific complications include late stomal stenosis,[32] severe peripheral neuropathy,[33] and Wernicke's encephalopathy.[34] There is also a very high incidence of symptomatic biliary disease developing within a few years postoperatively, so much so that routine cholecystectomy has been recommended at the time of gastric exclusion surgery.[35]

Careful patient selection, scrupulous attention to surgical technique and postoperative care, with prolonged follow-up, all contribute to successful weight reduction and minimize the complications of gastric exclusion surgery; yet no procedure is without risk, and the ideal technique remains unestablished.

Patient Selection

The need for caution is reflected by the guidelines for patient selection laid down by the Task Force of the American Society for Clinical Nutrition.[36] These are that surgery should only be performed in subjects who either are at least 100 lbs (45 kg) or 100% in excess of their ideal, or else have a significant, but less severe, degree of refractory obesity in combination with one or more associated serious medical conditions. In addition, subjects should have been substantially obese for at least three years in spite of making repeated attempts at nonsurgical weight loss. Clearly, patients are excluded if they are suffering from any serious underlying medical problems such as severe cardiorespiratory disease or malignancy. The Task Force also emphasized the importance of explaining the full implications of surgery to the patient and the need for long-term postoperative follow-up. An alternative approach is to apply the same criteria but only to offer gastric surgery as part of a program intended to minimize weight regain following substantial weight loss achieved by nonsurgical means.

INTRAGASTRIC AND EXTRAGASTRIC BALLOONS

Large, intragastric masses of foreign material, bezoars, are often remarkably well-tolerated, producing few symptoms other than weight loss.[37] This observation and the development of a gastric reduction operation provided the stimulus to evaluate the use of intragastric balloons as a technique producing weight loss in the assumption that a reduction in gastric capacity might alleviate feelings of hunger. In 1982, Nieben and Harboe described their preliminary experience in five obese women and reported promising weight loss when the intragastric balloons were inflated.[38] Unfortunately, these balloons were of limited durability and only remained effective for a few weeks. Others have encountered similar difficulties, but weight losses of up to 12 kg have been reported in the short term.[39] Various kinds of artificial bezoars have been tried, including semipermeable mammary implants that require regular refilling and therefore attached to a nasal catheter.[40] Even an extragastric balloon capable to compressing the stomach to a controlled degree has been described.[41] Possibly the most encouraging development is the Garren gastric bubble. This is cylindrical with a central channel and a one-way valve through which the balloon is filled with air by a cannula that can then be detached. The balloon is inspected endoscopically after one month and subsequently at three monthly intervals. Deflated balloons may pass painlessly in the stool or require removal from the stomach by endoscopy. One patient developed a small gastric ulcer. Otherwise, the initial experience of seventy subjects showed weight losses ranging up to 35 kg during a six-month period.[42] Although the gastric bubble is inexpensive, it is too early to judge its long-term efficacy, or indeed safety.[43]

Patient Selection

It seems doubtful that those intragastric balloons currently available will permanently control hyperphagic obesity. At present, their use should be restricted to centers of special expertise until further clinical information has been obtained regarding their efficacy and safety. In general terms, the same criteria should be applied as for the selection of subjects requiring gastric surgery. Possibly, however, those candidates most justifying this form of approach are subjects in whom gastric surgery itself is contraindicated.[8]

JAW WIRING

Jaw wiring for the treatment of obesity was first described twelve years ago.[44] Further experience confirmed that it was a safe, effective method of producing substantial weight losses,[45,46] and it can even be used in edentulous subjects.[47] Dental fixation prevents mastication and therefore restricts the patient to a liquid diet. This need not in itself produce weight loss; we have personal experience of subjects who have gained weight during a jaw wiring program. Most subjects, however, who adhere strictly to the regime can expect to lose about 2 kg per month after a rapid initial weight loss lasting for a month or so. In some subjects, actual fixation of the jaw is not important. Weight loss has been reported when the wires were broken or even replaced by rubber bands, which the subjects could remove voluntarily.[48] Possibly a major component of the effectiveness of a jaw wiring program is that some subjects may find the temptation to consume extra calories easier to resist when adhering to a liquid diet than when restricting conventional food stuffs.

Unfortunately, further experience revealed that weight regain was common.[49] In one study more than half the subjects finished up heavier than before their jaws had been wired, within a mean follow-up period of eight months.[50] It was accordingly argued that dental splinting could not be recommended. This discouraging study may partly be the consequence of patient selection, but even the most enthusiastic advocates of dental splinting accept that weight regain is a significant problem.[51] With the most scrupulous methods of follow-up, involving a complex program of dietary advice, behavioral modification, and exercise, the default rate following dental splinting was greater and the overall weight loss no better than that achieved by subjects not undergoing jaw wiring but otherwise receiving a similar treatment program.[52] For this reason, it has been suggested that jaw wiring should only be considered in combination with gastric surgery.[53,54] Such a joint program should reduce the hazards of operating on the most severely obese and at the same time, enhance the prospects of overall weight reduction.

JAW WIRING WITH A NYLON WAIST CORD

In 1981, Garrow and Gardiner reported an alternative method of preventing weight regain following jaw wiring.[55] They described the use of a nylon cord that was fitted around the waist of seven subjects who had lost a mean of 31.8 kg during dental splinting. The ends of the nylon cord were fused together by heat. During a follow-up period of 4–14 months, the mean weight regain was only 5.6 kilograms. Further experience with this approach has recently been described. The waist cord has been applied to twenty-nine subjects, three of whom had reduced without recourse to dental splinting. During the follow-up period, twelve subjects either did not tolerate the waist cord or preferred a gastric reduction operation. The remaining seventeen lost a mean of 42.2 kilograms. During a mean follow-up period of more than 32 months, the mean weight regain, has been 9.4 kilograms. This study would suggest that the waist cord enables about half the subjects undergoing jaw wiring to maintain most of their weight loss without recourse to gastric surgery.[56]

Patient Selection

At present, there appears to be no clear-cut way of determining which patients will regain weight after a jaw wiring regime. This aspect requires further medical evaluation. In the meantime, it is suggested that subjects should only be selected for a dental splinting program if they fulfill the following minimal guidelines. In otherwise healthy subjects, the body mass index (BMI) should be in excess of 40, although this figure can be reduced to 35 in subjects where there is a clear-cut associated medical condition for weight loss, such as hypertension, or the need for elective surgery. The procedure should be restricted to subjects between the age of 18 and 60, preferably 50. Before selection, all patients should have attended the special clinic that is responsible for their supervision during dental splinting for at least three months. During this time, they must fail to achieve satisfactory weight reduction, but likewise should not be selected if they gain weight while taking the dietary regime that will be recommended once the dental splints are removed. We, in addition, expect our subjects to be able to show their ability to adhere, at least in the short term, to a liquid regime by losing weight while taking the jaw wiring program immediately prior to dental fixation. As with gastric surgery, it is important that all subjects understand the need for continuing medical supervision during a weight maintenance program possibly involving the use of a nylon waist cord. They should be warned that in spite of these steps, when weight regain occurs, then the program should involve a gastric reduction operation. With this in view, they are reassessed by the surgeon and accepted as suitable candidates for gastric bypass surgery. Finally, in addition to no contraindication for surgery, there should be no contraindication for jaw wiring, either medical, for example epilepsy, or psychological, due to a severe personality disorder.

AN ADJUSTABLE WAIST CORD

In order to be effective, the nylon waist cord must be sufficiently tight to make the subject aware of its presence. It follows that unless the cord can be easily adjusted, it is valuable only in preventing weight regain, as it will become loose during weight reduction. The incorporation, however, of a simple plastic button provides a method whereby the length of cord can be adjusted without difficulty, thus permitting its use not only after, but also during periods of weight reduction. We have evaluated this approach in a treatment program involving alternative periods of a very low calorie diet and a high fiber natural diet combined with behavioral modification. Forty subjects who completed the initial period of a liquid regime achieved a mean weight loss of 7.7 kilograms. During a mean follow-up of twelve months, four subjects defaulted and five are impossible to categorize. Those fourteen subjects who continued to wear a waist cord throughout achieved a further weight loss of 4.8 kilograms. This contrasts significantly with seventeen subjects who cut off the cord and regained a mean of 6.6 kilograms.[57] Naturally, it could be argued that those who removed the cord had to do so because of weight regain and that those who did well would have succeeded without recourse to the cord. In an attempt to assess the importance of the cord itself, we are currently undertaking a further study in which subjects who have completed an eight-week period of liquid dieting are randomly allocated into two groups, only one of which receives a waist cord. The initial results are encouraging.

Patient Selection

A nylon waist cord has limitations. It should not be used in subjects who have a skin rash or a sensory neurological disturbance. It is least likely to prove beneficial in those with an apple-shaped abdomen or with a significant abdominal apron. Because of its safety, however, we now offer the waist cord to those subjects attending the clinic who have lost substantial weight irrespective of how weight loss was achieved. We believe that it provides an effective and safe method of helping some subjects to achieve permanency of weight reduction.

CONCLUSION

Each subject with a severe obesity problem provides a unique clinical challenge. The hazards of treatment must be weighed against the risks of obesity itself. The last one or two decades have seen the introduction of various medical and surgical stratagems producing effective, but not necessarily safe, weight loss. These not only include the medical regimes that have been described, but also such therapies as behavior modification pharmacotherapy and the use of very low calorie diets. That the overall results for the management of obesity remain disappointing reflects two outstanding problems. The first is an inability to accurately select for individual subjects, the treatment program that might be most effective and appropriate to their specific needs. The second is the difficulty in preventing weight regain. This takes on special importance in view of the increasing evidence that weight loss followed by weight regain may be more disadvantageous in the long term than unremitting obesity. It emphasizes that whatever treatment regime is recommended, long-term follow-up is mandatory.

REFERENCES

1. PAYNE, J. H. & DE WIND, L. T. 1969. Surgical treatment of obesity. Am. J. Surg. **118:** 141–147.
2. McGILL, D. B., S. R. HUMPHREYS, A. H. BAGGENSTOSS & E. R. DICKSON. 1972. Cirrhosis and death after jejunoileal shunt. Gastroenterology **63:** 872–877.

3. GORAL, R. & M. TUSZEWSKI. 1985. Long term results of jejunoileostomy for extreme obesity. Acta Chir. Scand. **151:** 151–158.
4. MUSTAJOKI, P., M. LEMPINEN, K. HUIKUIRI, R. PELKONEN & E. NIKKILA. 1984. Long-term outcome after jejunoileal bypass for morbid obesity. Int. J. Obesity **8:** 319–325.
5. GRIFFEN, JR., W. P., V. L. YOUNG & C. C. STEVENSON. 1977. A protective comparison of gastric and jejunoileal bypass procedures for morbid obesity. Ann Surg. **186:** 500–509.
6. HOCKING, M. P., M. C. DUERSON, J. P. O'LEARY & E. R. WOODWARD. 1983. Jejunoileal bypass for morbid obesity: late follow-up in 100 cases. N. Engl. J. Med. **308:** 995–999.
7. MASON, E. E. & C. ITO. 1967. Gastric bypass in obesity. Surg. Clin. North Am. **47:** 1345–1351.
8. DEITEL, M., M. A. BOJM, M. D. ATKIN & G. S. ZAKHARY. 1982. Intestinal bypass and gastric partitioning for morbid obesity: a comparison. Can J. Surg. **25:** 283–289.
9. FLICKINGER, E. G., W. J. PORIES, D. MEELHEIM, D. R. SINAR, I. L. BLOSE & T. THOMAS. 1984. The Greenville gastric bypass: Progress Report at 3 years. Ann. Surg. **199:** 555–562.
10. TORRES, J. C., F. CLEMENTA & R. N. GARRISON. 1983. Gastric bypass: Roux-en-Y gastrojejunostomy from the lesser curve. South. Med. J. **76** (10): 1217–1220.
11. HARTFORD, C. E. 1984. Near total gastric bypass for morbid obesity. Arch. Surg. (Chicago) **119:** 282–286.
12. THOMPSON, W. R., J. F. AMARAL, M. D. CALDWELL, H. F. MARTIN & H. F. RANDALL. 1983. Complications and weight loss in 150 consecutive gastric exclusion patients. Am. J. Surg. **146:** 602–612.
13. GOMEZ, C. A. 1981. Gastroplasty in intractable obesity. Int. J. Obesity **5:** 413–420.
14. SMITH, L. B., F. J. FRICKE & A. S. GRANEY. 1983. Results and complications of gastric partitioning: 4 year follow up of 300 morbidly obese patients. Am. J. Surg. **146:** 815–819.
15. JONES, K. B. 1984. Horizontal gastroplasty: a safe effective alternative to gastric bypass in the surgical management of morbid obesity. Am. Surg. **50**(3): 128–131.
16. MASON, E. E. 1982. Vertical banded gastroplasty for obesity. Arch. Surg. (Chicago) **117:** 701–706.
17. SHAMBLIN, J. R., J. W. SESSIONS & M. K. SOILEAU. 1984. Vertical staple gastroplasty: experience with 100 patients. South. Med. J. **77**(1): 33–36.
18. MAKAREWICZ, P. A., M. D. FREEMAN, H. BURCHETT & P. BRAZEAU. 1985. Vertical banded gastroplasty: assessment of efficacy. Surgery **98**(4): 700–707.
19. WILKINSON, L. H. & O. A. PELOSO. 1981. Gastric (reservoir) reduction for morbid obesity. Arch. Surg. (Chicago) **116:** 602–605.
20. SOLHAUG, J. H. 1983. Gastric banding: a new method in the treatment of morbid obesity. Curr. Sug. **40**(6):424–428.
21. BACKMAN, L. & L. GRANSTROM. 1984. Initial (1 year) weight loss after gastric banding, gastroplasty or gastric banding. Acta Chir. Scand. **150:** 63–67.
22. BASHOUR, S. B. & R. W. HILL. 1985. The gastro-clip gastroplasty: an alternative surgical procedure for the treatment of morbid obesity. Tex. Med. **81**(10): 36–38.
23. MESSMER, J. M., J. C. WOLPER & H. J. SUGERMAN. 1984. Stomal disruption in gastric partition in morbid obesity (comparison of radiographic and endoscopic diagnoses). Am. J. Gastroenterol. **79:** 603–605.
24. PELTIER, G., A. S. HEMRECK, R. E. MOFFAT, C. A. HARDIN & W. R. JEWELL. 1979. Complications following gastric bypass procedures for morbid obesity. Surgery **86:** 648–654.
25. BUCKWALTER, J. A. & C. A. HERBST. 1980. Complications of gastric bypass for morbid obesity. Am. J. Surg. **139:** 55–60.
26. MURPHY, K., J. D. McCRACKEN & K. L. OZMENT. 1980. Gastric bypass for obesity: results of a community hospital series. Am. J. Surg. **140:** 747–750.
27. GRIFFEN, W. P., A. A. BIVENS, R. M. BELL & K. A. JACKSON. 1981. Gastric bypass for morbid obesity. World J. Surg. **5:** 817–822.

28. MASON, E. E. 1981. Surgical treatment of obesity. *In* Major Problems in Clinical Surgery. 137–224. W.B. Saunders. Philadelphia.
29. LINNER, J. H. 1982. Comparative effectiveness of gastric bypass and gastroplasty: a clinical study. Ann. Surg. **117:** 695–700.
30. KNECHT, B. H. 1983. Mason gastric bypass: long term follow-up and comparison with other procedures. Am. J. Surg. **154:** 604–608.
31. TAYLOR, R. R., T. M. KELLY, G. ELLIOT, R. L. JENSON & S. B. JONES. 1985. Hypoemia after gastric bypass surgery for morbid obesity. Arch. Surg. (Chicago) **120:** 1298–1302.
32. WOLPER, J. C., J. M. MESSMER, M. A. TURNER & H. J. SUGERMAN. 1984. Endoscopic dilation of late stomal stenosis. Its use following gastric surgery for morbid obesity. Arch. Surg. (Chicago) **119:** 836–837.
33. MARYNIAK, O. 1984. Severe peripheral neuropathy following gastric bypass surgery for morbid obesity. Can. Med. Assoc. J. **131:** 119–120.
34. FAWCETT, S., B. YOUNG & R. HALLIDAY. 1984. Wernicke's encephalopathy after gastric partitioning for morbid obesity. Can. J. Surg. **27**(2): 169–170.
35. AMARAL, J. F. & W. R. THOMPSON. 1985. Gallbladder disease in the morbidly obese. Am. J. Surg. **149:** 551–557.
36. Task Force of the American Society for Clinical Nutrition. 1985. Guidelines for surgery for morbid obesity. Am. J. Clin. Nutr. **42:** 904–905.
37. DEBAKEY, M. & A. OCHSNER. 1938. Bezoars and concretions: a comprehensive review of the literature with an analysis of 303 collected cases and a presentation of 8 additional cases. Surgery **4:** 934–963; 1939. Surgery **5:** 132–160.
38. NIEBEN, O. G. & H. HARBOE. 1982. Intragastric balloon as an artificial bezoar for treatment of obesity. Lancet **i:** 198–199.
39. TAYLOR, T. V. & B. R. PULLAN. 1983. Initial experience with a free floating intragastric balloon in the treatment of morbid obesity. Gut **24,** T43: A979.
40. PERCIVAL, W. L. 1984. "The balloon diet" a noninvasive treatment for morbid obesity: Preliminary report for 108 patients. Can. J. Surg. **27**(2): 135–136.
41. BERSON, D. 1981. Adjustable gastric compression balloon: A new approach to surgery for morbid obesity. Obesity/Bariatric Med. **10** (2): 40–43.
42. GARREN, M., L. R. GARREN & F. GIORDANO. 1984. The Garren gastric bubble: a treatment for the morbidly obese. Endosc. Rev. **2:** 57–60.
43. HOLLAND, S., D. BACH & J. DUFF. 1985. Balloon therapy for obesity—when the balloon bursts. J. Can. Assoc. of Radiologists. **36:** 347–349.
44. GARROW, J. S. Dental splinting in the treatment of hyperphagic obesity. Proc. Nutr. Soc. **33:** 29A.
45. RODGERS, E., A. GOSS, R. T. D. GOLDNEY, R. BURNET, P. PHILLIPS, C. KIMBER & P. HARDING. 1977. Jaw wiring in the treatment of obesity. Lancet **i:** 1221–1223.
46. WOOD, G. D. 1977. The early results of treatment of the obese by a diet regimen enforced by maxillomandibular fixation. J. Oral Surgery **35:** 461–464.
47. GOSS, A. N. 1980. Treatment of massive obesity by prolonged jaw immobilization for edentulous patients. Int. J. Oral Surg. **9:** 253–258.
48. BJORVELL, H., K. HADELL, B. JONSSON, C. MOLIN & S. ROSSNER. 1984. Long-term effects of jaw fixation in severe obesity. Int. J. Obesity **8** (1): 79–86.
49. CASTELNUOVO TEDESCO, P., D. C. BUCHANAN & H. D. HALL. 1980. Jaw wiring for obesity. Gen. Hosp. Psychiatry **2:** 156–159.
50. DRENICK, E. J. & H. W. HARGIS. 1978. Jaw wiring for weight reduction. Obesity/Bariatric Med. **7** (6): 210–213.
51. HARDING, P. E. 1980. Jaw wiring for obesity. Lanet **i:** 534–535.
52. BJORVELL, H. & S. ROSSNER. 1985. Long term treatment of severe obesity: four year follow up of results of combined behavioural modification programme. Br. Med. J. **291:** 379–382.
53. FORDYCE, G. L., J. S. GARROW, A. E. KARK & S. F. STALLEY. 1979. Jaw wiring and gastric bypass in the treatment of severe obesity. Obesity/Bariatric Med. **8** (1): 14–17.
54. RAMSAY-STEWART, G. & L. MARTIN. 1985. Jaw wiring in the treatment of morbid obesity. N.Z. Surg. **55:** 163–167.

55. GARROW, J. S. & G. T. GARDINER. 1981. Maintenance of weight loss in obese patients after jaw wiring. Br. Med. J. **282:** 858–860.
56. GARROW, J. S. & J. D. WEBSTER. 1986. Long term results of treatment of severe obesity with jaw wiring and waist cord. Proc. Nutr. Soc. **45:** 119A.
57. SIMPSON, G. K., D. L. FARQUHAR, P. CARR, S. MCL. GALLOWAY, I. C. STEWART, P. DONALD, F. STEVEN & J. F. MUNRO. 1986. Intermittent protein-sparing fasting with abdominal belting. Int. J. Obesity. **10:** 247–254.

A New Approach to the Treatment of Obesity

A Discussion

BERNARD J. P. GUY-GRAND

Service de Médecine et Nutrition
Université Paris VI
Paris, France

During the last two or three decades, research in obesity has deserved growing interest, and much new data have appeared in an exploding way. The basic concepts, however, underlying what is now one of the major health problems in western countries are slowly emerging. These concepts will be stated in the closing remarks by Richard Wurtman. Indeed, it is hard to integrate basic data collected from many specific fields: epidemiology, energy metabolism, adipose tissue physiology, food intake, neuroendocrinology, neuropharmacology, and psychoanalysis. Obviously this progress in knowledge has not led, so far, to more successful treatment of obese patients. For the most part, in spite of some exceptions, everyone dealing with obese people agrees that the treatment of obesity remains a puzzling challenge: the conventional treatments for obesity have poor long-term efficacy, drastic procedures are often hazardous, and the prevalence of obesity is still increasing.

Among the numerous reasons that could account for such an unsolved challenge may be that the problem has been set in the wrong way. This was pointed out by John Garrow,[1] who estimated that until recently, obesity was not seriously treated. Considering the general literature,[2] it clearly appears that the most frequent goal has been to design a treatment and to test its efficacy in "the obese" in a simple symptomatic way, taking short-term weight loss as the only end point. A more fruitful approach would be to start with the obese patients and to try to provide them with a more or less specific treatment (if available) tailored to their specific needs. These needs are clearly not restricted to a standardized short-term weight loss, even if body weight is usually easy to measure and to record. We must, however, achieve more refined goals that are, in part, subjective and difficult to measure.

Thoroughly developed in the preceding papers of this volume is the concept that obesity is a complex symptom, poorly defined as an excess in body fat with related health hazards. It is becoming more and more recognized that obesity is a heterogeneous symptom, multifactorial in origin, and elicited by various etiologies. Therefore it is not surprising that the various techniques that have been used for a long time (TABLE 1) to treat more or less defined obese populations have ended in overall failure. It is just the result that we could expect when treatment is administered without any attempt at accounting for the prevailing pathophysiology at work in each case. Failure of one method in a given patient, however, does not necessarily indicate that another method will also fail. In other words, the old question about treatment for obesity should be replaced by a new one that considers treatments for different kinds of obesity. The clinician, faced with his patients, should find a treatment for each of them. It is far too early for a full

TABLE 1. Main Techniques Used in the Treatment of Obesity

Pharmacotherapy	Surgery
· Anorectic drugs	· Ileojejunal bypass
· Thyroid hormone	· Gastric surgery
· Thermogenic drugs	· Jaw wiring
· HCG[a]	· Adipectomy
Diets	Miscellaneous
· Low calorie	· Psychotherapy
· Low carbohydrate	· Hypnosis
· Low fat	· Acupuncture
· Fasting	· Self-help groups
· PSMF[b]	
Behavior Therapy	Physical Exercise

[a] HCG = human chorionic gonadotropin
[b] PSMF = protein sparing modified fast

answer. Some improvements in the classifications of obesity that can make possible a complete assessment of the therapeutic relevance of some currently used techniques are clearly needed. We can suggest, however, that formulating the question in this way will point future research into new directions that will enable it to solve many impending questions.

New developments in the understanding of physiological mechanisms determining body weight make it possible to consider the general aspects of the treatment of obesity in a way that would not have previously been possible. Body weight or fat stores in a given subject, whether obese or not, are set spontaneously at a given level and are considered as more or less precisely regulated.[3] The mechanisms by which such a regulation is achieved would raise a theoretical and experimental discussion that is clearly not in the scope of this paper. Limiting ourselves to the therapeutic relevance of this theory, we can only consider that this spontaneous setting of body fat stores results from (1) genetic factors,[4] poorly understood, but probably very important; (2) environmental factors, including familial, social, and nutritional determinants in addition to their psychological impact, seen most often as stressors, and (3) most importantly, the subtle interactions of both types of factors.[5]

Whatever parts of these factors may be active in a given subject, this spontaneous setting cannot be changed or reversed, (*i.e.* excess weight challenged), without some constraint necessary to impose an influence on the energy balance that would induce weight loss. Of course the nature of the constraint can vary greatly according to the techniques used. It can include a fair and moderate self-willed control of food intake (diets), a drastic restriction obtained by way of anatomic manipulations (surgery, jaw wiring), or the administration of drugs to reduce food intake or to increase the disposal of energy, or both.

Provided that the constraint is effective and a negative energy balance is achieved, weight loss starts, as depicted in FIGURE 1. Progressively, some counteracting factors take place, tending to decrease the rate of weight loss. The effectiveness and the nature of the resistance, metabolic or psychologic, or both, have been abundantly described previously in this volume. Finally, after some time has elasped, depending on many factors such as the magnitude of the energy deficit, the composition of the diet, the importance of the residual intake, the level of energy expenditure, and the effectiveness of the constraint and its duration, a new state of equilibrium is reached (step II), except when a severe and long-lasting starvation or semistarvation is imposed, overstepping the adaptive capabilities. It is important to recognize that in most instances, this new setting of body weight represents some kind of new compromise between what has and has not changed for the person in question. The new steady state may be or may not be located in the so-called normal range, depending on the various etiologies of obesity, on the amount of internal and external changes that have been possible to achieve, and on the duration and the severity of the constraint.

The leveling of the weight curve that occurs with all types of treatments is often interpreted as some kind of tolerance to the treatment, which would become progressively inefficient. This interpretation can be seriously challenged: it indicates only that the limit of action of the treatment has been reached. Indeed the counteracting factors are still at work, and the treatment just compensates for their pressure. Usually the new setting of body weight appears more enforced that spontaneous, as the end of the story will show.

When the constraint is relaxed,[6] the energy balance again becomes positive, weight regain occurs, and the patient relapses (step III, 2). Quite frequently all the weight that was lost initially is regained. Eventually more weight is gained (step III, 1), particularly in those patients who were active gainers when the treatment was started. Relaxing the constraint occurs very frequently with diets, particularly when they consist of severe restrictions incompatible with everyday life. Weight gain almost invariably occurs when drugs are withdrawn or when a surgical modification is relieved. Even with gastric surgery, some escape from the constraint can occur, with similar results.

Only when it is possible to maintain the constraint for an indefinite period of time (step III, 3) can the long-term maintenance of the initial weight loss be obtained, unless it should have been possible to cure some fundamental etiologic disturbance. In that respect, special attention has to be paid to the subset of the obese population with mood disturbances. For the most part, this eventuality seldom occurs today, and the frequency of the long-term maintenance of body weight loss appears rather weak, not exceeding 10–15% of the initial cohorts. There is a sharp contrast between step I, which has up to now deserved most of the attention of the scientific community, resulting in the availability of numerous

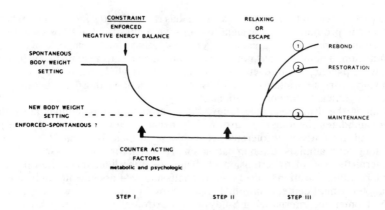

FIGURE 1. Shematic evolution in body weight in treated obese patients.

efficient techniques, and step III, which is certainly much more important and represents the true challenge in treating obese subjects. Long-term well-designed studies, however, evaluating the comparative effectiveness of different techniques in well-determined patients are lacking or impossible to perform.

The question now is, Which procedure could be both effective and safe for long-term (for life?) use? The candidates are few:

Diet and control of food intake, associated with educational programs and various kinds of psychological support (physicians, nutritionists, psychologists, and lay-led groups) is still useful, but far from successful in a large number of patients. It is probably best suitable for people with mild to moderate obesity without severe alterations in their feeding pattern (either quantitative or qualitative). This plan should consist of a gradual modification of eating habits to induce a moderate decrease in calorie intake compatible with everyday life.

Behavior therapy has been reported to have significant long-term results, but weight loss is generally modest. It can be associated with diets and incorporated in the program of self-help groups.

TABLE 2. Some Factors Likely to Affect Therapeutic Choices

Severity (hyperplasia)
Familial history
Fat distribution
Age at onset
Duration
Dynamic/static phase
Energy expenditure
Calorie intake
Eating pattern and its psychological significance
Somatic associated diseases
Depression
Expected benefits (somatic/psychologic/social)
Previous failures
Benefits of being fat
Tolerance to frustration
Realistic goal

Gastric surgery (J. Munro, this volume) has rather narrow indications. When it succeeds in promoting large weight loss in severe obesity by way of severe food restriction, it possibly shares with very low calorie diets the risk of chronic malnutrition, a point that has not been submitted, so far, to systematic evaluation. Untoward psychological reactions following large weight losses are less common following gastric restrictions than following severe long-lasting diets, but they can affect a significant number of patients.[7]

Among the drugs available today, the serotoninergic compounds are rather good candidates for long-term use, mainly because they have no addictive potency and are fairly well-tolerated. It would seem logical to consider seriously their long-term administration in patients more at risk for somatic disease, just as long-term therapy of hypertension, diabetes, or hyperlipidemias often includes long-term administration of drugs with serious and well-documented side effects. A long-term multicenter controlled trial is now in progress in western Europe (ISIS, Isomeride, International Study) with dextrofenfluramine, which has been shown to be quite a pure serotoninergic drug (C. Nathan, this volume), completely cleared of the confusing action of the *l* derivative. We will have an answer concerning its long-term efficacy and tolerance and also get some information on which obese persons are most responsive to this drug. They are probably not restricted to carbohydrate cravers (J. Wurtman, this volume), but could include other types of patients.[8]

One of the most important problems in the management of obesity is recognizing the type of obesity responsive to a given treatment. Although an ideal classification system is not available today, we are making progress in this recognition and classification process, which will be aided by a better understanding of the basic physiology and pathology of obesity. A fine and integrative analysis of the clinical semiology of obesity, however, is certainly a basis for the clinical recognition of the prevalent pathophysiology at work in each case. TABLE 2 includes an extensive list of some factors likely to affect therapeutic choices. An attentive medical, dietary, and psychological examination is often able to provide enough information. How to use these data, however, is far from clear. To comment in detail on the respective relevance of each of them is not in the scope of this discussion. Indeed, this information usually mixes together in various proportions that give rise to a large number of specific pictures. It would seem logical, however, to take into account most of the data in order to evaluate the feasibility and the adequacy of each available therapeutic strategy or to conclude that weight loss, but not the treatment of associated diseases or disturbances, is currently an impossibility.

REFERENCES

1. GARROWS, J. S. 1981. Treat obesity seriously. A clinical manual. Churchill Livingstone. London, England.
2. WING, R. R. & R. W. JEFFREY. 1979. Outpatient treatments of obesity: a comparison of methodology and clinical results. Int. J. Obesity **3:** 261–280.
3. STUNKARD, A. J. & E. STELLAR, EDS. 1984. EATING AND ITS DISORDERS. RAVEN PRESS. NEW YORK.
4. STUNKARD, A. J., T. I. SORENSEN, C. HANIS, T. W. TEASDALE, R. CHAKRABORTY, W. J. SCHULL & F. SHULSINGER. 1986. An adoption study of human obesity. N. Engl. J. Med. **314:** 193–198.
5. BOUCHARD, C. 1985. Inheritance of fat distribution and adipose tissue metabolism in metabolic complications of human obesities. J. Vague, P. Bjorntorp, B. Guy-Grand, M. Rebuffe-Scrive & P. Vague, Eds.: 87–96. Int. Congress Series Vol. 682. Excerpta Medica. Amsterdam-New York.
6. CRAIGHEAD, L. W., A. J. STUNKARD & R. O'BRIEN. 1981. Behavior therapy and pharmacotherapy of obesity. Arch. Gen. Psychiatry. **38:** 763–768.
7. HALMI, K. A., A. J. STUNKARD & E. E. MASON. 1980. Emotional responses to weight reduction by three methods: diet jenunoileal bypass and gastric bypass. Am. J. Clin. Nutr. **33:** 446–451.
8. STUNKARD, A. J. 1982. Appetite agents lower body weight set point. Life Sci. **30:** 2043–2055.

Effects of an Intragastric Balloon on Body Weight, Food Intake, and Gastric Emptying Rate[a]

ALLAN GELIEBTER, SANDRA WESTREICH,
DENNIS GAGE, RICHARD S. McCRAY, AND
SAMI A. HASHIM

St. Luke's-Roosevelt Hospital
New York, New York 10025
and
Touro College
New York, New York 10036

INTRODUCTION

A new procedure for treating obesity involves nonsurgical insertion of a balloon into the stomach. A gastric balloon was inserted into one of us (A. Geliebter, about 20% overweight) in 1983. It remained connected to a thin tube that was attached to a restraint kept in the nostril. It was inflated with 400 cc for one month (see FIGURE 1) and deflated for the next month. During the period of inflation, 4 lbs were lost, which were regained during deflation. Fasting glucose, insulin, and gastrin values remained normal. We then inserted a similar balloon in a morbidly obese patient.

METHOD

The patient was male, age 40, 6 feet in height, and weighed 485 pounds. Unknown to him, the balloon was inflated the first month and deflated the next. The patient was asked to eat ad libitum. Food intake and body weight were measured in a double-blind study. Solid meals consisting of macaroni and beef were provided weekly. Liquid meals (Sustacal), which were ingested by straw from a hidden reservoir were provided biweekly. The meals were served on an eating monitor that had a hidden scale below the food container and covertly recorded changes in weight. Gastric emptying of a liquid meal to which a radioactive tracer (150 μCi Technetium-99m sulfur colloid) had been added was measured. Using a gamma camera, the halftime for emptying the stomach was deter-

[a] This study was supported in part by the St. Luke's-Roosevelt Institute for Health Sciences and by NIH Grant AM 34702.

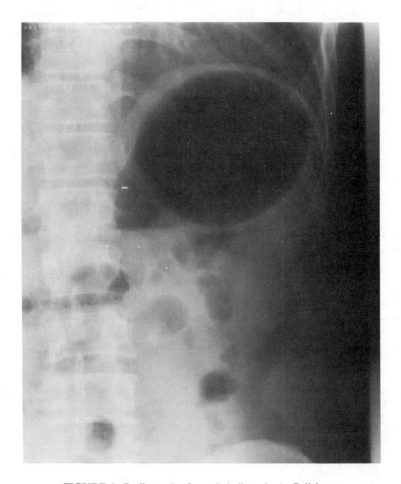

FIGURE 1. Radiograph of gastric balloon in A. Geliebter.

mined. Endoscopy was performed before insertion and after one month of inflation.

RESULTS

As shown in TABLE 1, the patient lost 5 lbs during the period of inflation and showed no weight change after the period of deflation. Side effects reported were occasional abdominal pain, nausea, and heartburn, especially in the first three days after insertion. Serum values of gastrin were elevated during balloon inflation. Mean intakes of solid meals were slightly depressed during balloon inflation as were liquid meals. Gastric emptying of a liquid meal was delayed during balloon inflation. Endoscopic appearance of the stomach was normal before insertion and after one month of inflation.

TABLE 1

	Balloon Period	
	Inflation	Deflation
Weight change (lbs)	-5	0
Solid meal intake (g)	256±56 (SE)	306±28
Liquid meal intake (g)	539	777±89
Gastric emptying half-time (min)	73	60
Gastrin levels (pg/ml)	1010	60
Endoscopy	normal	

CONCLUSION

The inflated balloon appeared to reduce total caloric intake as reflected in the weight loss and the nonsignificant trend seen in meal intakes. The effects on appetite and weight were modest. The same study is now underway with a larger group of subjects.

The balloon may be most effective in conjunction with a restrictive diet. Further studies are needed to parcel out the effects of a gastric balloon and diet. The consequences on body weight after balloon removal must also be assessed because body weight and food intake promptly increase in animals after balloon deflation.[1,2]

REFERENCES

1. GELIEBTER, A., S. WESTREICH, D. GAGE & S. A. HASHIM. 1986. Intragastric balloon reduces food intake and body weight in the rat. Am. J. Physiol. 251: R794–R797.
2. GELIEBTER, A., S. WESTREICH, S. A. HASHIM & D. GAGE. 1987. Gastric balloon reduces food intake and body weight in obese rats. Physiol. Behav. 39: 399–402.

The Effect of the 5-HT Releasing Drug d-Fenfluramine and the 5-HT Receptor Blocker, Metergoline, on Food Intake in Human Subjects

E. GOODALL[a] AND T. SILVERSTONE

Academic Unit of Human Psychopharmacology
Medical College of St. Bartholomew's Hospital
London, United Kingdom

INTRODUCTION

Animal evidence has shown that fenfluramine (FF) exerts its influence on food intake by way of a release of 5-hydroxytryptamine (5-HT) from presynaptic neurones and that it may have a selective effect on carbohydrate nutrients. In order to elucidate the role of 5-HT in human feeding, we have examined the effects of d-FF and metergoline (MTG), a 5-HT receptor blocker, on hunger and food intake in 14 healthy male volunteers.

METHOD

Subjects reported on four occasions at 0845 following an overnight fast. Thirty mg d-FF (or placebo) was administered at 0900 followed by 4 mg MTG (or placebo) at 1100 in the following combinations in random order at weekly intervals: d-FF + placebo, placebo + MTG, d-FF + MTG, and placebo + placebo. Subjective hunger and satiety were assessed hourly using visual analog scales (VAS). Food intake was measured from 1300 to 1500 using an automated food dispenser containing four snacks of known calorific value, prepared to each subject's preference. The percentage energy content derived from carbohydrate (CHO) and sweetness of the four snacks was varied to provide the following choices for each subject: low (22%) and medium (46%) nonsweet CHO, and medium (57%) and high (100%) sweet CHO.

RESULTS

d-FF significantly reduced hourly hunger ratings at 1200 (p < .05) and 1300 (p < .01) but not satiety ratings. These effects were not blocked by the addition of MTG. d-FF and MTG exerted differential effects on sweet and nonsweet food intake. d-FF significantly reduced intake of nonsweet food (FIG. 1) but did not affect sweet food intake (FIG. 2). MTG alone significantly increased sweet food

[a] Current address: Academic Unit of Human Psychopharmacology, St. John's Wing, Homerton Hospital, Homerton Grove, London, E.9, UK.

321

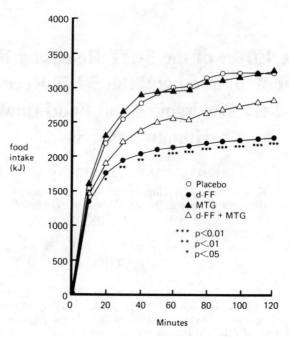

FIGURE 1. Mean cumulative nonsweet food intake (kJ) of 14 normal male volunteers following 30 mg *d*-FF (●), 4 mg MTG (▲), both drugs (△), and placebos (○).

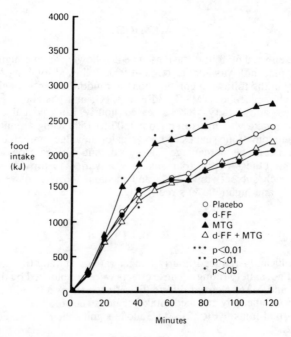

FIGURE 2. Mean cumulative sweet food intake (kJ) of 14 normal male volunteers following 30 mg *d*-FF (●), 4 mg MTG (▲), both drugs (△), and placebos (○).

322

intake (FIG. 2) but had no effect on nonsweet food (FIG. 1). When given together each drug attenuated the effect of the other (FIGURES 1 and 2).

DISCUSSION

These findings in humans parallel the animal evidence that 5-HT plays an important role in the regulation of food intake. The differential effects of *d*-FF on the intake of nonsweet and sweet food in human subjects is consistent with a recent animal study.[1] One explanation could be that the reinforcing taste of sweet food can override the anorectic effect of *d*-FF. The increase in sweet food intake following 5-HT receptor blockade by MTG and the reduction of this effect by *d*-FF is in keeping with Wurtman's observations on *d*-FF reduction of carbohydrate craving in obese women.[2] CHO craving is also seen in seasonal affective disorder, which might be due to a deficiency in 5-HT.[3] Similarly the antidepressant drug amitriptyline (which has some 5-HT receptor blocking properties) can cause a craving for sweet foods.[4]

REFERENCES

1. ORTHEN-GAMBILL, N. 1985. Sucrose intake unaffected by fenfluramine but suppressed by amphetamine administration. Psychopharmacology **87:** 25–29.
2. WURTMAN, J., R. WURTMAN, S. MARK, R. TSAY, W. GILBERT & J. GROWDON. 1985. *d*-Fenfluramine selectively suppresses carbohydrate snacking by obese subjects. Int. J. Eating Disorders **4:** 89–99.
3. ROSENTHAL, N. E. & M. M. HEFFERNAN. 1986. Bulimia, carbohydrate craving and depression; a central connection? *In* Food Constituents Affecting Normal and Abnormal Behaviors. Nutrition and the Brain, Vol. 7. R. J. Wurtman & J. J. Wurtman, Eds.: 139–166. Raven Press. New York.
4. PAYKEL, E. S., P. S. MUELLER & P. M. DE LA VERGNE. 1973. Amitriptyline, weight gain and carbohydrate craving, a side effect. Br. J. Psychiatry **123:** 501–507.

The Major Affective Disorder in Anorexia Nervosa and Bulimia

REINHOLD G. LAESSLE, SUSANNE KITTL,
ULRICH SCHWEIGER, MANFRED M. FICHTER, AND
KARL M. PIRKE

Max Planck Institute for Psychiatry
Munich, Federal Republic of Germany

In recent years, several lines of evidence have emerged suggesting that eating disorders in general, and bulimia in particular, are in some way linked to the major affective disorder.[1] Studies, however, on the phenomenological relationship between the two illnesses have shown inconsistent results, which might be partly due to the heterogeneity of eating disorders and shortcomings of a diagnostic assessment of affective disorders. We looked for depressive syndromes in subtypes of eating disorders using standardized assessment and DSM-III diagnostic criteria.

Characteristics of the study groups are depicted on TABLE 1. Diagnostic assessment was made using the National Institute of Mental Health Diagnostic Interview Schedule and the Eating Disorder Inventory. Sixty-three patients were interviewed as inpatients and 22 as outpatients, one year after hospital treatment.

DSM-III lifetime rates of affective disorders are depicted in FIGURE 1. The three bulimic groups differed significantly from the restrictors. The onset of the major affective disorder occurred significantly more frequently (in 72% of the patients) at least one year after onset of the eating disorder than before the eating disorder (9.4%). The rate of the current major affective disorder in the 63 inpatients with an active and severe eating disorder was significantly higher (31.7%) than in the outpatients whose eating disorder was in remission (4.5%).

In some contrast to previous results,[2] our data on temporal relationship indicate that the affective disturbance was likely to be secondary to an eating disorder. This is further supported by our finding a very low rate of depression in patients after treatment of the eating disorder. The higher frequency of major affective disorders in bulimics than in restrictors could partly be explained by the longer duration of illness in the bulimics. Our data are also consistent, however, with recent suggestions that bulimia is related to a more severe unspecific psychopathology and has a poorer prognosis. This view is further supported by our finding that in most patients developing bulimia after anorexia nervosa, the onset of major depression occurs only when bulimia is present.

REFERENCES

1. SWIFT, W. J., D. ANDREW & N. E. BARKLAGE. 1986. The relationship between affective disorder and eating disorders: A review of the literature. Am. J. Psychiatry **143** (3): 290–299.
2. HUDSON, J. F., H. G. POPE, J. M. JONAS & D. YURGELUN-TODD. 1983. Phenomenologic relationship of eating disorders to major affective disorder. Psychiatry Res. **9**: 345–354.

TABLE 1. Characteristics of 85 Patients with Eating Disorders

		Total Sample n = 85	AN-R (anorexia without bulimia) n = 19	AN-B (anorexia and bulimia) n = 18	BU-A (bulimia with a history of anorexia) n = 22	BUL (bulimia alone) n = 26
Age (years)	x̄	22.8	20.7	21.7	23.6	24.3
	(s)	(4.2)	(3.4)	(3.4)	(4.1)	(4.7)
Duration of illness (years)	x̄	5.4	1.9	4.6	7.8	6.5
	(s)	(4.2)	(1.9)	(3.3)	(3.9)	(4.5)
Weight maximum (% IBW[a])	x̄	107.8	96.4	109.9	109.8	113.3
	(s)	(17.7)	(13.5)	(15.6)	(20.6)	(17.9)
Weight minimum (% IBW)	x̄	72.9	65.7	65.2	68.8	86.7
	(s)	(13.0)	(9.9)	(5.0)	(9.2)	(11.0)

[a] IBW = ideal body weight.

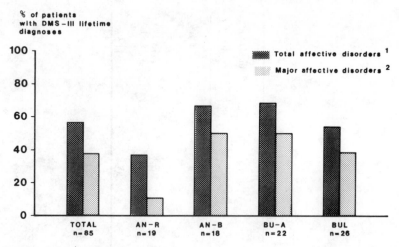

FIGURE 1. DSM-111 lifetime diagnoses of affective disorders in 85 patients with eating disorders. [1]Patients with at least one of the following diagnoses: major depression, bipolar, dysthymic, or atypical. [2]Major depression, bipolar.

Effects of *l*-Tryptophan on Food Intake and Selection in Lean Men and Women

L. A. LEITER,[a] N. HRBOTICKY,[b] AND G. H. ANDERSON[c]

[a] *Department of Medicine and Nutritional Sciences*
University of Toronto
Toronto, Ontario, Canada M5T 2R2

[b] *Department of Pediatrics*
The Research Centre
Vancouver, British Columbia, Canada V5X 4H4

[c] *Department of Nutritional Sciences*
University of Toronto
Toronto, Ontario, Canada M5S 1A8

The effects of the serotonin dietary precursor *l*-tryptophan (TRP) on energy and macronutrient specific appetites were studied in view of the known effects of serotonin on appetite regulation and macronutrient selection.[1,2] After a standardized breakfast (8:30 A.M.), normal weight subjects ($\pm 10\%$ reference table weight) took capsulated TRP or lactose placebo (PL) 45 minutes prior to a buffet-type lunch (12:00 noon). In the first study of 17 men, energy intake was reduced 13% by 2 g TRP over placebo (TABLE 1; $p < 0.001$). Study 2, in which 15 men received 3 levels of TRP, revealed that 2 or 3 g TRP, but not 1 g, suppressed food intake by at least 19% (TABLE 1; $p < 0.001$). In neither study was a TRP effect on macronutrient selection observed. By contrast, 14 women, uncontrolled for the menstrual cycle, did not suppress energy intake (TABLE 1; ns) but did decrease carbohydrate intake (expressed as a percentage of total energy, $\bar{x} \pm$ SEM) with 2 and 3 g TRP (PL = $40.7 \pm 1.0\%$, 1 g TRP = 39.9 ± 1.6, 2 g TRP = 38.8 ± 1.2, 3 g TRP = 36.6 ± 1.8; $p < 0.05$). These gender differences led to the examination of menstrual cycle effects of food intake and TRP metabolism under control conditions and following TRP loads. It was found that nine women consumed 20% more calories, carbohydrate foods, and desserts (all $p < 0.05$) during the luteal compared with the follicular phase of the menstrual cycle. In the follicular, but not the luteal phase, energy ($r = 0.78$) and carbohydrate ($r = 0.79$) intake suppression were correlated with plasma TRP ($p < 0.05$). TRP suppressed energy and CHO consumption in unrestrained but not restrained eaters (TABLE 2; $p < 0.05$). Plasma and urinary kynurenine, a metabolite of TRP, were higher during the luteal relative to the follicular phase ($p < 0.05$) after the administration of TRP, whereas urinary kynurenine alone was elevated during the luteal phase after placebo.

TABLE 1. Effects of Tryptophan on Energy Intake[a]

Study	Subjects	Placebo	1 g TRP	2 g TRP	3 g TRP
1	Men (n = 17)	1743 ± 84	—	1516 ± 96[b]	—
2	Men (n = 15)	1541 ± 73	1457 ± 62	1246 ± 53[b]	1236 ± 101[b]
3	Women (n = 14)	885 ± 72	867 ± 68	825 ± 74	795 ± 52

[a] Values (kcal) are mean ± SEM
[b] $p < 0.001$ versus placebo

TABLE 2. Energy and Carbohydrate Food Intakes in Restrained (R) and Unrestrained (NR) Eaters[a]

		Follicular		Luteal	
	Restraint	Placebo	TRP	Placebo	TRP
Energy	NR[b]	819 ± 88	612 ± 86	1006 ± 82	876 ± 68
(kcal)	R[c]	709 ± 109	863 ± 90	862 ± 85	902 ± 91
Bread	NR	74 ± 13	57 ± 27	86 ± 27	69 ± 19
(g)	R	54 ± 16	80 ± 12	77 ± 3	87 ± 15
Dessert	NR	61 ± 20	43 ± 16	85 ± 27	69 ± 19
(g)	R	44 ± 10	80 ± 12	77 ± 3	87 ± 8

[a] Values are means ± SEM.
[b] N = 5.
[c] N = 4.

CONCLUSIONS

TRP at or above 2 g decreased food intake in lean men but not women. Energy and carbohydrate consumption are higher during the luteal phase in women. The behavioral effects of TRP in women are influenced by the menstrual cycle and the degree of eating restraint. The metabolic disposal of TRP is also influenced by the menstrual cycle.

REFERENCES

1. BLUNDELL, J. E. 1984. Serotonin and appetite. Neuropharmacology 23: 1537–1551.
2. ANDERSON, G. H., E. T. S. LI & N. T. GLANVILLE. 1984. Brain mechanisms and the quantitative and qualitative aspects of food intake. Brain Res. Bull. 12: 167–173.

Treatment of Seasonal Affective Disorder with *d*-Fenfluramine

D. O'ROURKE, J. WURTMAN, A. BRZEZINSKI,
T. ABOU-NADER, P. MARCHANT, AND R. J. WURTMAN

Clinical Research Center
Massachusetts Institute of Technology
Cambridge, Massachusetts 02142

Of the eight million Americans who suffer a major depressive episode each year, about 10% are thought to have a specific vulnerability to a seasonally induced depression that recurs annually in the fall and winter. This depression has been termed seasonal affective disorder (SAD).[1] SAD appears to have seasonal light triggers causing both the onset of the depression and its amelioration during the following spring and summer. Symptoms that occur in conjunction with the depression can mimic physical illness. These include, along with the alterations in mood, increased appetite, particularly for carbohydrates; weight gain; hypersomnia; increased fatigue; social withdrawal; and impaired cognitive functioning. With the advent of spring and summer, the depression lifts and the individual feels well, at times even hypomanic.

The therapeutic efficacy of full-spectrum light in relieving the depression of SAD has been demonstrated,[1] and it has been suggested that the hormone melatonin might be involved in the etiology of the disease. Carbohydrate craving and hyperphagia have been documented in SAD patients during their depressive phase.[2] Studies at our institution have shown that *d*-fenfluramine reduces carbohydrate craving in some obese individuals without increasing the incidence or severity of depression.[3] We present preliminary data suggesting that abnormalities in serotonin-mediated brain neurotransmission may be an important factor in the etiology of this seasonal depression.

Seven subjects who met the diagnostic criteria for both bipolar II affective illness and for seasonal affective disorder were studied at the Massachusetts Institute of Technology Clinical Research Center, between the fall of 1985 and spring of 1986. The study was designed to measure mood, food intake, plasma melatonin levels, motor activity, and behavior. Food intake was measured during forty-eight-hour periods of the fall and spring. Subjects were allowed to choose unlimited amounts of six different isocaloric meal items; three were high in protein and three high in carbohydrate. They also could take, between meals, unlimited numbers of isocaloric snacks, chosen from among five that were high in protein and five high in carbohydrate. (These were dispensed, and the patients' choices recorded by a computer-driven refrigerated vending machine.)

Subjects were treated with *d*-fenfluramine (15 mg twice daily), a drug that enhances serotonin-mediated neurotransmission, or its placebo, for three weeks, using a double-blind crossover study design. Activity levels were assessed by wrist-activity monitors worn on the same days that food intake was measured. Mood states and behavior were evaluated periodically by clinical interviews and psychometric tests, including the beginning and end of each treatment period. For this purpose, the Hamilton depression scale and its SAD addendum (N. Rosenthal, personal communication) were used. Calorie and nutrient intakes were mon-

TABLE 1. Mood Scores and Caloric Intakes at Conclusion of Treatment, in the Fall and in the Spring[a]

| | Fall | | Spring |
	Placebo	Fenfluramine	No Treatment
Mood Scores	19 ± 4	8 ± 2	1 ± 0
Total kcal	2630 ± 280	1720 ± 340	1780 ± 280

[a] Data are expressed as mean and SEM.

itored by the computerized food intake measurement system mentioned above.[2] Measurements, made in the fall, of subjects who had received d-fenfluramine or its placebo, were compared with those on the same subjects in the spring, when they were symptom-free.

d-Fenfluramine, but not placebo, was associated with a remission of all symptoms in four of the seven subjects. A fifth subject's calorie and nutrient intakes returned to normal levels after fenfluramine (but not placebo), but his depression ratings did not return to normal levels. The two remaining subjects responded to placebo; one of them also experienced a therapeutic response to fenfluramine. (Melatonin levels and activity measurements are currently being evaluated.)

The effectiveness of d-fenfluramine treatment (TABLE 1) suggests that serotonin might be involved in the disturbances of mood and food intake associated with this type of depression. Moreover, the treatment of depression with a drug that ameliorates both appetitive and mood disturbances has an advantage over many currently available serotoninergic antidepressants, which are often associated with increased appetite and weight gain.

REFERENCES

1. ROSENTHAL, N., D. A. SACK, C. GILLIN, A. LEWY, F. GOODWIN, Y. DAVENPORT, P. MUELLER, D. NEWSOME & T. WEHR. 1984. Seasonal Affective Disorder. Arch. Gen. Psychiatry 41: 72–80.
2. ROSENTHAL, N., D. A. SACK, C. J. CARPENTER, B. L. PARRY, W. S. MENDELSON & T. A. WEHR. 1985. Antidepressant effects of light in seasonal affective disorders. J. Psychiatry 142: 2, 606–608.
3. WURTMAN, J., R. WURTMAN, S. MARK, R. TSAY, W. GILBERT & J. GROWDON. 1985. d-Fenfluramine selectively suppresses carbohydrate snacking by obese subjects. Int. J. Eating Disorders 4: 89–99.

Obesity Types in Stone Age Art

A Study in Icono-Diagnosis

ANNELIESE A. PONTIUS

Department of Psychiatry
Harvard Medical School
Boston, Massachusetts 02115

Medical pattern detection, icono-diagnosis,[1-4] is applied to those kinds of prehistoric art that consistently depict a characteristic deviation from the usual appearance of the human body, the meaning of which has largely remained undeciphered (TABLE 1). By means of icono-diagnosis specific heuristic questions can be raised that are otherwise overlooked, because prehistory leaves no records of communication other than its art. Hundreds of Stone Age figures from ancient Europe are a case in point. Inasmuch as there is a pattern of the geographic distribution of two distinct types of obesity depicted in such figures, and inasmuch as present-day research in obesity also distinguishes between these two types[5] and also points to factors potentially shared by the two sets of problems,[6-8] it is tempting to propose testable hypotheses. In Stone Age figures, abdominal obesity prevails in present-day Romania and Lower Austria ("venuses" of Willendorf), whereas there is mostly gluteal obesity depicted in present-day France,[9] Spain, Greece, Czechoslovakia, and Western Ukraine[10] (TABLE 2). Normal appearance of the female body tends to appear in areas with a prevalence of abdominal obesity. Such geographically patterned distribution appears to offer some support for modern findings[5] linking abdominal obesity and its distinct fat cell receptors with pathological deviation (which can coexist with normalcy), whereas gluteal obesity and its specific fat cell receptors are not linked with disease. Thus, in light of the large number of Stone Age figures with gluteal obesity, and given their consistent geographical distribution over hundreds of years, it is hypothesized that gluteal obesity served survival during periods of scant nutrition (40% of X rays of tooth enamel from Aurignacian skeletons of southern France implicate starvation or illness[11]).

Special factors that can thus be implicated to have contributed to gluteal obesity or to have favored the survival of persons genetically so inclined, comprise the following ones: fluctuations in climate (temperature),[7] and food[6] or water[8] supplies. These factors would favor the survival of those genetically predisposed people who could store reserve energy in gluteal-femoral fat cells in a physiological way. Such a storage would be advantageous for both men and women, particularly those of child-bearing age, benefiting the fetus and the breast-fed child. Indeed, most Stone Age figures are female with gluteal obesity. Certain Stone Age male figures, however, are also depicted with gluteal obesity. Indeed, gluteal obesity persists to this day in both sexes and in all ages in certain African regions where cyclical drought and famine are common (analogous to the camel's hump.) Thus, in regions where storage of reserve energy is advantageous, hormonal factors are not exclusively implicated in gluteal (femoral) obesity. Furthermore, the Stone Age figures with abdominal obesity (TABLE 2) are all females, whereas presently, abdominal obesity is prevalent mostly in males of a sedentary life style, different from Stone Age hunters.

TABLE 1. Icono-Diagnosis;[1-4] Medical Pattern Detection in Prehistoric Art With Heuristic Implications

Prehistoric Population	Prehistoric Art Form, so far Undeciphered	Depiction of Medical Pattern or Function
Easter Island,[1] South Pacific	1000 stone giants (made A.D. 1150–1650)	twelve signs of leprosy in reversed, over-corrected form (as leprosy is experienced as a threat)
Classic Maori[2] (New Zealand)	hundreds of wooden carved boards depicting humans	eight signs of pseudo-hypoparathyroidism in direct form (as signs of tetany seizures were probably considered sacred)
Cook Islands,[3] South Pacific	numerous wooden statues (fisherman's gods), traditionally placed on canoe prow	twenty signs of full Crouzon's malformation in direct form (as signs are nonthreatening)
Nazca,[4] Peru	hundreds of huge geoglyphs up to 70 km long; most are unusual geometrical patterns; a few are figurative	nine characteristics of these patterns, if used by people to move along these outlines render them specifically effective for practicing unique frontal lobe system functioning: the unexpected switching of the plan of action during an ongoing activity; such exercises fostered survival specifically in Nazca environment.
Europe (from France to Western Ukraine)	hundreds of female Stone Age art figures ("venuses"); appearance differs consistently with geographic location	two types of obesity: abdominal and gluteal (including hips and thighs); aside from normal body depiction, these may offer clues to specific geographical area climate, food and water supply, and medical conditions

TABLE 2. Distribution of Two Types of Obesity in European Paleolithic Art[a]

Geographic Location (Culture)	No Obesity	Gluteal	Abdominal
Spain			
Central Anatolia		3	
Greece			
Macedonia (Anza II)		3	
Thessaly	3	1	
East Crete (Gournia)	2		
Hungary			
Tisza River (southeast)	3		
Bulgaria			
Sophia		1	
Sulica		1	
Barets		1	
Blagoevo	4		
Yugoslavia			
Vinča	4	10	
Donja Branjevina (north)		3	
Deronja (north)		5	
Rudnik (southwest)		1	
Czechoslovakia			
Moravia, Strelice (central)		1	
Russia			
Dniester Valley		1	
Sebatinovka, North Moldavia, West Ukraine		4	
Sipintsi, West Ukraine		4	
Bilcze Zlote, West Ukraine		1	
Bernovo Luka, (Proto Cucutani), West Ukraine		1	
Romania			
Cernavoda (Hamangia) (east)			2
Vidra (north)			2
Sultana (south)			1
Cernica (south)			1
Lower Austria			
Willendorf			1
	16	41	7

[a] Female statues (stone, bone) of European Paleolithic art (c. 7000 B.C. to 3500 B.C.) based on Gimbutas' (1982) depictions, wherever clearly visible, adding one "venus" of Willendorf (of which numerous examples exist in the Vienna Ethnographic Museum.) Note that non-obese female figures were found mostly in areas also depicting gluteal, but not abdominal, obesity. Leroi-Gourhan et al.[9] depict several female figures with mostly gluteal obesity found in France that are not included in Gimbutas' book and are not counted here.

Thus, an unequal interaction of three factors is hypothesized. Of primary importance seems to be a combination of ecological and genetic factors (where natural selection can be implicated), whereas hormonal factors play merely a secondary role. If this analysis of body configuration of Stone Age figures is valid, then specific questions arise about the times and lives of our ancestors in particular geographical regions (TABLE 2) during the Stone Age with its great change toward agriculture and urbanization. In turn, insights gained about the ancients can heuristically cross-fertilize present-day obesity research.[5,7]

REFERENCES

1. PONTIUS, A. A. 1969. Easter Island's stone giants: a neuropsychiatric view. Percept. Mot. Skills **28:** 207–212.
2. PONTIUS, A. A. 1973. Maori art and pseudo-hypoparathyroidism—a medical contribution to prehistoric anthropology. J. Am. Med. Women's Assoc. **28:** 231–237.
3. PONTIUS, A. A. 1978. Nazca's prehistoric fostering of frontal lobe functions. Proceedings 2nd International Meeting on Human Ecology, 1977. Vienna. Arch. Oecologiae Hominis (Vienna). 135–143.
4. PONTIUS, A. A. 1983. Icono-diagnosis: a medical humanistic approach, detecting Crouzon's malformation in Cook Islands' prehistoric art. Perspect. Biol. Med. **27:** 107–120.
5. KOLLATA, G. 1985. Why do people get fat? Science **227:** 1549–1558.
6. LAMBERT, J. B., S. V. SIMPSONS, C. B. SZPUNAR & J. E. BUIKSTRA. 1984. Ancient human diet from inorganic analysis of bone. Acc. Chem. Res. **17:** 298–305.
7. HIMMS-HAGEN, J. 1984. Thermogenesis in brown adipose tissue as an energy buffer. N. Engl. J. Med. **311:** 1549–1558.
8. STREET-PERROTT, F. A. & N. ROBERTS, Eds. 1983. Variations in the global water supply. 331–345. Reidel. Boston.
9. LEROI-GOURHAN, A., G. BAILLOUD, J. CHAVAILLON & A. LAMING-EMPERAIRE. 1968. La Préhistoire. Presses Universitaires de France. Paris.
10. GIMBUTAS, M. 1982. The goddesses and gods of old Europe. University of California Press. Berkeley, CA.
11. BRENNAN, M. U., 1986. Cited in R. White. 1986. Dark caves, bright visions. Life in Ice Age Europe. Am. Museum Natural History & W. W. Norton. New York. p. 77.

Macronutrient Intake and Mood during Weight-Reducing Diets

ULRICH SCHWEIGER, REINHOLD LAESSLE, AND
KARL M. PIRKE

Max Planck Institut for Psychiatry
Munich, Federal Republic of Germany

Reports about mood changes during weight loss are controversial. It has been suggested that mood changes might be associated with alterations of relative macronutrient intake, which are frequent in weight-reducing diets. This hypothesis is supported by the finding that brain serotonin synthesis is linked to relative carbohydrate intake by modulation of the flow of its precursor, tryptophan, into the brain, which can be predicted by the molar ratio of tryptophan to the sum of all large neutral amino acids (TRP/LNAA). High carbohydrate intake typically leads to high TRP/LNAA and decreased serotonin synthesis, whereas low carbohydrate intake leads to low TRP/LNAA and low serotonin synthesis.[1]

Eighteen normal weight young women participated in the study. They were healthy and ate largely unrestricted before and during the control period. Subjects were followed for a four-week control period and a six-week diet period. Both diet groups were instructed to restrict caloric intake to approximately 1000 kcal. The mixed diet group received additional instructions to eat equal amounts of all foods and to maintain an intake of 500 g meat or fish per week. The vegetarian group was instructed to avoid meat, fish, and poultry and to restrict milk, milk products, and eggs, and to consume a diet based on vegetables, salad, fruit, and whole meal products. Participants rated mood daily on a visual analog scale. During the second week of the control phase, subjects spent 24 hours at the hospital. Blood was collected every two hours. Plasma amino acids were determined by high-performance liquid chromatography. Nutritional diaries were evaluated using German food tables.

The carbohydrate proportion of caloric intake rose significantly ($p < 0.05$) in the vegetarian group during the diet, whereas the protein proportion increased significantly in the mixed diet group ($p < 0.05$). The fat portion decreased in both groups. There was a significant group × phase interaction in global mood score that did not differ between groups during the control phase but differed during the last three weeks of the diet. Average global mood scores were significantly higher during the last three weeks of dieting, meaning that mood was worse in the mixed diet group (FIG. 1). The average global mood score during the last three weeks of the diet correlated significantly ($r = -0.52$; $p < 0.05$) with the carbohydrate proportion of the total caloric intake (FIG. 2). There was an equally significant correlation between the 24 hour average of TRP/LNAA and global mood ($r = -0.52$; $p < 0.05$).

Data demonstrate that mood during weight-reducing diets can be differentially influenced by their composition. Both diets were relatively mild, and endocrine data (not shown) yielded no evidence that either of them was particularly stress-

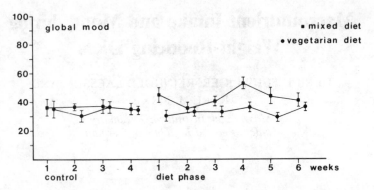

FIGURE 1. Global mood (percent of maximum score) during control and diet phase. Mean ± SEM. High scores indicate bad mood.

ful. The significant negative correlation between relative carbohydrate intake and mood scores (meaning that mood worsened with decreasing carbohydrate proportions of caloric intake) suggests that group differences cannot be attributed to differences between a vegetarian and a mixed diet per se, but are related to differences in carbohydrate intake. The significant negative correlation between mood scores and TRP/LNAA (meaning that low TRP/LNAA ratios are associated with worsened mood) indicate a possible mechanism for this interaction. Low carbohydrate intake, which results in low TRP/LNAA, may prompt mood deteri-

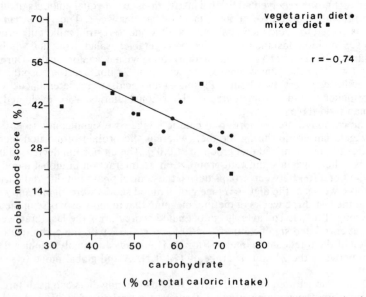

FIGURE 2. Correlation between carbohydrate intake (percent of total caloric intake) and global mood (percent of maximum score) during the last three weeks of dieting.

oration by way of impairment of central serotonergic functions due to reduced brain tryptophan availability.

REFERENCE

1. WURTMAN, R. J., F. HEFTI & E. MELAMED. 1981. Precursor control of neurotransmitter synthesis. Pharmacol. Rev. **32:** 315–335.

The Effect of Active Weight Loss Achieved by Dieting versus Exercise on Postheparin Hepatic and Lipoprotein Lipase Activity

MARCIA L. STEFANICK, BARBARA FREY-HEWITT,
CRAIG A. HOOVER, RICHARD B. TERRY, AND
PETER D. WOOD

Stanford Center for Research in Disease Prevention
Stanford, California 94305

Postheparin hepatic (HLA) and lipoprotein lipase (LPLA) activities were studied in moderately overweight ($27.8 \pm 4.3\%$ body fat, mean $\pm$ SD), sedentary men, aged 30–59, before, and seven months after, randomization to control status (C; N = 41) to a weight-loss program involving moderate caloric restriction without exercise (D; N = 38), or exercise, primarily running, without dieting (E; N = 43). At seven months, during active weight loss, caloric intake, as determined by seven-day food records, was decreased ($p < 0.001$) from baseline in D, relative to C (-362.3 kcal) and E (-360.0 kcal), but was unchanged in E relative to C (-2.4 kcal). Exercisers were running 41.1 ± 20.1 miles per month and had increased their daily living activity level, whereas D and C remained sedentary.

At the seven-month point, both D and E had achieved significant ($p < 0.01$) weight loss (-7.9 kg and -3.2 kg, respectively), relative to C, primarily by reducing fat mass (-5.9 kg and -3.0 kg), as determined by hydrostatic weighing. D lost significant ($p < 0.01$) nonfat mass (-1.9 kg), relative to C, whereas nonfat mass was not reduced in E. Percent body fat was thereby reduced ($p < 0.01$) in D (-4.5%) and E (-2.4%) versus C. Finally, compared to E, D lost more ($p < 0.01$) fat (-3.0 kg) and nonfat (-1.7 kg) mass and showed greater reduction in percent body fat (-2.1%).

Postheparin lipase activity was determined from blood collected 15 minutes after injection of 75 U/kg body weight sodium heparin, using the method of Krauss *et al.*,[1] which involves calculation of HLA following inhibition of LPLA by protamine sulfate. Mean HLA was reduced from baseline (7.7 ± 2.9 mU/ml/min) in both D (-0.84; $p < 0.01$) and E (-0.59; $p < 0.05$), relative to C. By contrast, LPLA was elevated from baseline (2.4 ± 1.5 mU/ml/min) in E (0.62, $p < 0.01$), but not in D (0.36, $p = 0.10$). Changes in HLA and LPLA did not differ significantly between D and E. ΔHLA correlated ($p < 0.01$) with ΔLPLA (Spearman's rho) in D ($r = -0.76$), E ($r = -0.55$) and C ($r = -0.48$).

TABLE 1 and TABLE 2 present the Spearman's correlations for all three groups for changes in HLA and LPLA, respectively, with changes in body composition. Significant positive associations were found between changes in HLA and fat mass in both D and E and for changes in HLA with total weight change in E and percent body fat change in D. None of the body composition changes related to LPLA changes in D, whereas a significant negative relationship was found between changes in LPLA and fat mass in E.

TABLE 1. Hepatic Lipase Activity Changes: Spearman's rho Correlations

	Dieters (N = 38)	Exercisers (N = 43)	Controls (N = 41)
Δ Total weight (kg)	0.29	0.36[a]	0.04
Δ Fat mass (kg)	0.43[b]	0.30[a]	−0.06
Δ Nonfat mass (kg)	−0.09	0.14	−0.02
Δ Percent body fat	0.38[a]	0.23	−0.06

[a] $p < 0.05$
[b] $p < 0.01$

TABLE 2. Lipoprotein Lipase Activity Changes: Spearman's rho Correlations

	Dieters (N = 38)	Exercisers (N = 43)	Controls (N = 41)
Δ Total weight (kg)	−0.25	−0.17	0.03
Δ Fat mass (kg)	−0.20	−0.30[a]	−0.14
Δ Percent body fat	−0.08	−0.27	−0.16
Δ Nonfat mass (kg)	−0.14	0.07	0.22

[a] $p < 0.05$

   In summary, active weight loss by dieting or exercise resulted in decreased HLA in overweight men, whereas LPLA was elevated only when weight loss was achieved by exercising. Furthermore, ΔHLA correlated significantly with body fat changes in D and E, whereas ΔLPLA correlated with fat weight changes in E only. It appears that negative calorie balance resulting in fat loss, whether it is achieved by decreasing caloric intake or increasing energy output, brings about reduction in hepatic triglyceride lipase activity. By contrast, the data presented here suggest that loss of body fat by increased energy expenditure differs from that achieved by moderate caloric restriction, with respect to associated changes in lipoprotein lipase activity in adipose and/or skeletal muscle.

REFERENCE

1. KRAUSS, R. M., R. I. LEVY & D. S. FREDRICKSON. 1974. Selective measurement of two lipase activities in postheparin plasma from normal subjects and patients with hyperlipoproteinemia. J. Clin. Invest. **54**: 1107–1124.

Body Composition in Obese Males

A. N. VASWANI, S. H. COHN, K. J. ELLIS, J. YEH, AND
J. F. ALOIA

Department of Medicine
Winthrop University Hospital
Mineola, New York 11501
and
Brookhaven National Laboratory
Upton, New York 11973

INTRODUCTION

A number of techniques are available to evaluate body composition, from simple measurement of skinfold thickness to an elaborate underwater weighing technique to determine lean body mass and estimate fat mass. Measurement of body composition is useful in evaluating the impact of dietary or drug manipulations on various compartments of body composition.[1]

METHODS

Eight healthy obese men who were at least 20% above their ideal body weight were age-matched with nine nonobese subjects. Body composition studies were done as follows. Total body water (TBW) was determined from a blood sample taken three hours after the patient drank 50 μCi of tritiated water mixed with orange juice. The coefficient of variation for the measurement of TBW with this technique is less than one percent. Total body potassium (TBK) was determined by counting ^{40}K in the 54 detector Brookhaven Whole Body Counter. This facility, with its on-line computer, corrects for body size and the internal location of the naturally occurring isotope of potassium (^{40}K). The precision and accuracy of this technique is ±3% in the Alderson Phantom.[2] Total body nitrogen (TBN) was determined by prompt gamma neutron activation.[3] In addition to nitrogen, the gamma rays from the neutron capture provide a way to measure hydrogen. The use of total body hydrogen (TBH) as an internal standard reduces the error due to the effect of body size and shape. Total body nitrogen is determined by the formula: TBN = K × N/H × TBH, where K is a constant determined from irradiation of an Alderson Phantom, containing known amounts of nitrogen and hydrogen, and where N/H is the corrected ratio for the differences in thickness between the patient and the Alderson Phantom.

RESULTS

See TABLE 1.

CONCLUSIONS

We conclude that obese males not only have increased body fat, as compared to normal subjects, but also have increased parameters of lean body mass. The

TABLE 1. Comparison of Body Composition in Obese and Nonobese Men

Group	Age (yrs)	Wt (kg)	Ht (m)	TBW (L)	TBK (g)	TBN (kg)	TBF[a] (by TBN)	SKF[b] (kg)
Control	40.1 ±8.0	74.80 ±2.92	1.76 ±0.05	44.18 ±3.33	142.6 ±16.2	1.85 ±0.16	16.42 ±2.56	12.36 ±1.30
Obese	37.9 ±9.2	111.76 ±16.53	1.78 ±0.09	52.72 ±4.54	162.2 ±10.7	1.96 ±0.24	44.00 ±12.98	32.35 ±7.93
p	ns	<0.005	ns	<0.005	<0.005	<0.01	<0.005	<0.005

[a] TBF = total body fat
[b] SKF = skinfold

increase in lean tissue may be an adaptive phenomenon to support the increased fat mass, and conforms to the concept of increased metabolic rate in obese individuals. There is no direct method to estimate or determine total body fat. Indirect methods of TBF measurement are either cumbersome or imprecise. Estimation of TBF by skinfold thickness underestimated the body fat content when compared to other techniques, such as neutron activation analysis or determination of lean body mass by TBK.

REFERENCES

1. Ashok, N. Vaswani, David Vartsky, Kenneth J. Ellis, Seiichi Yasumura & Stanton H. Cohn. 1983. Effects of caloric restriction on body composition and total body nitrogen as measured by neutron activation. Metab. Clin. Exp. **32:** No. 2, 185–188.
2. Cohn, S. H., C. S. Dombrowski, H. R. Pate *et al.* 1969. A whole-body counter with an invariant response to radionuclide distribution and body size. Physics Med. Biol. **14:** 645–658.
3. Vartsky, D., K. J. Ellis & S. H. Cohn. 1979. *In vivo* measurement of body nitrogen by analysis of prompt gammas from neutron capture. J. Nucl. Med. **20:** 1158–1165.

Summary and Forecast

RICHARD J. WURTMAN

Massachusetts Institute of Technology
Cambridge, Massachusetts 02139

Why do people become obese, and why do they remain so? Primarily because they eat too many calories in relation to the number that they expend.

For a minority of obese people, as Dr. Eric Jequier describes, this behavioral problem may be exacerbated by a metabolic defect that causes them to use too little of their food energy producing heat (by facultative thermogenesis), an adaptation that, Dr. Peter J. Brown suggests, may once have had survival value. Obesity may also be influenced by cultural factors, as in the tendency of American children to spend long hours sitting (and nibbling) in front of the television, or the propensity of fast-food restaurants to treble the calories in a hamburger by coating it with mayonnaise and cheese. Moreover, as Dr. Benjamin Caballero and Dr. George Cahill have proposed, the obese state, once established, may be stabilized by secondary metabolic changes that the obesity itself generates, as in resistance to insulin's effects on plasma amino acids and glucose.

For most obese people, however, the accumulation of excess weight and adipose tissue most likely signifies a prolonged, and often, insidious process: excessive consumption of calories, during a sufficient number of days, above and beyond those used for muscular or metabolic work.

This inappropriate eating behavior is generally attributed to the failure of hypothetical regulatory mechanisms, like the two outlined below (FIGURES 1 and 2), which are thought to keep energy intake and output in balance. Dr. William Bennett objects, rightly, that explanations of obesity as the reflection of caloric imbalances may be nothing more than tautologies, because obesity could also be defined as the state in which calories eaten chronically transcend calories burnt. If there is nothing characteristic (and pathologic) about the way obese people eat, and if, as he documents, attempts to treat obesity by reducing caloric intake are often met with little long-term success, then attributing obesity to overeating might indeed be tantamount to saying nothing at all.

But is this, in fact, the case? Is it established that there is nothing peculiar about the eating behaviors of obese people, and that therapies designed to treat such peculiarities, once they have been identified, invariably fail in the long run? Probably not. Optimism that such peculiarities in eating behavior can be identified, explained, and ultimately treated underlies the topics of this volume. At present, we have only fragmentary knowledge of what (and when) obesity-prone people tend to eat while they are becoming obese or, even later, when they are maintaining their excess weight. Apparently, there are fewer than a handful of publications that provide actual measurements of what preobese or obese people have eaten when they were allowed to choose among the kinds of meal and snack foods that they normally consume, unconstrained by the watchful and perhaps judgmental eye of an investigator. Information abounds on what obese people say they eat, as reported in questionnaires; attempts, however, to correlate these remembrances with on-line measurements of actual food intake affirm that whereas many obese people accurately describe what they eat at meals, they

343

invariably underreport their consumption of the snacks that not infrequently provide most of their excess calories.

Clearly, everyone will agree that, if the study of how people become and remain obese is a serious science, it is essential that its practitioners routinely measure what obese people actually eat and use such measurements to evaluate hypotheses about obesity's causes. As described at this *Annal*, the few such measurements that do exist have already allowed recognition of one distinctive subgroup of obese people, the carbohydrate cravers, who derive most of their

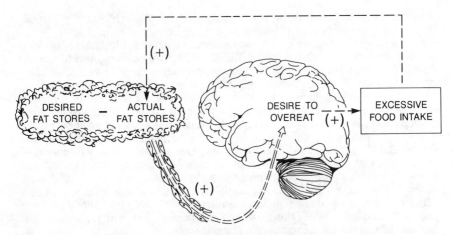

FIGURE 1. Peripheral model for the development of obesity. The model assumes the existence of a system that regulates the extent of the body's fat stores. When these stores are low, as in an adult who has been obese since childhood, who has an excessive number of adipocytes, and who has lost weight, a signal is generated indicating the difference. The chemical that carries the signal travels by way of the blood stream to the brain, where it modifies brain composition (*i.e.*, neurotransmitter release) and function, causing the individual to overeat. Prolonged overeating subsequently increases actual fat stores to their desired level, whereupon body weight again stabilizes, providing suggestive evidence that its set point has been attained.

This model suffers from the fact that no substance has been identified that is released from fat cells into the blood stream and that modifies neurotransmission or other relevant functional properties of the brain. Moreover, the model would predict that the desire to overeat would be continuous, so long as body weight was below its presumed set point, and that foods containing any of the macronutrients would be chosen, since all are able to be converted to fat in the body. Studies of the actual eating behaviors of obese people, however, indicate that, for many, the periods of excessive food intake are discontinuous and tend to be characterized by preferences for a particular macronutrient.

excess calories by eating carbohydrate-rich, protein-poor snacks in the mid-afternoon or evening, and who consume normal amounts of carbohydrates, proteins, and calories at mealtime. Recognition that many obese people exhibit this eating disorder has already led to formulations about its underlying mechanisms and to proposals for its treatment, as discussed by Dr. John Blundell, Dr. C. Nathan, and Dr. Silvio Garattini. (Not all obese people are carbohydrate-cravers, and not all carbohydrate-cravers are obese; many successfully use techniques like exercising

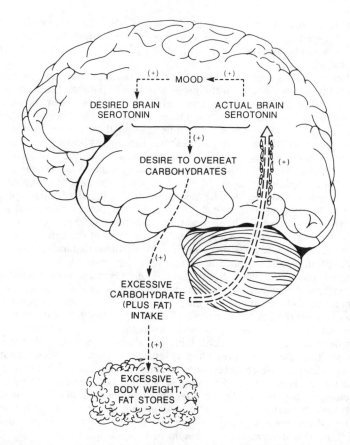

FIGURE 2. Brain model for the development of obesity. The model assumes the existence of a system that controls the rate of food intake and the macronutrient composition of the food, by regulating the release of serotonin at brain synapses. The number of serotonin molecules released per unit time depends on the firing frequency of the serotoninergic neurons and the amount of transmitter that each neuron releases per firing. This quantity is increased when the individual consumes a carbohydrate-rich, protein-poor meal or snack. The carbohydrate elicits the secretion of insulin, which increases the plasma tryptophan ratio, that is, the ratio of the plasma tryptophan concentration to the summed concentrations of the other plasma amino acids that compete with tryptophan for brain uptake. This increase, in turn, raises brain tryptophan levels and accelerates the production of serotonin from tryptophan.

If serotonin-mediated neurotransmission, at a particular time of day or year, is less than the brain desires, the individual perceives the motivation to eat carbohydrates; their ingestion restores desired serotoninergic neurotransmission within 15–60 minutes, thus terminating the carbohydrate craving. This persistently excessive consumption of carbohydrate-rich snacks is, according to the model, a major factor contributing to the accumulation of excessive body weight and fat stores, especially if the dietary carbohydrates chosen for snacking also happen to be rich in fats.

Although the signal that generates the excessive food intake arises within the brain, the shutoff signal is peripheral, that is, the plasma tryptophan ratio, defined above. The signal increases as the consequence of carbohydrate intake. The model further predicts that changes in mood (*e.g.,* in seasonal or other depressions) may predispose one to excessive or skipping meals to avoid gaining weight.) It seems likely that, as more investigators actually measure what and when obese people eat, additional subgroups of obese patients will be identified with distinctive eating patterns that identify their particular caloric excess.

So, when is the statement "people are obese because they eat too much," simply a definition, and when is it the progenitor of a hypothesis? It becomes the latter when applied to subgroups whose eating patterns have been shown to be both distinctive and excessive. For such patients the statement becomes, "these people are obese because they eat too much," and the hypotheses it spawns concern why they eat the way they do and whether their obesity would be controlled if they stopped eating that way. Consider this analogy: the statement, "the patient's blood has too little oxygen, because he breathes too infrequently" is little more than a definition; however, the statement, "the patient is hypoxic and breathes too infrequently because he has a disease that impairs his perception of depressed blood oxygen levels" constitutes a testable hypothesis about the pathogenesis of the hypoxia and the likelihood that it will respond to particular types of treatments, for example, those increasing the sensitivity of the carotid body. Do many obese people manifest distinct behavioral syndromes that include the excessive consumption of certain foods at certain times? Probably.

Ultimately, understanding the pathogenesis of obesity requires solving a formidable conceptual problem: determining whether the body's weight or, perhaps, its fat content actually are regulated, and, if so, how this regulation operates and how it may be disturbed in obese people. (The fact that body weight can be quite stable over long periods of time in no way proves that it is regulated: the level of water in a deep lake is also relatively stable, but this does not mean that the lake has the power to cause a rainstorm when its level falls below some desired range.) It also means attempting to determine whether a circulating substance exists whose plasma levels vary with, for example, the mass of the adipose tissue, and whether changes in these levels can affect the composition and function of the brain and, thus, behavior. (A circulating compound with these properties would be an essential component of any system that regulated metabolic phenomena, including those that determine body weight or composition.)

Once the hypothetical regulatory system is understood, it may then become possible to identify components that possibly are disturbed and to design drugs or other treatments that may be able to correct these disturbances. As discussed by several authors in this volume, a favorite current formulation of obesity is that it does, in fact, arise from a particular kind of regulatory defect, a faulty set point for the desired body weight. The brain presumably defends this elevated set point, so that weight reduction usually is futile, most commonly being followed by weight regain, back to predieting levels. Is this formulation supported by compelling evidence that elevated set points characterize the obese state (or for that matter, that set points for body weight exist in normal people)? This *Annal* provides little evidence in support of either hypothesis.

Two very different kinds of regulatory systems might exist that would protect normal individuals against the development of obesity. One of these, defined above, would regulate body weight or perhaps body fat content. The other would control food intake, perhaps the amount of food consumed per meal or per day, its

---

carbohydrate intake if the individual has learned, consciously or unconsciously, that his subjective state is improved by carbohydrate consumption. In this situation, the dietary carbohydrate is being used as a drug.

caloric content, or its proportions of various nutrients. The first system would include the second; that is, hunger for calories, and thus food intake would be increased if the phenomenon being regulated, body fat content, fell too low. The second system would govern short-term appetitive responses to variations in plasma composition and could operate entirely independent of the first. There is no *a priori* reason that food intake need be coupled at all to body weight or composition: its regulation could just as well be for nutritional goals, for example, to provide appropriate proportions of proteins and carbohydrates (and sufficient calories) to keep plasma composition within a healthy range.

Both hypothetical regulatory systems would operate by sensing some key circulating compound. In the former case, the concentration of this compound would depend on the mass of the body (or of a component, *e.g.,* the adipose tissue); in the latter, its concentration would be affected by eating. In the first case, the development and persistence of obesity would ultimately have a peripheral metabolic basis; in the latter, the cause would be behavioral and triggered not by something previously learned (as proposed in the food-as-a-reward theory of obesity), but by some inappropriate property of the brain mechanisms that control food intake (and perhaps also exacerbated by metabolic phenomena, like insulin resistance.) A genetic propensity to obesity, as proposed by Dr. Albert Stunkard and his colleagues, could operate by disturbing brain mechanisms underlying either type of regulatory system.

It should be noted at this point that no circulating chemical has ever been identified whose plasma level depends on body mass or fat stores, or the state of fullness of these fat stores, much less one whose variations also affect the language of the brain, neurotransmitter production, or release. (Moreover, it has yet to be demonstrated that any dietary lipid or lipid metabolite affects synaptic transmission, with the lone and probably irrelevant exception of the choline-containing phospholipids, whose consumption can enhance acetylcholine synthesis.) The lack of such a known chemical signal is a strong argument against the hypothesis that the brain senses and regulates body mass or composition, and that the failure of such regulation underlies obesity.

A system whose malfunction led to obesity could also operate, as stated above, by sensing a circulating compound whose concentration was predictably altered by eating (*e.g.,* the amino acids or choline), and which also affected brain neurotransmission. Alternatively, a system might monitor inputs from a peripheral sensory receptor (*e.g.,* for taste or one sensing gastric distension) that was activated by eating. Normally, eating would stop when enough of the circulating compound (or a sufficiently persistent sensory signal) had reached the brain to modify transmission across a key synapse in the chain of neurons responsible for the desire to eat. (As Dr. Jerrold Bernstein describes, drugs that interrupt this chain can have the opposite effect, producing obesity in people with no prior history of this problem.)

At this point, it becomes relevant to return to the data available on how obese people, and those who are in the process of becoming so, actually eat. As discussed above, only fragmentary data are available concerning this question; this information, however, does not support the view that fat people are always hungry, or that their hunger is for all foods, independent of macronutrient composition, as would be expected if the motivation to overeat was to refill partly empty fat stores. By contrast, one large subgroup of obese people, the carbohydrate cravers, have a very distinctive pattern of eating, consuming excess calories only at particular times of the day (or the year, for the seasonally depressed group described by Dr. Norman Rosenthal), and then almost exclusively in the form of carbohydrate-rich, protein-poor snacks. Apparently, their capacity to regulate food intake is normal most of the time, and explicitly so at mealtime. But then something happens to them at predictable times of day or year, so that an immediate need for dietary carbohydrates is allowed to override their otherwise functional mechanism that regulates their food intake.

Several of our authors have offered speculations as to why the mechanisms that normally control food intake intermittently fail in these patients: current explanations relate to the diversity of behavioral processes that involve serotonin-releasing brain neurons, a diversity that allows eating to become hostage to entirely different functions. The serotonin-releasing neurons respond to food intake, making and releasing more of their neurotransmitter after carbohydrates are consumed. These neurons not only affect the appetite, but also influence subjective feelings such as those included in the term *mood*. Hence, carbohydrate craving may, in some people, reflect a desire for the psychopharmacologic effects of the food, and not its taste or its nutritional value, a hypothesis consistent with the fact that most antidepressant drugs share with dietary carbohydrates the ability to enhance serotoninergic neurotransmission. Eating carbohydrates may make them feel better.

Such speculations can be useful if they generate testable hypotheses and, especially, if they contribute to the development of possible treatments for obesity. One such hypothesis has been described in this volume by Dr. D. O'Rourke. He found that drugs that selectively facilitate serotoninergic neurotransmission might be expected to ameliorate both carbohydrate-craving (and weight gain) and the affective symptoms of people with seasonal depression.

Other hypotheses are sure to follow if future studies identify additional subgroups of obese people with distinctive eating patterns or with other characteristic behavioral symptoms. The possibility that medical science will be able not only to classify obesity syndromes, but also to design specific treatments for each, as it has done for hypertension, depression, and other diseases involving the nervous system, is one that excites us all.

Index of Contributors